Disorders of the Patellofemoral Joint
Fourth Edition

Disorders of the Patellofemoral Joint
Fourth Edition

John P. Fulkerson, M.D.
Orthopaedic Associates of Hartford, P.C.
Farmington, Connecticut

Contributing Authors:
David A. Buuck, M.D.
Scott F. Dye, M.D.
Jack Farr, II, M.D.
William R. Post, M.D.

LIPPINCOTT WILLIAMS & WILKINS
A **Wolters Kluwer** Company
Philadelphia · Baltimore · New York · London
Buenos Aires · Hong Kong · Sydney · Tokyo

Acquisitions Editors: James Merritt and Robert A. Hurley
Developmental Editor: Eileen Wolfberg
Production Editor: Robin E. Cook
Manufacturing Manager: Benjamin Rivera
Cover Designer: David Levy
Compositor: Lippincott Williams & Wilkins Desktop Division
Printer: Maple Press

© 2004 by LIPPINCOTT WILLIAMS & WILKINS
530 Walnut St.
Philadelphia, P 19106 USA
LWW.com

Printed in the USA

Library of Congress Cataloging-in-Publication Data

Fulkerson, John P. (John Pryor)
   Disorders of the patellofemoral joint / John P. Fulkerson ; contributing authors,
David A. Buuck ... [et al.]—4th ed.
     p. ; cm.
   Includes bibliographical references and index.
   ISBN 0-7817-4081-9
    1. Patellofemoral joint—Diseases. 2. Patellofemoral joint—Wounds and injuries. I.
Buuck, David A. II. Title.
   [DNLM: 1. Knee Joint. 2. Patella. 3. Joint Diseases. 4. Knee Injuries. 5.
Patella—injuries. WE 870 F964d 2004]
   RD561.F85 2004
   617.5′82—dc22

                       2003065907

10 9 8 7 6 5 4 3 2 1

Contents

Foreword

The patellofemoral joint represents one of the most challenging musculoskeletal systems to understand and manage within the entire field of orthopaedic surgery. Despite the vast numbers of patients who develop symptoms of patellofemoral dysfunction and undergo treatment each year, controversy remains as how best to return these knees to full asymptomatic physiologic function. Often, the worst patients are those who have had multiple surgical procedures for initial symptoms that were only mild intermittent anterior knee pain.

The knee functions as a kind of biologic transmission whose purpose is to accept and redirect a range of biomechanical loads without structural or supraphysiological failure. The ligaments represent sensate adaptive linkages, the menisci sensate bearings, and the muscles' cellular and molecular engines. The patellofemoral joint represents a large slide bearing within this biologic transmission that is frequently subjected to the greatest biomechanical forces, both in compression and tension, of any human joint. Because of this harsh biomechanical environment, it is common for symptoms of patellofemoral dysfunction to develop, and once initiated, to persist. Complaints of anterior knee pain, in particular, are extremely common, and may arise from a variable mosaic of pathophysiologic events within overloaded innervated patellofemoral tissues such as the patellar bone and particularly the peripatellar synovium and fat pad. These sensitive tissues, in intimate contact with the patellofemoral joint, are highly vulnerable to mechanical impingement. The patellofemoral joint can be notoriously unforgiving of treatment that does not respect the special biomechanical and biologic nature of this joint. Therefore, it is best to approach the patient with patellofemoral problems with meticulous evaluation and a substantial degree of gentleness in therapy.

From an evolutionary standpoint, the patella is a rather late development within the vertebrate knee, appearing approximately 65 million years ago, in a design that is well over 300 million years ancient. Only in the past 3 million years or so has the human knee had to function in full extension, as our hominid ancestors began to walk upright with a bipedal gait. The human lumbosacral spine, which was evolutionarily designed as well, for quadrupedal locomotion, is now also functioning in an upright position and shares a similar high frequency of dysfunction with the patellofemoral joint, perhaps for similar reasons.

Over the past two decades, John Fulkerson has been an academic and clinical leader in the field of patellofemoral problems. Through this classic textbook, now in its fourth edition, he shares with us his vast experience and expertise in managing these often most difficult patients. In this text he wisely points out the myriad possible underlying factors that can account for patellofemoral dysfunction, including such subtle, occult, but genuine pathology as retinacular neuromas, that cannot be imaged by any current modality. Also in this new addition, the inherently safe and frequently effective physical therapy taping techniques of McConnell are recommended. Patients with an initial presentation of anterior knee pain—often due to transient osseous and soft tissue overload—frequently will respond positively to simple load restriction within their functional envelope, and a safe, pain-free rehabilitation program that can obviate the need for surgical intervention altogether. In the more difficult patient with established symptomatic degenerative arthrosis or recurrent patellar dislocation, Dr. Fulkerson provides rational, tested guidelines to treatment.

The patellofemoral joint, however, has not yet revealed all of its secrets. There is still much to discover about this special musculoskeletal system, including determining actual *in vivo* joint reaction forces, and discovering why some patients are asymptomatic despite obvious radiographically identifiable structural abnormalities, such as advanced chondromalacia, substantial malalignment, and even established degenerative arthrosis. When these mysteries are eventually explained, the principles discovered would be broadly applicable to the field of orthopaedic surgery.

Scott F. Dye, M.D.
Associate Clinical Professor of Orthopaedic Surgery
University of California, San Francisco

Preface

With the help of Jean Yves Dupont, we organized the International Patellofemoral Study Group in 1995. This created a worldwide forum for inquisitive scholars of the patella every other year. Between this opportunity to share information and the rapid transfer of ideas electronically, knowledge of the patellofemoral joint has advanced more rapidly than ever during the past decade.

Thus, the fourth edition of *Disorders of the Patellofemoral Joint* steps well beyond the third edition and ventures into new concepts of patellofemoral pain genesis, control and stabilization. Resurfacing, realignment, and arthroscopic techniques for the treatment of patellofemoral diseases have become increasingly refined. The importance of homeostatic balance, rest, and nonoperative therapy is clearer than ever.

This complex patellofemoral joint, so easily examined and prominent yet so confounding to clinicians, continues to pose unique challenges. To stimulate broader research efforts and education regarding patellofemoral problems, we have recently formed the Patellofemoral Foundation. Between the International Patellofemoral Study Group and the Patellofemoral Foundation, there is new hope for patients with chronic or disabling patellofemoral dysfunction. This edition is another step toward a brighter future for the many patients who suffer with patellofemoral pain.

John P. Fulkerson
October 5, 2003

Acknowledgments

I wish to thank all of those who have contributed their energy, time, and ideas to this fourth edition of *Disorders of the Patellofemoral Joint*. Most of all, I thank my wife, Lynn, for her patience and support during the countless hours required for the production of this edition. Eileen Wolfberg and Donna Wasowicz have been my backbone support in the processing and management of the manuscript and I am extremely grateful to both of them.

I would also like to acknowledge Phoebe Fulkerson, Susan Brust and George Barile for their excellent illustrations. Thanks also to Charlotte Massie for illustrations and ideas on rehabilitation. Appreciation as well to all of my fellows, residents, and medical students, past and present, for their interest and enthusiasm; and Ron Grelsamer, Jean Yves Dupont, Jenny McConnell, Bill Post, Dave Buuck, Jack Farr, and Scott Dye for their contributions to the book. Finally, I want to thank Jim Merritt for challenging me to tackle this edition, and Bob Hurley for helping to bring this to fruition.

John P. Fulkerson

Disorders of the Patellofemoral Joint

Fourth Edition

1
Normal Anatomy

*"You made all the delicate, inner parts of my body, and knit
them together in my mother's womb. Thank you for making me
so wonderfully complex! It is amazing to think about. Your
workmanship is marvelous—and how well I know it!"*

—*Psalm 139:13–14 (Living Bible).*

EMBRYOLOGY

According to Walmsley (1) and later confirmed by Gray and Gardner (2), the patella's anlage is distinguishable within the quadriceps condensation by close aggregation of rounded cells in the 20-mm embryo or at 7.5 weeks of gestation (Fig. 1.1). By 30 mm, it is clearly a cartilaginous anlage (1–3). In the embryo, the knee develops in a position of 90 degrees of flexion, before motor units exist to induce movement (1). This means that the patella initially conforms to the distal aspect of the femoral condyles that will articulate with the tibial plateaus instance. The patella acquires a free articular surface by the formation of a primitive joint plate in common with the distal femur. The subsequent mechanical behavior of the patella molds it and determines, to some extent, its ultimate shape.

The patella increases in relative size up to the sixth month of fetal life (1), after which it increases at the same rate as the other bones of the lower extremity. Initially, the medial and lateral patellar facets are equal in size. However, by the 192-mm stage (23 weeks' gestation), the patella has already acquired lateral facet predominance, a characteristic of the adult patella and one that plays a key role in understanding disorders of this joint.

Development of the trochlear surface of the femur, the surface that articulates only with the patella, is particularly fascinating. Several authors (1, 4, 5) are in agreement that very early in fetal life, and before movement has occurred, the general adult and *human* form of the femoral trochlea has been achieved. Langer (5) puts this as early as the 24-mm (8 weeks' gestation) stage. At this stage, the lateral facet extends more proximally, is more prominent anteriorly, and has greater transverse width; in short, all the essential characteristics of the adult. This is even more striking because this development is not in contact with or in response to the patella but to the quadriceps mechanism.

It would appear that the form of the trochlea is primary and genetically determined. Furthermore, the general forms of both parts of the patellofemoral joint are determined before they are in use. There is, however, at least one exception to this that may be important. Ficat and Hungerford (unpublished data) examined ten stillborn fetuses and did not identify a ridge separating the medial facets, a characteristic of adult patellae. This ridge has been present in several postmortem knee specimens from children between 3 and 8 years of age, which have become available. It would appear that this subdivision of the

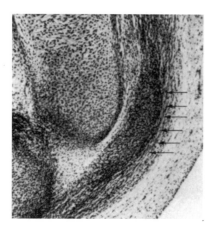

Figure 1.1. Sagittal section through the center of the knee of a 20-mm fetus (8 weeks' gestation). The anlage of the patella is clearly visible (*arrows*). Reprinted with permission from Walmsley R. The development of the patella. J Anat 1939–1940;74: 360–370.

medial facet is a secondary characteristic, presumably in response to the forces and constraints applied during early life. There is little doubt that form follows function and that the final shape of both the patella and the femoral trochlea will be modified by use.

PATELLAR MORPHOLOGY

Dye (6) has noted that amphibians and some reptiles do not have osseous patellae. However, lizards, birds, and mammals do. One must speculate, then, based on this observation, that a bony patella is important in terrestrial existence. Several standard anatomy texts contain significant omissions regarding the complex patellar form, the details of which are important to a full understanding of the function and pathology of the patella. The peripheral borders of the patella form a vague triangle, slightly wider than high, with the apex pointing distally (Fig. 1.2, A and B). DeVriese (7), in his anthropologic studies, failed to find any notable racial differences, with limits for lengths varying from 47 to 58

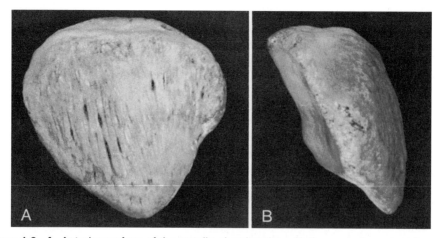

Figure 1.2. A, Anterior surface of the patella showing the cribriform roughened surface with multiple vascular orifices. **B,** The lateral view of the patella shows its general configuration and particularly the sloping base into which the quadriceps inserts.

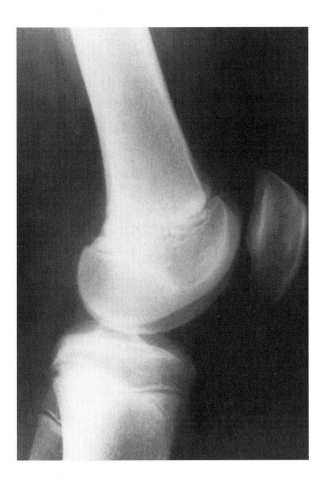

Figure 1.3. The "Cyrano" long-nosed patella. Reprinted with permission from Grelsamer RP, Proctor CS, Bazos AN. Evaluation of patellar shape in the sagittal plane. Am J Sports Med 1994;22(1):61.

mm and for width, from 51 to 57 mm. Vallois (8) developed his patellar index [I = (width × 100/length)], which nearly always exceeds 100. The variations are slight, from 100 (Native American) to 106.2 (Madagascar native).

Whereas width and height are remarkably constant, thickness is quite variable, ranging from 2 to 3 cm as measured in the equatorial plane between the median ridge and the superficial cortex. This measurement on average of 2.5 cm does not include the articular cartilage, which also attains its maximal height at the same level. Variations in both bone and cartilage thicknesses within a given patella determine its particular surface contour that can only be fully appreciated on review of serial sections.

Grelsamer et al (9) studied 564 patients and noted three different patellar shape patterns when analyzing overall patellar length compared with length of the articular surface. They described the "Cyrano" long-nosed patella, in which the distal nonarticular portion of the patella is particularly long (Fig. 1.3).

Anterior Surface

Slightly convex in all directions, the anterior surface is divided into three parts. The rough superior third, the base of the triangle, receives the insertion of the quadriceps tendon. The superficial portion of this tendon continues over the anterior surface to form the deep fascia, which is densely adherent to the bone. The middle third reveals numerous vascular orifices and is crossed by numerous vertical striations, giving a fuzzy or bristled appearance as seen on the axial radiograph. The inferior third terminates in a V-shaped point, which is enveloped by the patellar tendon.

Posterior Surface

This side of the patella can be divided into two parts. The inferior portion, which is nonarticulating, represents a full 25% of the patellar height. This inferior surface, forming the apex of the rough triangle of the patella, is dotted with vascular orifices whose vessels pass through the densely adherent infrapatellar fat pad. The superior, or articular, portion of the posterior surface is completely covered by hyaline cartilage (Fig. 1.4) and makes up approximately 75% of the height of the patella. This articular cartilage, reaching a 4- to 5-mm thickness in its central portion, is the thickest in the body.

Articular Surface

Roughly oval in shape, the articulating portion of the patella is divided into lateral and medial facets by a vertical ridge (Fig. 1.5). The median ridge is oriented in the longitudinal axis of the patella and has roughly the same degree of prominence throughout. The two facets that it separates may be roughly equal in size, but, in general, the lateral facet predominates. Wiberg (10) described the different facet configurations of the patella,

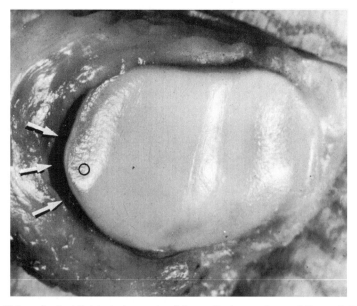

Figure 1.4. This reflected light photograph of the articular surface of the patella shows not only the surface contour but particularly the odd facet (*o*). The extraarticular portion of the patella is completely covered with soft tissue. The cuff of synovium surrounding the articular surface is also shown (*arrows*).

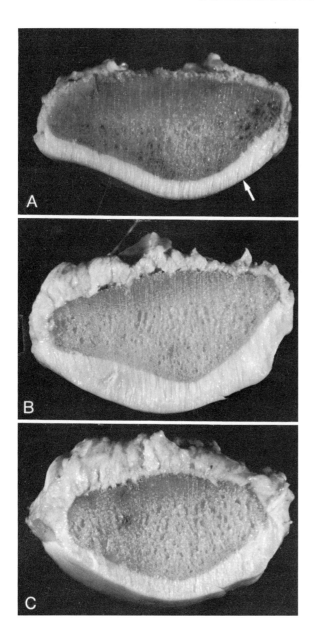

Figure 1.5. Serial cross-sections through the 90-degree **(A)**, 60-degree **(B)**, and 30-degree **(C)** contact zones. The articular cartilage is shown inferiorly with the medial border of the patella to the right. The variations in cartilage thickness and in subchondral configuration are particularly evident. The secondary ridge between the odd and medial facets is very apparent in the 30- and 60-degree sections but not evident in the 90-degree section. The *arrow* in **A** shows the junction between the medial facet and the odd facet, even though no ridge is seen at this level.

which range from medial/lateral facet equality to extreme lateral facet prominence, sometimes referred to as the Wiberg "hunter's cap" patella. Kwak et al (11) described variations of patellofemoral surface geometry in 1997. Staubli et al (12, 13) have pointed out that the articular cartilage surface geometry does not line up with the underlying bone structure. Inferences about congruity based on standard radiographs, therefore, may not always be correct, and magnetic resonance imaging may be necessary to fully appreciate these relationships in patients (Fig. 1.6).

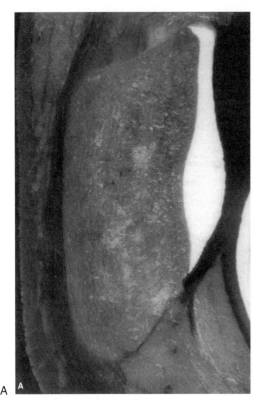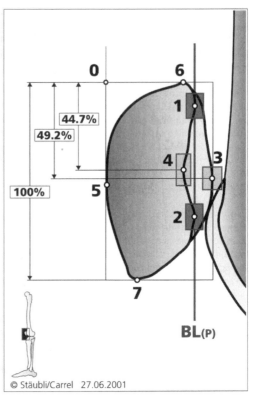

A   B

Figure 1.6. A, A cryosection of the patella shows different bony and articular cartilage surface geometry. **B,** These measurements confirm relative differences of bone-cartilage incongruities. Reprinted with permission from Staubli HU, Bosshard C, Rauschning W. Patellofemoral joint in the sagittal plane: articular surface geometry and osseous anatomy. Sports Med Arthrosc Rev 2001;9(4):288–294.

Medial Facet

This portion of the articular surface shows the greatest anatomic variation. It is subdivided into the medial facet proper and a much smaller "odd" facet along the medial border of the patella (Figs. 1.4, 1.5). This odd facet is separated from the remainder of the medial facet by a small vertical ridge. We have labeled this the "secondary ridge" in that it is less prominent than the median ridge and may develop after birth in response to functional loads applied to the knee. The secondary ridge runs obliquely in a generally longitudinal sense, being closer to the median ridge proximally than distally. It is also more prominent distally than proximally on most specimens (Fig. 1.5, A to C). This ridge conforms to the curve of the lateral border of the medial condyle with the knee in full flexion, whereas the median ridge conforms to the straight medial border of the lateral condyle. This feature has often been overlooked in anatomy textbooks and articles on the patella. One possible reason for this is the fact that this secondary ridge is often purely cartilaginous (Fig. 1.5) and, not always being reflected in subchondral bone, may not be apparent on tangential radiographs of the patellofemoral joint (Fig. 1.7, A and B). There is considerable individual variation in the prominence of the secondary ridge. Also, the odd facet may be in nearly the same plane as the

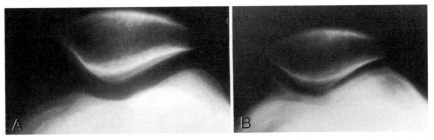

Figure 1.7. A, Axial radiograph of the patellofemoral joint in 30 degrees of flexion. **B,** Same joint with radiopaque contrast added. Note the demonstration of the secondary ridge separating the odd and medial facets, not evident on the plain film.

remainder of the medial facet or assume as much as a 60-degree angle to it. The odd facet may be slightly concave or flat. The remainder of the medial facet also shows great variation but is usually flat or slightly convex. The surface configuration of the articular surface is determined not only by the underlying subchondral bone but also by variations in thickness of the patellar cartilage itself. This makes determination of the patellofemoral articular cartilage condition difficult on any patellofemoral radiographs or imaging studies that do not also employ contrast media, computed tomography, or magnetic resonance imaging.

Lateral Facet

Both longer and wider, the lateral portion of the articular surface is concave in both vertical and transverse planes. Some authors (14, 15) have described three transverse segments on the articular surface, which are delineated in the adult by the presence on both medial and lateral facets of two transverse ridges at the junction of each third. These ridges supposedly isolate three segments of different functional significance as the lower, middle, and upper thirds of the patella are progressively brought into contact (in this order) with the femur during flexion. Emery and Meachim (16) and Ficat (17) have drawn attention to a subtle, relatively constant ridge separating the middle and lower thirds. It is more often present on the lateral facet (Fig. 1.8). Because of varied cartilage thickness of the lateral facet (thicker toward the central ridge), one must be careful about an appearance of lateral facet incongruity (Fig. 1.9), using established radiographic criteria, not visual impression, to determine whether alignment is normal.

Base of the Patella

The proximal margin of the patella forms a triangle with its apex directly posteriorly. It is inclined distally from posterior to anterior, merging with the anterior surface of the patella. Anteriorly, the surface is very irregular and receives the insertion of the quadriceps tendon with the rectus femoris anteriorly, the vastus medialis and lateralis in the midportion, and the intermedius posteriorly. Posteriorly, there is a small free section between the tendon insertion and the insertion of the synovium at the posterior margin. Often there is a small peripatellar fat pad that fills this space, although at the level of the quadriceps insertion, this fat pad is often nonexistent.

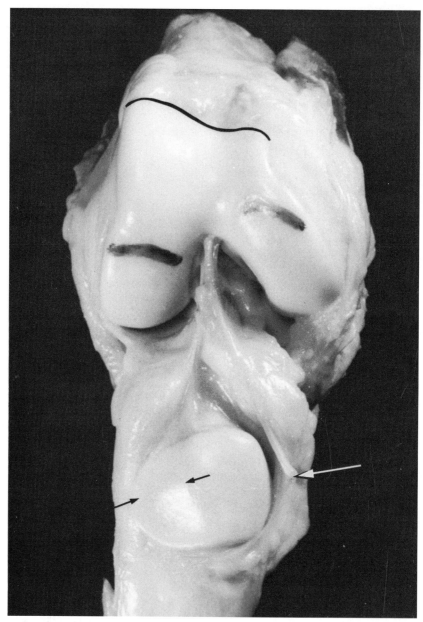

Figure 1.8. Distal femur from the front with the knee in 90 degrees of flexion. The lateral trochlear facet can be seen protruding more anteriorly than the medial. The medial and lateral trochlear condylar junctions have been marked with India ink. The ligamentum mucosum can be seen inserting into the anterior border of the intercondylar notch just anterior to the femoral attachment of the posterior cruciate. The light reflected from the patella shows the transverse ridge often present on the lateral facet (*small arrows*). A well-developed plica synovialis mediopatellaris is also evident (*large arrow*).

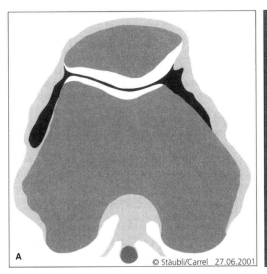
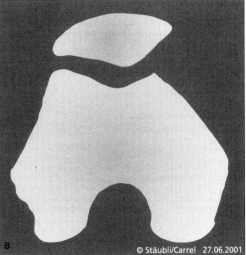

Figure 1.9. These transverse images demonstrate how an impression of patellofemoral incongruity may be possible despite perfect articular alignment. Reprinted with permission from Staubli HU, Durrenmalt U, Porcellini B, Raushning W. Articular cartilage surface and osseous anatomy of the patellofemoral joint in the axial plane. Sports Med Arthrosc Rev 2001;9:282–287.

Apex of the Patella

The distal pole forms a rounded projection that receives the attachment of the patellar tendon.

Paramedian Borders

These are roughly vertical at the level of the articular surface of the patella but then become thinner and run obliquely distally and toward the midline to converge at the apex of the patella. The medial border is considerably thicker than the lateral border, whereas both sides receive the attachment, from posterior to anterior, of the synovium, the joint capsule, the patellofemoral retinaculum, and the quadriceps expansion (the vastus medialis descending more distally than the lateralis). The lateral border receives a fibrous retinaculum, which is composed of two major layers. The superficial oblique lateral retinaculum reflects anterior to the patella and blends with the expansion, whereas the deep transverse lateral retinaculum inserts directly into the lateral patella.

OSSEOUS STRUCTURE

A transverse section of the patella (Fig. 1.10) through the middle of the articulating surface gives a view similar to what one can see using computed tomography or magnetic

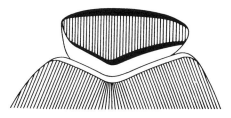

Figure 1.10. Osseous structure of the patellofemoral joint.

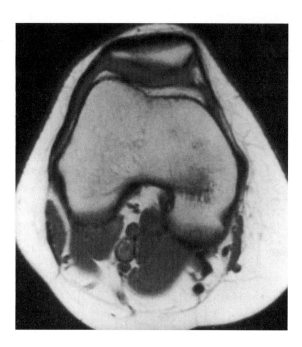

Figure 1.11. Magnetic resonance imaging can discriminate osseous, retinacular, and cartilaginous structures.

resonance imaging (Fig. 1.11). Magnetic resonance imaging (Fig. 1.11) differentiates osseous, cartilaginous, and retinacular structures. Subchondral bone outlines the medial and lateral facets. The lateral line is generally thicker, suggesting greater loading. Subchondral bone density is maximal at the proximal lateral facet (18). The medial line rarely reaches the medial margin of the patella, often dwindling near the junction of the medial and odd facets. Between these two layers of compact bone, the trabeculae of cancellous bone are aligned more or less parallel to each other and perpendicular to the coronal plane of the patella, therefore slightly oblique vis-à-vis the articular facets. The trabeculae of the femur are aligned perpendicular to the articular facets of the femoral trochlea.

TROCHLEAR SURFACE OF THE FEMUR

The articular portion of the anterior surface of the distal femur, which articulates with the patella, has been referred to variously as the patellar facets of the femur, the patellar groove, the femoral sulcus, and the trochlea. The term *trochlea* is chosen here because of its conciseness and lack of confusion with the articular surface of the patella. The trochlear surface of the femur is divided into two facets: medial and lateral. Proximally, they are in continuity with a shallow groove conforming to the contours of the distal patellar articular surface. Curving distally and posteriorly, this groove deepens to become the intercondylar notch.

Lateral (External) Trochlear Facet

This extends more proximally, is larger overall, and projects further anteriorly than the medial facet in most people. The cartilage covering is significantly thinner on the femur than on the patella, being approximately 2 to 3 mm. It is also thinner on the medial facet than on the lateral. The trochlea represents only one part of the femoral pulley with

respect to the patella, albeit the most functional part. In full extension with the quadriceps tightened, the patella articulates with the supratrochlear fat pad of the femur and in
full flexion with that portion of the medial and lateral femoral condyles that articulates
with the tibial plateaus in full extension (see Chapter 2).

The lateral trochlea facet provides a buttress to lateral patellar subluxation and helps
to maintain the patella centered in the trochlea during normal knee function from 15-
degree knee flexion into full flexion. There is substantial variability in trochlear depth,
however. A flat lateral trochlea is common in patients with lateral patellar instability.

Supratrochlear Fossa

This is situated on the anterior surface of the femur immediately proximal to the
trochlear facet. It is slightly depressed and almost triangular in shape. Medially, it is subtly delineated by the rounded anteromedial distal femoral metaphysis. Laterally, the border is more sharply defined by the anterolateral metaphyseal ridge that runs into the
superolateral border of the trochlea. At this juncture, there is often a small tubercle to
which the capsule attaches. This fossa, dotted with vascular channels, is covered with a
prefemoral fat pad. At the lateral margin, an area marked by thickened, fibrotic, blanched
synovia appears as a fibrocartilaginous extension of the lateral facet. This is the site of
contact with the patella under full forced extension (quadriceps setting) (Fig. 1.12).
Because the lateral trochlear facet extends both more proximally and more anteriorly than
the medial, the superior trochlear border runs obliquely posteriorly and distally from lateral to medial (Fig. 1.8). The cartilaginous border of the lateral facet terminates subtly,
which perhaps favors lateral displacement of the patella at the end of extension. The prox-

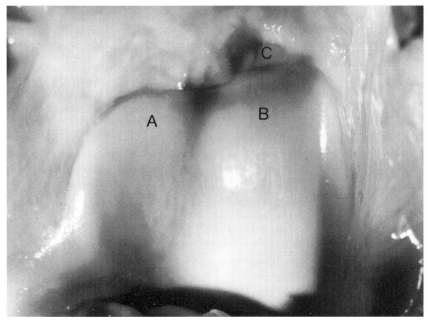

Figure 1.12. Trochlear and supratrochlear fat pad of the femur: **A,** Medial facet. **B,** Lateral
facet. **C,** Supratrochlear tubercle, the site of patellar pressure with the knee in full extension.

imal cartilaginous border of the medial facet is, by contrast, more marked and can form an abrupt convex ridge that has the potential to cause difficulties at the moment of patellar engagement in the trochlear groove as flexion proceeds (19). However, this is not frequently the case because the patella usually enters the trochlear sulcus from a characteristic obliquely lateral position. This pattern has been demonstrated consistently using computed tomography.

Trochlear Condylar Junctions

The condylar surface is separated from its corresponding trochlear surface by a slight groove. This corresponds to the impression of the meniscus at full extension, which explains its secondary appearance in the adult. These indentations are delineated anteriorly by a subtle ridge. Because of the medial condyle's smaller size, greater distal projection, and greater obliquity, the trochlear condylar junctions are asymmetric (Fig. 1.8). The medial ridge is directed convexly, anteriorly, and laterally and is less well developed than the lateral ridge.

SYNOVIUM OF THE PATELLOFEMORAL JOINT

The synovial limits of the patellofemoral joint are essentially the synovium of the anterior portion of the knee and consist of the suprapatellar pouch, the middle portion or peripatellar part, including the lateral recesses and the inferior portion or the infrapatellar fat pad.

Suprapatellar Pouch

Although this pouch can remain isolated and independent of the synovial cavity, there is generally a wide communication with the knee joint proper (20). The proximal extent is variable, but averages 4 to 5 cm from the proximal articular border of the femur. The synovium covers the anterior surfaces of the femur from which it is separated by the prefemoral fat pad. Anteriorly, the synovial pouch is covered by the extensor apparatus. The synovium is densely adherent to the central cartilaginous insertion of the quadriceps femoris distally, but separated from the medial and lateral vasti by a small quantity of fat. The superior reaches of the sac receive the insertion of aberrant fibers of the vasti, referred to as the tensor synovialis. These anatomic facts become important at the time of synovectomy. The distal aspect of the pouch usually communicates widely with the synovial cavity of the knee joint proper. This communication is marked by vestigial fibrous remnants of the embryonic diaphragm that separate the two cavities and more or less involute in the course of the development of the knee. This fibrous ring, the plica synovialis suprapatellaris, is particularly noticeable at the sides and as it approaches the lateral aspects of the patella, approximately 1.5 cm above the base.

Peripatellar Synovium

Here the synovium blends imperceptibly superiorly with the suprapatellar pouch and laterally and medially into the respective recesses. A small synovial fold or fringe less than 1 cm wide surrounds the patella. This is generally less evident at the level of the quadriceps femoris insertion into the patella proximally but is a definite structure laterally, medially, and inferiorly. This middle synovial region represents the true synovium of

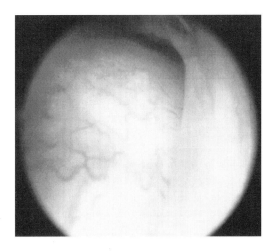

Figure 1.13. Medial infrapatellar plica as seen with an arthroscope.

the patellofemoral joint. Medially and laterally, where the synovium is reflected from the respective condylar coverings to the undersurface of the quadriceps expansion, a synovial fold can be palpated to appreciate synovial thickness in disease. This area of synovium is not only the most exposed but also the most accessible. Both the lateral and medial recesses decrease in height from anterior to posterior to become continuous with the suprameniscal synovium. Medially, there is a plica synovialis mediopatellaris (21), a synovial pleat starting from the medial alar fold and running toward the medial part of the plica synovialis suprapatellaris (Fig. 1.13). This may become apparent during arthroscopy and can, in some cases, produce symptoms similar to those in a patient with patellar articular cartilage degeneration. Hughston and Andrews (22) described plical inflammation in association with chondromalacia and Patel (23, 24) later described the arthroscopic anatomy of plicae. He noted three plicae: the infrapatellar plica (or ligamentum mucosum), the medial patellar plica (or shelf), which most often catches under the medial patella, and the suprapatellar plica. Jackson et al (25) and Dandy (26) emphasized the clinical importance of the medial patellar plica (shelf). Broom and Fulkerson (27) pointed out that plica irritation is frequently associated with abnormal patella mechanics. In fact, one must consider the possibility that an abnormally prominent medial infrapatella plica could result from chronic patellar malalignment developmentally, with excess mesenchymal filling of a medial potential space, later to become a hypertrophic plica.

Infrapatellar Synovium

The infrapatellar fat pad is covered by a true synovial layer and, in turn, covers the extraarticular portion of the posterior patellar surface. The fat pad extends superiorly to merge with the peripatellar fold on both sides of the patella. The superior extent of the fat pad is often past the midpoint of the articular surface of the patella. Posteriorly, it extends into the ligamentum mucosum, which inserts into the anterior border of the intercondylar notch. This bell-shaped ligament, narrow at its femoral attachment, broad as it flows into the fat pad, is delineated medially and laterally by alar folds that merge into the fat pad (Fig. 1.8). Inferiorly, the ligamentum mucosum may form a thin vellum separating the medial and lateral tibiofemoral compartments. In full extension, with the patellar tendon under tension, the fat pad bulges anteriorly on each side of the tendon, giving the false impression of separate medial and lateral pads. This impression is accentuated in patella alta and genu recurvatum, both conditions reducing the space for the fat pad between the extensor apparatus and the femoral condyles. The fat pad may hypertrophy under conditions of recurrent injury and may be the source of symptoms (28).

SOFT-TISSUE STABILIZERS

The patella is the central pole, the crossroad for the converging retinacular elements, ligament, muscle, tendon, and capsule (Fig. 1.14), of the extensive synovial expansion. The patellofemoral articulation cannot tolerate a tightly closed capsular cuff, which explains why the capsule, often poorly defined, does not play its habitual stabilizing role. By contrast, the stabilizer system, comprising ligaments and tendons, is remarkably effective. The patella is solidly anchored to the knee, in both the transverse and the longitudinal directions, by a cruciform soft-tissue system in which it is possible to distinguish both active and passive elements.

Passive Stabilizers

Inferiorly, the patellar tendon limits the proximal ascent of the patella from the tibia. This flattened tendon is 3 cm wide at its insertion into the apex of the patella and 2.5 cm wide at its insertion into the tibial tubercle. It is 5 to 6 cm long and 7 mm thick. Its orientation is roughly in the long axis of the lower extremity but often slightly oblique laterally from proximal to distal, which adds to the tendency toward lateral displacement of

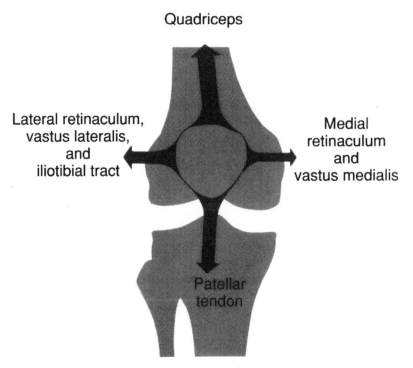

Figure 1.14. Schematic diagram shows the basic orientation of the forces and constraints applied to the patella during function.

the patella. Components of the peripatellar retinaculum interdigitate with the patellar tendon medially and laterally.

The *lateral peripatellar retinaculum* (29) comprises two major components: the superficial oblique retinaculum and the deep transverse retinaculum. The *superficial oblique retinaculum* is rather thin and runs superficially from the iliotibial band to the patella, as shown in Figures 1.15 and 1.16, A. On reflection of the superficial oblique retinaculum, there is a much denser *deep transverse retinaculum* (Fig. 1.16, B), which comprises three major components. The *epicondylopatellar* band portion, also known as the lateral patellofemoral ligament, was originally described by Kaplan (30). It provides superolateral static support for the patella, and its width correlates with patellar shape (31). The midportion of the *deep transverse retinaculum* courses directly from the iliotibial band to the patella and has a dense, fibrous attachment to the patella. This is the primary support structure for the lateral patella. There is also another band, the *patellotibial band*, which provides some distal inferior support for the lateral patella. This band has also been called

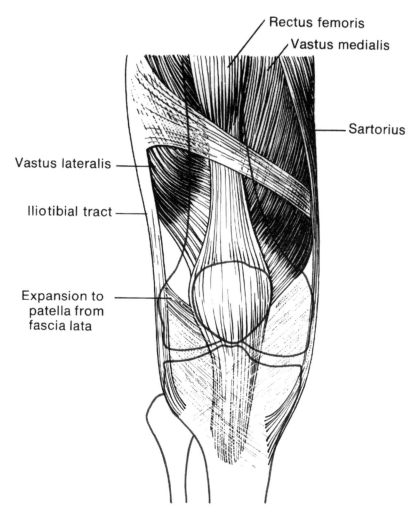

Figure 1.15. The superficial portion of the extensor apparatus.

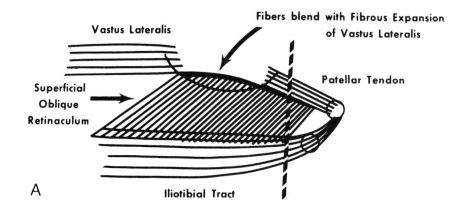

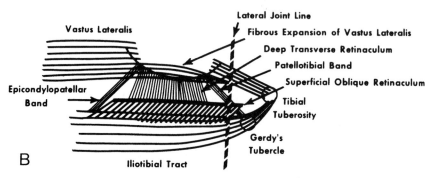

Figure 1.16. A, Lateral view of the extensor mechanism shows the orientation of the elements making up the lateral retinaculum. **B,** Components of the deep lateral retinaculum. Reprinted with permission from Fulkerson JP, Gossling HR. Anatomy of the knee joint lateral retinaculum. Clin Orthop 1980;153:183–188.

the lateral meniscopatellar ligament but is probably more appropriately described by its insertion on the tibia as the patellotibial band. On flexion of the knee, these lateral retinacular bands are drawn posteriorly along with the iliotibial band placing a lateral displacement force on the patella that would cause progressive tilting of the patella except that the medial stabilizers are also tightening and provide a counteracting force. When the medial stabilizers have been stretched, however, the static lateral stabilizers create lateral tilt and displacement of the patella, which may lead to subluxation, excessive tilt, dislocation, or excessive lateral pressure syndrome. Balance between the medial and lateral static stabilizers, therefore, is very important in maintaining appropriate alignment of the extensor mechanism within the femoral trochlea. There is stronger retinacular support laterally than medially.

Medially, capsular condensations form a tough fibrous layer that inserts into the superior two-thirds of the posterior part of the medial border of the patella. This medial *patellofemoral ligament* links the patella to the medial femoral epicondyle and passively limits lateral patellar excursion. Inferiorly, the *medial meniscopatellar ligament* inserts into the inferior third of the medial border of the patella, connecting the patella to the anterior part of the medial meniscus. This ligament is buried in the margins of the fat pad but can be palpated when the patella is put under load.

Above the patella is the central quadriceps tendon expansion of the quadriceps muscle (32). This thick (>9 mm) band of rectus femoris and vastus intermedius tendons can become inflamed or overused like any other tendon. It can be a source of anterior knee pain. This region also provides plentiful tendon graft for cruciate ligament reconstruction. There is much more fibrocartilage at the central quadriceps tendon insertion than at the patellar tendon insertion into the tibia (33), possibly related to the greater absolute size of the central quadriceps tendon compared with the patellar tendon (Fig. 1.17).

The patellar tendon, the central quadriceps tendon, and the medial and lateral retinacula are the passive elements of soft-tissue stabilization. They, along with the bony confines of the trochlea and the active stabilizers, define the limits of patellar excursion. Strictly speaking, however, both the medial and lateral retinacula are partially affected by

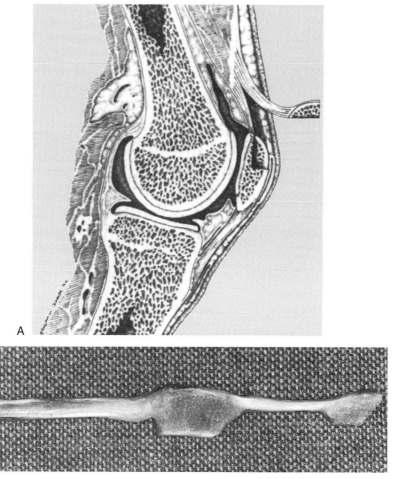

Figure 1.17. A, Central quadriceps tendon is far thicker than the patellar tendon and can provide an alternative tendon graft for cruciate ligament reconstruction. Tendinitis and overuse can occur in this region. Partial thickness central quadriceps tendon is also an excellent alternative cruciate reconstruction graft. (From Fulkerson J, Langeland R. An alternative cruciate reconstruction graft: The central quadriceps tendon. Arthroscopy 1995;11(2):252–254, with permission.) **B,** Central quadriceps tendon. (Courtesy of Rolf Langeland, University of Connecticut School of Medicine, Farmington, CT.)

active stabilizers to some extent. Most of the lateral retinaculum, for instance, originates in the iliotibial band that provides both active and passive stabilization of the patella.

Active Stabilizers

The four main muscular elements of the quadriceps fuse distally into the quadriceps tendon, which can still be identified as three separate layers at their insertion into the patella (Fig. 1.18). Superficially, the rectus femoris inserts into the anterior portion of the top of the patella, as well as the superior third of the anterior surface. The most superficial fibers continue over the anterior surface of the patella to operate a continuous bridge of tough fibrous tissue ending in the patellar tendon. These represent a direct tibial insertion of the quadriceps. In the midportion, the vasti medialis and lateralis unite in the midline to form a solid aponeurosis that inserts into the base of the patella just posterior to the insertion of the rectus femoris. The vasti insertions also continue medially and laterally into their respective borders of the patella. Medially, the muscle fibers and fibrous insertion descend more distally than on the lateral side. Koskinen and Kujala (34), however, have noted more proximal insertion of the vastus medialis in patients with patellar dislocation. The vastus intermedius inserts via a broad, thin tendon into the base of the patella, posterior to the other vasti but anterior to the capsule. Medially and laterally, these insertions reinforce the respective patellofemoral ligaments.

There is some evidence (35) that the rectus femoris may initiate extension of the knee, but contributions from the vastus medialis and lateralis become important only during the latter part of knee extension. This work has suggested independent functioning of different quadriceps components and has supported rehabilitation efforts that emphasize selective strengthening of the vastus medialis to increase dynamic medial support of the patella.

Although the presence of a vastus medialis obliquus has been well accepted by most orthopedic surgeons, little attention was paid to the vastus lateralis insertion into the patella until description of the vastus lateralis obliquus in 1987 by Hallisey et al (36). In this study, it was noted that there is an anatomically distinct group of vastus lateralis

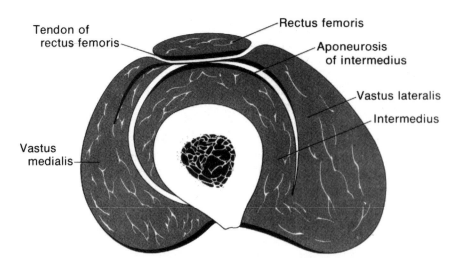

Figure 1.18. This cross-sectional view of the distal femur shows the orientation of the four individual components of the quadriceps. The fascial orientation remains constant as they insert into the proximal, medial, and lateral borders of the patella.

fibers separated from the main belly of the vastus lateralis by a thin layer of fat. This muscle group interdigitates with the lateral intermuscular septum before inserting into the patella. Vastus lateralis obliquus fibers are important because they provide a direct lateral pull on the extensor mechanism by virtue of interdigitation with the lateral intermuscular septum. In addition, this relatively small muscle may be released at the time of lateral retinacular release without detaching the main vastus lateralis tendon. Lateral dynamic support of the patella, then, is very important in understanding patellar balance in the trochlea. Figure 1.19, A and B illustrates the vastus lateralis obliquus photographically and diagrammatically.

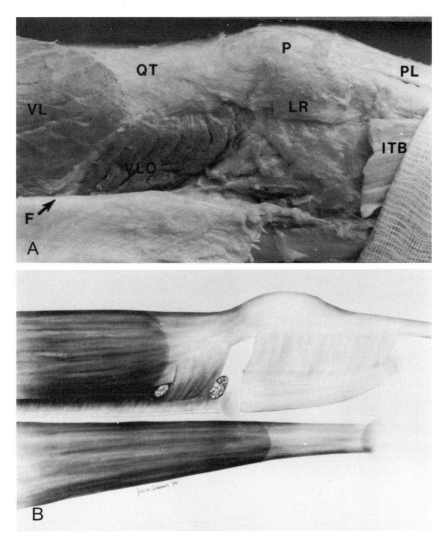

Figure 1.19. A, This photograph shows the lateral musculoretinacular structures that support the patella. *VL,* vastus lateralis; *QT,* quadriceps tendon; *P,* patella; *PL,* patellar ligament (tendon); *VLO,* vastus lateralis obliquus; *LR,* lateral retinaculum; *ITB,* iliotibial band; *F,* fat between VL and VLO. **B,** The same structures in diagrammatic form. Reprinted with permission from Hallisey M, Doherty N, Bennett W, Fulkerson J. Anatomy of the junction of the vastus lateralis tendon and the patella. J Bone Joint Surg 1987;69A:545.

VASCULAR ANATOMY OF THE PATELLOFEMORAL JOINT

Arterial Supply

The patellofemoral joint enjoys a rich vascular anastomosis, receiving arterial input from the medial and lateral sides both superiorly and inferiorly (Fig. 1.20). Superiorly, the lateral superior genicular artery passes through the insertion of the lateral intermuscular septum and sends a branch to the superolateral border of the patella. This branch anastomoses anteriorly and through the quadriceps insertion with branches of the *medial superior genicular artery* approaching the superomedial aspect of the patella. Distally, the *medial inferior genicular artery* approaches the patella and sends anastomosing branches both superiorly, paralleling the medial border of the patella, and laterally, behind the patellar tendon, to anastomose with the *lateral inferior genicular artery*. The *anterior tibial recurrent artery* also approaches the inferolateral border of the patella. In fact, the fat pad is an important source of blood supply entry into the patella (37). The six named arterial components of the patellar circulation anastomose freely around the patella, forming a peripatellar circle.

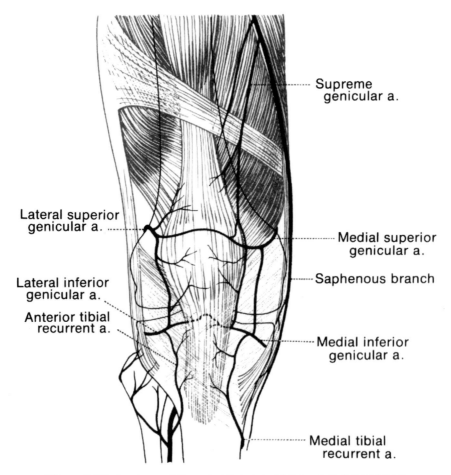

Figure 1.20. Anatomy of the arterial supply of the patellofemoral joint.

Outside this anastomotic peripatellar system, which richly supplies the anterior or patellar portion of the patellofemoral joint, there also exist two other deep anastomotic systems coming from the same superior and inferior genicular arteries that form the blood supply to the femur and tibia underneath the synovial coverings. These two arcades then irrigate the synovium and epiphyses of the tibia and femur. It is evident, then, that the patellofemoral joint is supplied on its two sides by six peripheral vascular sources from the same origin, which anastomose on two levels—one superficial and the other deep. This anatomic distribution of arterial blood supply demonstrates a remarkable vascular unity, particularly with regard to the patella, which receives branches from all directions, with the peripatellar circle providing entry into the patella itself through two principal routes: one through the middle third of the anterior surface and the other at the level of the inferior extraarticular portion of the posterior surface (38).

Venous Drainage

Transpatellar venography was carried out in a series of patients by injection of contrast medium directly into the cancellous bone of the patella, demonstrating the distribution of the venous drainage of the patella. This phlebography reproduces the general vascular peripatellar framework that has just been described on the arterial side and permits several comments. The richness of the venous elements of small caliber sometimes hinders interpretation of the phlebograms and the identification of the principal drainage pathways. The inferior pole of the patella appears to be the veritable vascular hilus of this bone (Fig. 1.21, A and B). The vascular penetration of the anterior surface seems to be much more the accessory system. The two principal drainage routes consist of, in the first instance, the *popliteal vein*, the midportion of which is usually well visualized, and sec-

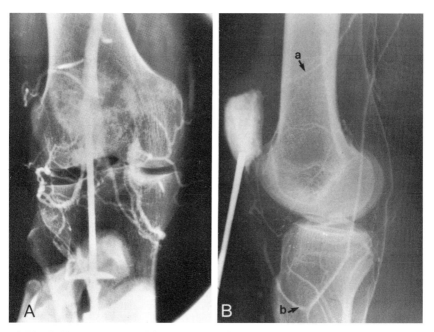

Figure 1.21. A, Transpatellar phlebogram, anterior view. **B,** Transpatellar phlebogram, lateral view: *a*, superior venous circle. Popliteal not well visualized; *b*, inferior venous circle.

ond, the *internal saphenous vein*. One discovers, in general, the same kind of picture as the arterial input, but the anterior recurrent tibial veins are not always visualized. When carrying out phlebography, one should always observe the medullary circulation by taking a radiographic film 15 minutes after the injection of opaque material, by which time all material should have cleared the bone unless intraosseous stasis exists. Thus, the patella is not a bone that is poorly vascularized as some have written, but, on the contrary, is well nourished and well drained by multiple ports of entry, both anteriorly and posteriorly, and supplemented by a rich anastomotic system.

Functional Aspects of the Vascular Supply

The intramedullary pressure that prevails is similar to that found at other points in the body and averages between 10 and 15 mm Hg. The bone blood flow is controlled by various systemic and local factors that influence bone blood flow in general, particularly the sympathetic system. This vascular system both determines and is influenced by joint function. Much as the architectural anatomy of the bone structures is modeled according to the functional constraint of the joint itself, so the vascular anatomy is also influenced by joint function. The vascular anatomy demonstrates the relative independence of the patellofemoral joint in that it possesses its own true vascular tree. However, there is some interdependence with the femorotibial articulation because the deep anastomotic branches also participate in nutrition of the femoral and tibial epiphyses, anastomosing with the posterior network as well. Pathologic conditions of the vascular system can affect the entire knee or simply one of its components, such as the patellofemoral compartment.

REFERENCES

1. Walmsley R. The development of the patella. J Anat 1939–1940;74:360–370.
2. Gray DJ, Gardner E. Prenatal development of the human knee and superior tibiofibular joints. Am J Anat 1950; 86:235–287.
3. Bernays A. Die entwicklungsgeschichte des kniegelenkes des menschen. Morph 1878;JB:4.
4. Grynflet E. Note sur le developpement de l'articulation du genou chez l'homme. Montpellier Med 1904;1: 613–624.
5. Langer M. Uber die entwicklung des kniegelenkes. Z Gesamte Anat 1929;89:83–101.
6. Dye SF. An evolutionary perspective of the knee. J Bone Joint Surg 1987;69A:976.
7. DeVriese B. La signification morphologique de la rotule basee sur des recherches antropologiques. Bull Mem Soc Anthrop (Paris) 1913;4:316.
8. Vallois H. La valeur morphologique de la rotule chez les mammiferes. Bull Mem Soc Anthrop (Paris) 1917;18 January.
9. Grelsamer RP, Proctor CS, Bazos AN. Evaluation of patellar shape in the sagittal plane. A clinical analysis. Am J Sports Med 1994;22(1):61.
10. Wiberg G. Roentgenographic and anatomic studies on the femoro-patellar joint. Acta Orthop Scand 1941;12: 319–10.
11. Kwak SD, Colman W, Ateshian G et al. Anatomy of the human patellofemoral joint articular cartilage surface curvature analysis. J Orthop Res 1997;15:468–472.
12. Staubli H, Bosshard C, Rauschning W. Patellofemoral joint in the sagittal plane: articular surface geometry and osseous anatomy. Sports Med Arthrosc Rev 2001;9(4):288–294,
13. Staubli HU, Durrenmatt U, Porcellini B, Raushning W. Articular cartilage surface and osseous anatomy of the patellofemoral joint in the axial plane. Sports Med Arthrosc Rev 2001;9:282–287.
14. De Palma AF. Diseases of the Knee. Philadelphia: JB Lippincott; 1954.
15. Watanabe M. In Helfet A, ed. Disorders of the Knee. Philadelphia: JB Lippincott; 1974, p. 147.
16. Emery IH, Meachim G. Surface morphology and topography of patello-femoral cartilage fibrillation in Liverpool necropsies. J Anat 1973;116:103–120.
17. Ficat C. La degenerescence du cartilage de la rotule. De la chondromalacie a l'arthrose. Semin Hosp (Paris) 1974;50:3201–3209.

18. Eckstein F, Muller-Gerbl M, Putz R. Distribution of subchondral bone density and cartilage thickness in the human patella. J Anat 1992;180(pt 3):425–433.
19. Outerbridge RE. The etiology of chondromalacia patellae. J Bone Joint Surg 1961;43B:752–757.
20. Paturet G. Traite d'anatomie humaine. Paris: Masson et Cie; 1951.
21. Ilino S. Normal arthroscopic findings in the knee joint in adult cadavers. J Jpn Orthop Assoc 1939;14:467–523.
22. Hughston J, Andrews J. The suprapatellar plica and internal derangement. J Bone Joint Surg 1973;55A:1318.
23. Patel D. Arthroscopy of the plical-synovial folds and their significance. Am J Sports Med 1978;6:217.
24. Patel D. Plica as a cause of anterior knee pain. Orthop Clin North Am 1986;17(2):273.
25. Jackson R, Marshall D, Fujisawa Y. The pathological medial shelf. Orthop Clin North Am 1982;13(2):307.
26. Dandy D. Arthroscopy in the treatment of young patients with anterior knee pain. Orthop Clin North Am 1986;17(2):221.
27. Broom M, Fulkerson J. The plica syndrome: a new perspective. Orthop Clin North Am 1986;17:279–281.
28. Hoffa A. The influence of the adipose tissue with regard to the pathology of the knee joint. JAMA 1904,43:795.
29. Fulkerson JP, Gossling HR. Anatomy of the knee joint lateral retinaculum. Clin Orthop 1980;153:183–188.
30. Kaplan E. Some aspects of functional anatomy of the human knee joint. Clin Orthop 1962;23:18.
31. Reider B, Marshall L, Koslin B, Girgis FG. The anterior aspect of the knee joint. J Bone Joint Surg 1981;63A(3):351–356.
32. Fulkerson J, Langeland R. An alternative cruciate reconstruction graft. Arthroscopy 1995;11(2): 252–254.
33. Evans EJ, Benjamin M, Pemberton DJ. Fibrocartilage in the attachment zones of the quadriceps tendon and patellar ligament of man. J Anat 1990;171:155–162.
34. Koskinen SK, Kujala UM. Patellofemoral relationships and distal insertion of the vastus medialis muscle: A magnetic resonance imaging study in nonsymptomatic subjects and in patients with patellar dislocation. Arthroscopy 1992;8(4):465–468.
35. Wheatley M, Jahnke W. Electromyographic study of the superficial thigh and hip muscles in normal individuals. Arch Phys Med Rehabil 1951;32:508.
36. Hallisey M, Doherty N, Bennett W, Fulkerson J. Anatomy of the junction of the vastus lateralis tendon and the patella. J Bone Joint Surg 1987;69A:545.
37. Shim SS, Leung G. Blood supply of the knee joint. A microangiographic study in children and adults. Clin Orthop 1986;208:119–125.
38. Scapinelli R. Blood supply of the human patella. J Bone Joint Surg 1967;49B:563–570.

2

Biomechanics of the Patellofemoral Joint

"If we select any object from the whole extent of animated nature, and contemplate it fully and in all its bearings, we shall certainly come to this conclusion: that there is Design in the mechanical construction, Benevolence in the endowments of the living properties, and that Good on the whole is the result."

—Sir Charles Bell (1774–1842)
(The Hand, Its Mechanism and Vital Endowments as Evincing Design, Ch 1.)

BIOMECHANICS

Ultimately, health and disease of the patellofemoral joint must be understood in biomechanical terms. In carrying out its functions, the patella must accommodate the forces that normal activity brings to bear on this joint. The capacity to accommodate these forces may be reduced by abnormalities of anatomy or disease or overcome by injury or overloading. Alterations of the joint caused by aging may also have an adverse effect. Understanding the failure to meet the mechanical demands of daily activity requires an understanding of how load is transmitted across the patellofemoral joint, how that joint is stabilized, and how the two parts of the joint move in relation to one another during function. It is not necessary to be an engineer or a mathematician to understand the basic mechanical principles governing the patellofemoral joint that play an important role both in pathology and rehabilitation.

FUNCTIONS OF THE PATELLA

Some authors believe that the patella is not very important in extensor mechanism mechanics (1–3) and, therefore, readily recommend patellectomy. Others, on the contrary, attribute to the patella a more prominent role (4–8), recommending its preservation whenever possible.

Perhaps the patella's most important function is facilitating extension of the knee by increasing the distance of the extensor apparatus from the axis of flexion and extension of the knee. Throughout the entire range of motion, the patella increases the force of extension by as much as 50% (9). Hyaline cartilage, with its very low compressive stiffness and coefficient of friction (10), is indispensable for transmitting the quadriceps force around the distal femur to the tibia. This function is underlined by the existence of a superior patella in the tendon of the intermedius muscle in some mammals that function with the knee in extreme flexion (11).

The patella acts as a guide for the quadriceps tendon in centralizing the divergent input from the four muscles of the quadriceps, transmitting these forces to the patellar tendon. This decreases the possibility of dislocation of the extensor apparatus and controls the capsular tension of the knee. The patella also protects the cartilage of the trochlea as well as the condyles by acting as a bony shield.

Most authors seem to have taken for granted an essential function of the patella, the loss of which results in patients seeking treatment. One of the capital characteristics of hyaline cartilage is its absence of a nerve supply. Healthy cartilage allows the transmission of forces to subchondral and cancellous bone in such a way that the pain threshold of the richly innervated bone is not surpassed. It is also well known that tendons are capable of withstanding great tensile loads, but not high friction or compression. The presence of the patella in the extensor apparatus protects the tendon from friction and permits the extensor apparatus to tolerate high compressive loads.

Finally, the patella plays a role in the aesthetic appearance of the knee. This can be appreciated in the patellectomized knee in which the flattened ends of the condyles are easily visible with the knee flexed. Of all these functions, the most important role of the patella is in extension of the knee. Patellectomy results in weakened extension of the knee or even incomplete knee extension. Some muscle atrophy inevitably follows patellectomy despite sustained and intensive physical therapy.

STATICS

Statics is a useful engineering tool to describe forces acting on a body in equilibrium. Using mathematical calculations to analyze the forces applied to the knee joint in various positions of flexion, one can calculate minimal compressive loads that cross the patellofemoral joint for a given degree of flexion. This exercise has been carried out by numerous authors (4, 7, 12–20), with considerable divergence of quantitative values. This is not surprising because any determination of net patellofemoral contact force will depend on many factors, including body weight, quadriceps force, angle of flexion, rotation, and individual anatomic variations.

Calculation of Patellofemoral Compression

The patellofemoral joint reaction (PFJR) force is equal and opposite to the resultant of the quadriceps tension (M_1) and patellar tendon tension (M_2) acting perpendicular to the articular surfaces (Fig. 2.1). The PFJR force increases with increasing flexion on two accounts: first, as the angle between the patellar tendon and the quadriceps becomes more acute and the resultant vector increases; second, as knee flexion increases, the effective lever arms of the femur and the tibia increase, requiring greater quadriceps power to resist the flexion moment of body weight (Fig. 2.2). Some authors have used the entire length of the femur in carrying out their calculations. Bandi (4) pointed out, however, that during normal activities requiring knee flexion under load, hip flexion is also present, thus bringing the center of gravity forward and shortening the femoral lever arm. This difference in calculation alone results in nearly halving the calculated PFJR force (Fig. 2.3).

Earlier authors, including those of the first edition of this book, made the incorrect assumption that quadriceps force (M_1) equaled patellar tendon force (M_2), viewing the

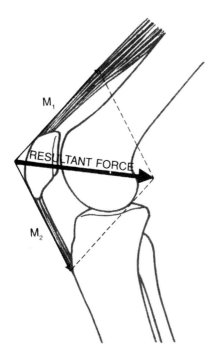

Figure 2.1. Compressive forces on the patellofemoral joint are determined by the resultant of flexion as schematized.

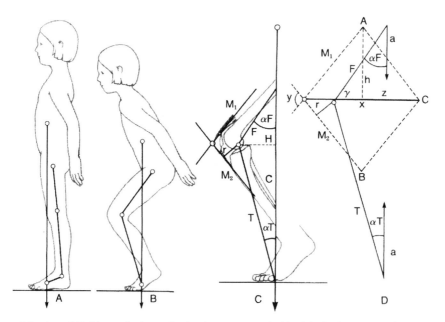

Figure 2.2. A and **B,** Normally, knee flexion is accompanied by hip flexion that shifts the center of gravity forward, reducing the length of the lever arm working on the patellofemoral joint. **C,** Diagram from which numerical calculation of M_1 and M_2 can be made as long as angle of flexion and body weight are known (see text). **D,** Diagram from which resultant patellofemoral joint reaction can be calculated once M_1 and M_2 are determined (see text). Redrawn from Bandi W. Chondromalacia patellae and femoro-patellare arthrose. Helv Chir Acta 1972;1(suppl):3–70.

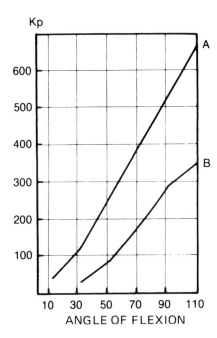

Figure 2.3. Graph shows the total compressive load applied to the patellofemoral joint with changing knee flexion. **B,** Taking into account both associated hip flexion and the changing length of R with the varying degrees of flexion. **A,** Same calculation using entire length of femur in equation. The graph shows 0 degrees for full extension, although in actually carrying out mathematical manipulation from the formula, it is necessary to use 180 degrees for the position of full extension (see text). Adapted from Bandi W. Chondromalacia patellae and femoropatellar arthrose. Helv Chir Acta 1972;1(suppl):3–70.

patellofemoral joint as a frictionless pulley. This has now been shown to be incorrect, and the ratio M_1/M_2 does not equal 1 throughout most of the range of motion. Maquet (21) pointed out the complex relationship between M_1 and M_2 through the static force analysis of line drawings of the lateral view of the knee in several angles of flexion. The essential findings of his original work have been experimentally confirmed by several authors (18–20, 22, 23). The most comprehensive analysis was published recently by Ahmed et al (20). Potentially, the extensor mechanism could be viewed as a frictionless pulley or as frictionless contact. The frictionless contact concept best fits the experimental data. The ratio of M_1/M_2 is shown in Figure 2.4. Huberti et al (19) and Ahmed et al (20), using a direct method of measuring M_1 but a buckle transducer for M_2, obtained quantitatively different but qualitatively similar results to those of Buff et al (18). From a knowledge of M_1 and M_2, body weight, angle of knee flexion, extensor lever arm, flexor lever arm, and angle of quadriceps tendon/patellar tendon, the PFJR can be calculated according to the formula:

$$\text{PFJR} = \sqrt{F_q^2 + F_p^2 + 2FqFp\cos\gamma}$$

Although the ratio of M_1/M_2 increases steadily with increasing knee flexion under normal weight bearing, both the patellar tendon force (M_2) and PFJR increase with increasing flexion (Fig. 2.4).

Although mathematical manipulations are necessary to arrive at quantitative figures for a given situation, analyzing particular qualitative factors will facilitate an understanding of patellofemoral mechanics. For the same degree of knee flexion, the center of gravity may be shifted forward, having the effect of reducing the flexion moment arm. An example of this is the movement in rising from a chair. Some sports, notably skiing, may shift the center of gravity backward, increasing this moment arm considerably and increasing the PFJR force. Bandi (4) calculated the PFJR according to degree of knee flexion, but more recent studies (18, 19) permit more accurate determination of the PFJR force.

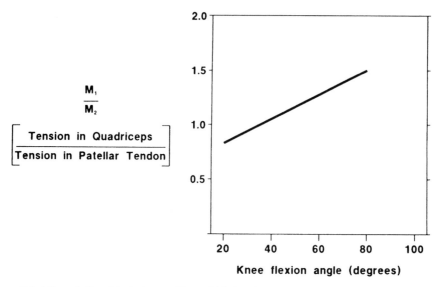

Figure 2.4. The relationship between M_1 and M_2 has been extrapolated from several authors. Reprinted with permission from Buff HU, Jones LC, Hungerford DS. Experimental determination of forces transmitted through the patello-femoral joint. J Biomech 1988;21:17–23, and Huberti HH, Hayes WC, Stone JL, Shybut GT. Force ratios in the quadriceps tendon and ligamentum patellae. J Orthop Res 1984;2:49–54. Quadriceps tension becomes relatively more prominent with increasing knee flexion.

One should not be fooled, however, into thinking that *in vitro* models used in many biomechanical studies give more than a superficial view of the mechanical factors affecting the patellofemoral joint. Most models do not take into account retinacular tensions or the effect of acceleration and deceleration. They do, however, give some appreciation of the severalfold multiplication of body weight across the articulation and potential concentration of these loads on patellar cartilage when the knee is in particular positions.

Reilly and Martens (17) calculated the highest PFJR force for level walking to be 0.5 times body weight. In contrast, with stair climbing and descending, the PFJR force reached 3.3 times body weight. Hungerford and Barry (24) showed that extending the knee against the weight of a 9-kg boot attached to the foot produced a peak PFJR force at 36 degrees of knee flexion. Huberti and Hayes (25) extrapolated contact forces of 4600 N (approximately 6.5 × body weight) on the patella, again emphasizing the magnitude of patellar contact pressures that can occur over very small surface areas.

Dye (26–28) introduced the concept of an "envelope of function," which can apply to many musculoskeletal systems but is very helpful in understanding stresses applied to the patellofemoral joint and surrounding structures. Function normally goes on within a zone of homeostasis, the outer limit of which is defined as the envelope of function by Dye. Stresses beyond this limit may cause loss of tissue integrity and, presumably, pain or tissue damage. Thus, an individual may create a painful condition by simply applying too much load with too much frequency (Fig. 2.5). Alternatively, if too little load is applied

Figure 2.5. The Dye envelope of function theory (from Dye S et al, Op Tech Sports Med 1999;April 17(2):51–52).

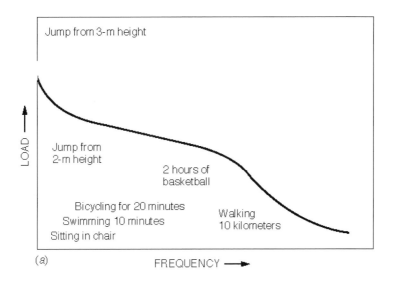

Jump from 3-m height

Jump from
2-m height

2 hours of
basketball

Bicycling for 20 minutes

Swimming 10 minutes

Sitting in chair

Walking
10 kilometers

LOAD

FREQUENCY

(a)

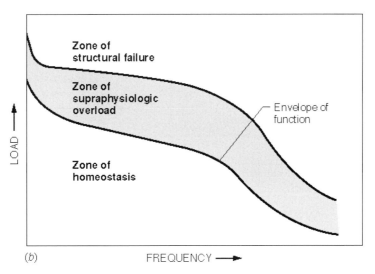

Zone of
structural failure

Zone of
supraphysiologic
overload

Envelope of
function

Zone of
homeostasis

LOAD

FREQUENCY

(b)

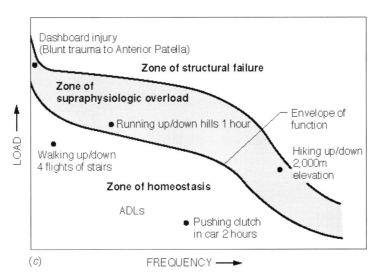

Dashboard injury
(Blunt trauma to Anterior Patella)

Zone of structural failure

Zone of
supraphysiologic overload

Envelope of
function

● Running up/down hills 1 hour

Hiking up/down
2,000m
elevation

●

Walking up/down
4 flights of stairs

Zone of homeostasis

ADLs

● Pushing clutch
in car 2 hours

LOAD

FREQUENCY

(c)

to the knee for an extended period of time (e.g., bed rest for a month), loss of tissue homeostasis manifested, for example, by disuse atrophy of muscle, can occur.

The Dye theory is helpful in explaining patellofemoral pain in patients with apparently normal patellofemoral alignment and function but also applies to patients with abnormal mechanical function (such as malalignment). When there is abnormal alignment, unit loads on one part of the patellofemoral joint (such as the lateral facet in patients with the Ficat excessive lateral pressure syndrome) may be extremely high such that realignment to redistribute and equalize forces may become necessary to get load distribution back into the envelope of function for that patient.

PATELLOFEMORAL CONTACT AREAS

The absolute PFJR is only one part of the equation in understanding the mechanics of the patellofemoral joint in health and disease. The second essential part is to understand what is happening to the patellofemoral contact area. Although the PFJR is steadily increasing with increasing flexion, so is the patellofemoral contact area. Under normal loading conditions, this is not sufficient to maintain a constant unit load, but it is helpful.

Staubli et al (29) provided some wonderful tomographic images depicting the "mismatch" between cartilage and bone congruity is patellofemoral articulation. Congruity between patella and trochlea may be perfect with regard to articular cartilage, yet bony surfaces may be apparently incongruous (Fig. 2.6).

Wiberg's classic article (30) on the patellofemoral joint contains a great deal of information concerning the contact areas, which seems to have been lost by many subsequent authors. His technique of serially sectioning cadaveric knees frozen in various degrees of flexion posed three problems: (a) only one position could be used per joint, (b) the patellofemoral joint was not loaded, and (c) the method necessitated reconstruction of the contact area from the serial sections, making them difficult to visualize. The essentials of his work, however, have been confirmed.

Goodfellow et al (31) reported a method that allows multiple contact prints per cadaver knee under a load qualitatively but not quantitatively simulating normal knee flexion (Fig.

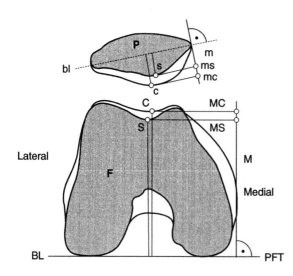

Figure 2.6. Staubli's documentation of the differences between osseous and chondral anatomy at the articular level: diagram of the measurement technique on magnetic resonance arthrotomograms for the patella (*P*) and femoral trochlea (*FT*) in the axial plane. *F*, femur; *P*, patella; *PFT*, posterior femoral tangent; *B1*, baseline patella; *BL*, baseline femur; *m*, medial tangent patella; *mc*, distance of median cartilage ridge (*c*) of patella to *m*; *ms*, distance of subchondral bony prominence (*s*) to *m*; *M*, medial tangent femur; *MC*, distance of deepest part of surface concavity of intercondylar sulcus (*C*) to *M*; *MS*, distance of deepest part of osseous concavity of femoral trochlea (*S*) to *M*.

2.7, A). In this technique, the area of articular contact was delineated by dyeing noncontact cartilage using a technique described by Greenwald and Haynes (32) and modified by Deane (33). This model demonstrated that after 30 degrees of flexion and under static conditions, patellar stability is determined by the resultant of force perpendicular to the articular surfaces. The congruence of the surfaces in all degrees of flexion contributes to stability under load in the same way that Hsieh and Walker (34) have shown for the tibiofemoral joint. To come out of contact, the patella has to work "uphill" on the trochlea against the resultant of force applied by the quadriceps and patellar tendon forces.

The patella first begins to glide onto the articular surface of the trochlea at approximately 10 degrees of knee flexion. The controlling factor is the length of the patellar tendon. In patella alta, greater flexion will be necessary before the patella reaches the relatively stable seating of the trochlea. As the patella first begins to glide onto the articular cartilage of the trochlea, the contact print shows why the transition from lateral femoral condyle to femoral metaphysis is smooth, whereas the medial condyle presents a definite step of varying degrees of prominence. Pressure from the patella molds the lateral femur, whereas the median ridge does not come in contact with the patella under the usual circumstances. The 20-degree contact print (Fig. 2.7, B) shows the smooth zone of contact extending from near the secondary ridge between the medial and lateral facets to near the lateral border of the patella. The continuous nature of this contact encompassing the medial and lateral facets is characteristic of the contact up to 90 degrees of flexion. Although one can speak of separate medial and lateral facets, there is not a corresponding separate zone of contact for each facet but rather a band of contact on the patella that moves proximally with increasing knee flexion (Fig. 2.7, C). In 1995, Singerman et al (35) confirmed this pattern of proximal patellar load-bearing shift with increasing knee flexion. In normal alignment, the lateral to medial contact area ratio is 1.6:1.0, with mean pressure the same on both facets (36).

The contact zone reaches the proximal patellar border by 90 degrees of flexion, with the contact area increasing as the contact zone moves proximally and as knee flexion proceeds (Fig. 2.7, D). Thus, in the first 90 degrees of flexion, virtually all the patellar articular cartilage, with the exception of the odd facet, is brought into load-bearing contact with femoral articular cartilage. As this contact band has been moving up the patella, it has also been steadily increasing in area (Fig. 2.7, E–G). Considering the earlier demonstration of the increasing load with progressive flexion, this would appear to be a sophisticated mechanism for maintaining a relatively constant unit load. Figure 2.8 shows area comparisons for varying degrees of flexion for four knees in which these measurements were carried out. Aglietti et al (37) found a similar quantitative increase in patellofemoral contact area with increasing flexion.

By 135 degrees of flexion, the contact pattern has changed drastically. The central ridge and medial facet now lie free in the intercondylar notch, completely out of contact (Figs. 2.8, 2.9). The entire odd facet engages the lateral border of the medial condyle. This area of the medial condyle contacts the medial tibial spine in full extension, and it is also the classic site for osteochondritis dissecans (6, 22, 38). The lateral patellar facet covers a large part of the lateral condyle of the femur, whereas the medial condyle is not covered. It should be noted that the lateral contact area on the femur corresponds to the tibial contact area on the femur with the knee in full extension. Eckstein et al (39) noted that subchondral bone density maxima correspond to this part of the patella, being greatest at the proximal lateral facet.

In passing from the 90-degree contact pattern to the 135-degree pattern, the zone of contact has passed over the ridge separating the medial and odd facets (40).

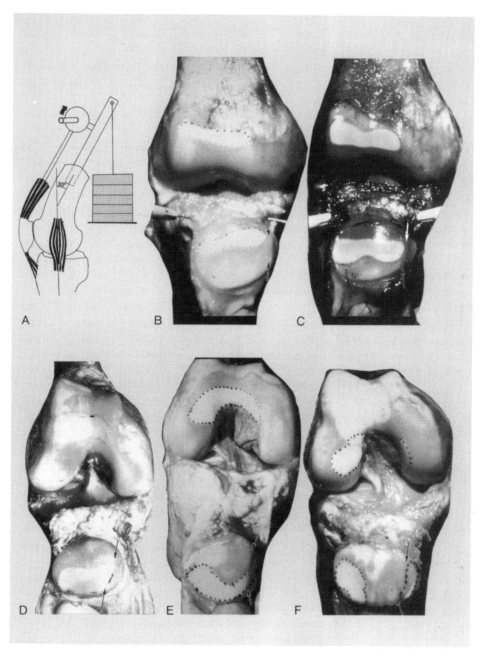

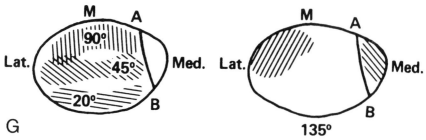

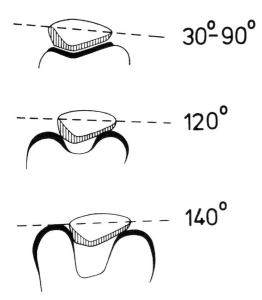

Figure 2.8. Shifting of load-bearing surface on patella with increasing knee flexion. Reprinted with permission from Hehne HJ. Biomechanics of the patellofemoral joint and its clinical relevance. Clin Orthop 1990;258:73–85.

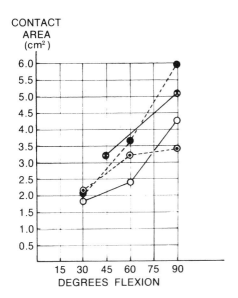

Figure 2.9. Graph shows unit area of contact in relationship to increasing knee flexion for four individual specimens. Compare the increasing surface area with increasing flexion to Figure 2.7; this comparison demonstrates the increasing compressive load with increased flexion.

Figure 2.7. A, Method of applying force to the patellofemoral joint for the contact studies. **B** to **F,** Patellofemoral contact areas for increasing degrees of flexion: **B,** 20 degrees; **C,** 60 degrees; **D,** 90 degrees; **E,** 120 degrees; **F,** 135 degrees (see text). In all photographs, the knee is seen from the front with the lateral side on the reader's left. *Arrows* delineate the secondary ridge separating the medial and odd facets. **G,** Areas of articular contact on the patella with increasing knee flexion. Reprinted with permission from Hungerford DS, Barry M. Biomechanics of the patellofemoral joint. Clin Orthop 1979;144: 1. Note that in early knee flexion, the area of contact is distal on the patella, but the contact area moves proximal on the patella with increasing flexion.

Patellofemoral contact has been characterized up to 90 degrees of flexion by congruence between the patellar and the trochlear facets. Even the contact between the odd facet and the lateral border of the medial condyle is normally characterized by congruence grossly, but Fujikawa et al (41) noted that the femoral trochlea angle was slightly greater than the patellar facet angle at every region of contact between the patella and the femur. However, in passing from 90 to 135 degrees, the convex ridge of cartilage, which is normally thick, comes into apposition with convex femoral articular cartilage, which suggests the possibility of high unit load. This transition takes place, however, in the proximal patella where the ridge is normally not very prominent. This may account for the fact that not every patella shows pathology in this area. Also, retropatellar contact stress is reduced past 70 degrees of knee flexion because of direct force transmission to the patellar tendon (36).

From an observation of the contact prints alone, one could come to the conclusion that the area available for load bearing decreases after 90 degrees of flexion. However, a look at the femur after 90 degrees of flexion shows a broad band of unstained cartilage proximal to the site of patellar contact (Fig. 2.7, C to E). After 90 degrees of flexion, the posterior surface of the quadriceps tendon is brought into contact with the trochlear facets of the femur. Goymann and Mueller (15) have referred to this as the "turn-around" of forces. Once the quadriceps tendon comes into a load-bearing relationship with the femur, the actual compression forces are divided between the extensive "tendofemoral" contact and the patellofemoral contact. This would appear to be another sophisticated means of maintaining constant unit load in situations in which total load is increasing.

DYNAMICS

In full extension, the patella articulates with the supratrochlear fat pad. Normal knee valgus creates an angle between the line of pull of the quadriceps and the patellar tendon, the so-called "Q angle" (Fig. 2.10). Hvid and Andersen (42) showed that the Q angle correlates with internal hip rotation. The "screw home" mechanism of the tibiofemoral joint in terminal extension (whereby the tibia rotates externally in relation to the femur) further lateralizes the tibial tubercle. With the quadriceps contracted and the knee fully extended, the patella is free from the confines of the femoral trochlea. The pull of the quadriceps then produces a valgus vector (Fig. 2.11), which is resisted by the medial patellar retinaculum (Fig. 2.12) (36) and the vastus medialis. It is dangerous, however, to focus too much on the Q angle. The clinician must recognize that this is only *one* of many factors affecting patellar balance. An increased Q angle provides *no* direct correlation with patellofemoral pain, any more than correcting a high Q angle ensures consistent relief of pain.

With the knee fully extended and the quadriceps flaccid, the distal patella rests at the proximal trochlea. Setting the quadriceps produces 8 to 10 mm of proximal movement of the patella. This proximal movement is limited by the patellar tendon. In most cases, the proximal movement has a definite lateral component, although Moller et al (43) found no difference in vastus medialis and lateralis contraction by electromyography in patients with symptomatic subluxation and chondromalacia. Stein et al (44) stated, however, that the patella moves medially with normal ambulation, and this is consistent with clinical observations. Hefzy and Yang (45) also noted medial translation of the patella in the first 40 degrees of knee flexion.

Observing the course of flexion of the patella, beginning from a position of forced full extension, can bring out some of the dynamics associated with various pathologic condi-

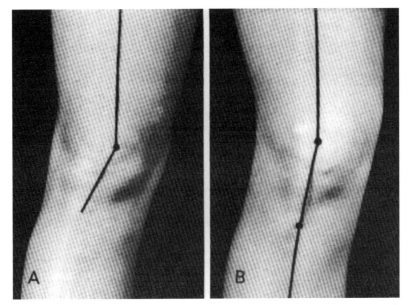

Figure 2.10. A, Q angle is demonstrated with the knee in full extension. **B,** Knee is flexed 30 degrees in this photograph. The tibia has rotated medially, nearly completely neutralizing the Q angle. The patellar tendon is lined up with the anterior border of the tibia. Note also in **B** how the fat pad bulge has disappeared and the patella has increased in prominence as it is lifted away from the axis of flexion by the trochlea.

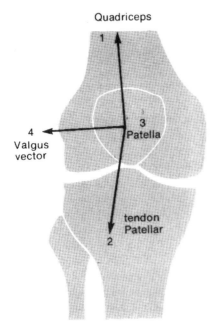

Figure 2.11. The Q angle imposes a valgus vector on the terminal degrees of extensor movement.

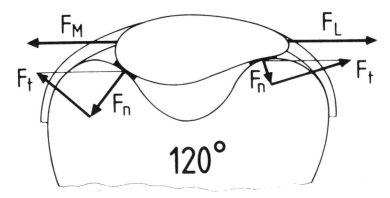

Figure 2.12. The medial retinaculum produces medial support for the patella and significant medial joint reaction force. Reprinted with permission from Hehne HJ. Biomechanics of the patellofemoral joint and its clinical relevance. Clin Orthop 1990;258:73–85.

tions. Van Eijden et al (46) pointed out that there is a linear relationship between the angle of knee flexion and movement of the patella and patellar tendon with respect to the tibia. During the first 20 degrees of flexion, the tibia derotates. This significantly decreases the Q angle and also decreases the lateral vector. The patella is drawn into the trochlea, and the first articular contact is made by 10 degrees of knee flexion. The patella enters the trochlea from a slightly lateral position. This course of patellar movement can be followed nicely with the help of serial computed tomography or magnetic resonance imaging slices of the patella during progressive knee flexion. From 20 to 30 degrees of flexion, the patella becomes more prominent as it is lifted away from the axis of rotation of the knee by the prominence of the femoral trochlea (4). Beyond 30 degrees, the patella begins to settle into the deepening trochlear groove. Instability beyond 30 degrees is less common, and many patellofemoral pain problems are associated with abnormal patellar tracking in the first 30 degrees of knee flexion. Also, if static alignment of the patella is excessively tilted to the lateral side, flexion of the knee will cause posterior movement of the iliotibial band, and the lateral retinaculum will experience abnormally elevated tension as the patella is drawn into the trochlea by medial retinacular pull (Fig. 2.13).

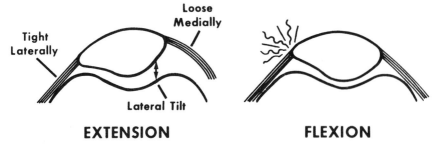

Figure 2.13. With knee flexion, the medial retinaculum tightens and pulls the patella into the trochlea. If the lateral retinaculum is shortened and tightened, there will be lateral retinacular strain and excessive lateral facet pressure. Reprinted with permission from Fulkerson JP. The etiology of patellofemoral pain in young active patients. Clin Orthop 1983;179:129–133.

Csintalan et al (47) have noted that women have higher mean contact pressure stresses at 0 and 30 degrees of knee flexion, raising speculation about subtle structural differences of patellofemoral contact in men and women. Do such factors pertain to different incidences of patellofemoral pain between men and women?

Many factors, including geometric characteristics of contact surfaces (20), are brought into play to maintain relatively constant unit loads. Cartilage thickness and subchondral bone (48) quality will affect the patellar response to stress. Analytical stereophotogrammetry (49, 50) now permits cartilage thickness determinations *in vitro* to an accuracy of 90 mm. Rotation of the femur (51) during knee extension also affects patellar tracking. The whole complex system of adaptation to maintain constant unit load, therefore, must be considered to understand biomechanical function of the patellofemoral joint. Perhaps newer techniques, such as stereophotogrammetry (52), will permit us to understand better the complex interaction between knee kinematics and patellofemoral contact pressure. In any meaningful model, however, retinacular forces (53) must be considered. Consider, for example, the contact pressure consequences of a medial patellofemoral ligament reconstruction (Fig. 2.14). Pulling the patella medial may have inordinate contact stress effects.

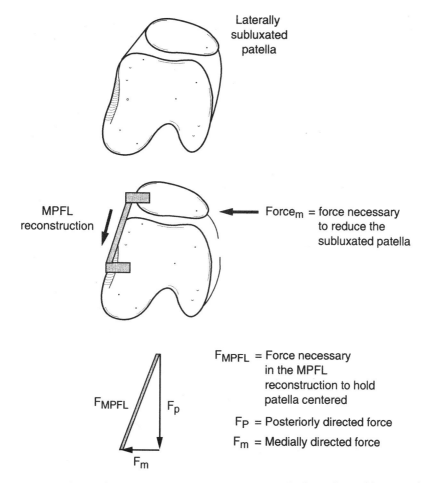

Figure 2.14. The force of any reconstruction used to "normalize" patella tracking must be considered carefully to be sure that the "corrective" procedure does not cause adverse articular contact stress consequences.

KNEE EXTENSION AGAINST RESISTANCE

Normal activities (walking, running, climbing and descending stairs, squatting, jumping) all load the knee in a standardized, physiologic way. Under all these circumstances, with body weight applied from above, the flexor lever arm, quadriceps tension, patellar tendon tension, PFJR force, and patellar contact area are all increasing with increasing knee flexion. However, there is another way in which the patellofemoral joint is loaded, namely, by applying a weight or resistance to the ankle against which the patient must extend. Free weights, many home exercise machines, and isokinetic testing equipment can overload the patellar articular surface substantially unless one uses extreme caution.

Under these circumstances, the weight moves further from the center of rotation as knee extension proceeds. Thus, quadriceps and patellar tendon tension steadily increase with decreasing knee flexion. Because the PFJR is a function not only of the absolute quadriceps and patellar tendon forces, but also of the angle between them, the PFJR force under these loading circumstances first increases with progressive knee extension and then decreases. However, this PFJR force is falling on a steadily decreasing contact area.

These loading circumstances were experimentally evaluated by Hungerford and Barry (24). Calculating the absolute values, they used $M_1 = M_2$, which only changes the numerical results slightly. The quantitative aspects of their work are still valid and show that resistance against a 9-kg boot equals contact stress of flexion under body weight at approximately 55 degrees of flexion. From there to 30 degrees of flexion, pressure exceeds the contact stresses of body weight by several orders of magnitude. Thus, extension exercises against even modest weight can generate enormous cartilage contact stress. If the cartilage is already damaged, this can produce further increase in symptoms and accelerate pathologic changes. Understanding these concepts is essential so that methods of rehabilitating the quadriceps that may be damaging to the joint itself are not employed.

Cohen et al (54) used computer simulations on cadaver knees to show that patellofemoral contact forces were not significantly higher during open-chain compared with closed-chain exercises, but emphasized again the importance of avoiding repetitive loading to more proximal patella lesions at higher flexion angles.

In general, it may be safer to avoid isokinetic exercise in the rehabilitation of most patients with patellar imbalance or articular disease. If isokinetic exercise is used, it must be carefully supervised with monitoring of the range of motion, antishear, and higher speeds (less chance of overloading defective cartilage).

LAW OF VALGUS

This is an aspect of the physiology and biomechanics of the patellofemoral joint that is so important for understanding both normal and abnormal function of the knee that we feel compelled to treat it as a separate section and elevate it to the level of a "law." The physiologic valgus of the lower extremity is a characteristic only of those animals that walk on their hind legs, being most pronounced in humans. Bringing the lower extremity to the midline reduces the work required for maintaining balance. A quadruped normally, whether walking or running, is supported by one extremity on each side of his/her body.

The physiologic valgus in the biped is then important and necessary. However, it has its effect on the knee.

The physiologic valgus per se would not necessarily dictate that the forces would have a valgus vector except for the fact that the muscles follow the longitudinal axis of the femur, giving a Q angle facing laterally. From the soft-tissue point of view, the lateral stabilizers are considerably stronger and more fibrous than the medial counterpart. It is not exactly clear why this should be so, but it is anatomically evident. We do not mean to imply that we find these facts to represent a morphologic failure. In fact, the patellofemoral joint is a remarkable design to fulfill the demands imposed on it. It also in many ways appears to be *a priori* because the design is present in the fetus long before there is any apparent mechanical need for it. However, understanding valgus helps the understanding of nearly all the pathophysiology involved in this joint and also how one might restore the delicate balance that is compatible with symptom-free function.

Morphologically, the "law of valgus" finds expression in the predominant lateral trochlear surface. This predominance is evidenced in both size and anterior projection. Also, the most frequently discovered patellar form (Wiberg Type II) has a definitely larger lateral facet than medial facet. Rather than consider this a dysplastic form, it seems to be one that is normal for the joint and capable of properly modulating the forces that pass through it. The lateral soft-tissue elements reinforced by the fascia lata are balanced by similar medial soft-tissue stabilizers. The congruence of the contact surfaces offers further stability, which, however, decreases in terminal extension. The orientation of the lateral trochlear facet offers further impediment to lateralization. This is the stage in which disorders of the patellofemoral joint will be played. We will see the tremendous importance of this setting as each of the acts unfolds.

ABNORMAL BIOMECHANICS

Even minor alterations in the knee joint can profoundly affect patellofemoral contact loading and retinacular stresses. Heino Brechter and Powers (55) have pointed out that increased contact stress causes pain and pain is probably relieved by balancing patellofemoral contact. Structural tilt of the patella will eventually result in adaptively shortened lateral retinaculum, which can abnormally increase loading of the lateral facet while reducing and distorting load on the distal medial facet of the patella. There is normally a broad distribution of contact along the distal patella at 30 degrees of knee flexion. Flatow et al (56) showed a dramatic reduction of contact area with simulated lateral tilt (5 degrees) and lateral translation (5 mm) of the patella. It is evident that even minor alterations of patellofemoral alignment can create peak loads on articular cartilage, which will eventually lead to pathologic changes in the joint. Distal tethering of the patella (Fig. 2.15), as well as mediolateral imbalance, will cause abnormal peak stresses on articular cartilage. Removing hamstring tendons for knee reconstruction may also create subtle imbalance in the extensor mechanism by altering pelvic balance slightly.

Hagena et al (57) studied retropatellar forces after posterior cruciate ligament (PCL) rupture. Presumably related to the resulting posterior tibial translation after PCL rupture, these researchers noted elevated retropatellar contact pressures in PCL-deficient knees, which may have long-term implications for patellofemoral degeneration after PCL rupture.

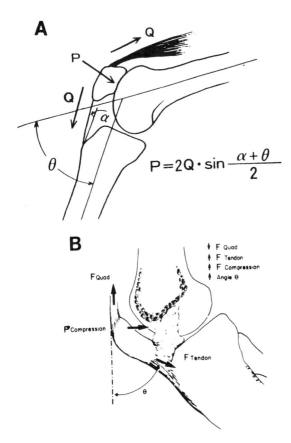

$$P = 2Q \cdot \sin \frac{\alpha + \theta}{2}$$

Figure 2.15. An infrapatellar contracture will grossly increase patellofemoral focal loading and retraction of the distal pole. Reprinted with permission from Paulos L, Ownorowski D, Greenwald A. Infrapatellar contracture syndrome. Am J Sports Med 1994;22:440–449.

REFERENCES

1. Brooke R. The treatment of fractured patella by excision. A study of morphology and function. J Bone Joint Surg 1937;24:733.
2. Freehafer A. Study of the function of the patella. Clin Orthop 1962;25:163.
3. Hey Groves EW. Note on the extension apparatus of the knee joint. Br J Surg 1937;24:747.
4. Bandi W. Chondromalacia patellae and femoro-patellare arthrose. Helv Chir Acta 1972;1(suppl):3–70.
5. Bandi W, Brennwald J. The significance of femoro-patellar pressure in the pathogenesis and treatment of chondromalacia patellae and femoro-patellar arthrosis. In Ingwersen I, ed. The Knee Joint. New York: American Elsevier Publishing; 1974.
6. Baumgartl F. Das Kniegelenk. Berlin: Springer-Verlag; 1964.
7. Ficat P. Pathologie Femoro-Patellaire. Paris: Masson et Cie; 1970.
8. Kaufer H. Mechanical function of the patella. J Bone Joint Surg 1971;53A:1551.
9. Steindler A. Kinesiology of the Human Body. Springfield, IL: Charles C Thomas; 1955.
10. Mow V, Holmes M, Lai W. Fluid transport and mechanical properties of articular cartilage: A review. J Biomech 1984;17:377–394.
11. Vallois H. La valeur morphologique de la rotule chez les mammiferes. Bull Mem Sec Anthrop (Paris) 1917;January 18.
12. Bouillet R, Van Gaver P. L'arthrose du genou. Etude pathologique et traitement. Acta Orthop Belg 1961;27:7.
13. French PR. The patello-femoral joint. J Bone Joint Surg 1959;41B:857.
14. Furmaier A. Beitrag zur mechanik der patella and des kniegelenks. Arch Orthop Unfallchir 1953;46:78.
15. Goymann V, Mueller HG. New calculations of the biomechanics of the patellofemoral joint and its clinical significance. In The Knee Joint, International Congress Series no. 324. Amsterdam: Excerpta Medica; 1974.
16. Lacreuse M. Contribution d la dynamique rotulienne (thesis). Paris, 1961.
17. Reilly DT, Martens M. Experimental analysis of the quadriceps muscle force and patello-femoral joint reaction force for various activities. Acta Orthop Scand 1972;43:126–137.

18. Buff HU, Jones LC, Hungerford DS. Experimental determination of forces transmitted through the patello-femoral joint. J Biomech 1988;21:17–23.
19. Huberti HH, Hayes WC, Stone JL, Shybut GT. Force ratios in the quadriceps tendon and ligamentum patellae. J Orthop Res 1984;2:49–54.
20. Ahmed A, Burke D, Hyder A. Force analysis of the patellar mechanism. J Orthop Res 1987;5(1):69–85.
21. Maquet P. Biomechanics of the Knee. Berlin: Springer-Verlag; 1976.
22. Perry J, Antonelli D, Ford W. Analysis of knee-joint forces during flexed-knee stance. J Bone Joint Surg 1975;57A:961–967.
23. Van Eijden TN, Weijs WA. Forces acting on the patella during maximal voluntary contraction of the quadriceps femoris muscle at different knee flexion/extension angles. Acta Anat (Basel) 1987;129:310–314.
24. Hungerford DS, Barry M. Biomechanics of the patellofemoral joint. Clin Orthop 1979;144:9–15.
25. Huberti HH, Hayes WC. Patellofemoral contact pressures. The influence of Q-angle and tendofemoral contact. J Bone Joint Surg 1984;66A:715–724.
26. Dye SF. The knee as a biologic transmission with an envelope of function. Clin Orthop 1996;325:10–18.
27. Dye SF, Staubli HU, Beidert RM, Vaupel GL. The mosaic of pathophysiology causing patellofemoral pain: therapeutic implications. Op Tech Sports Med 1999;7:46–54.
28. Dye SF. Patellofemoral pain current concepts: An overview. Sports Med Arthrosc Rev 2001;9:264–272.
29. Staubli HU, Durrenmatt U, Porcellini B, Rauschning W. Articular cartilage surfaces and osseous anatomy of the patellofemoral joint in the axial plane. Sports Med Arthrosc Rev 2001;9(4):282–287.
30. Wiberg G. Roentgenographic and anatomic studies on the femoro-patellar joint. Acta Orthop Scand 1941;12:319–410.
31. Goodfellow JW, Hungerford DS, Zindel M. Patello-femoral mechanics and pathology: I. Functional anatomy of the patello-femoral joint. J Bone Joint Surg 1976;58B:287.
32. Greenwald AS, Haynes DW. Weight-bearing areas in the human hip joint. J Bone Joint Surg 1972;54B:157.
33. Deane G. Contact print studies in the human knee joint. Thesis, University of Surrey, Surrey, England, 1970.
34. Hsieh HH, Walker PS. Stabilizing mechanisms of the loaded and unloaded knee joint. J Bone Joint Surg 1976;58A:87–93.
35. Singerman R, Berilla J, Davy DT. Direct in vitro determination of the patellofemoral contact force for normal knees. J Biomech Eng 1995;117:8–14.
36. Hehne HJ. Biomechanics of the patellofemoral joint and its clinical relevance. Clin Orthop 1990;258:73–85.
37. Aglietti P, Insall JM, Walker PS, Trent PA. A new patella prosthesis. Clin Orthop 1975;107:175–187.
38. Aichroth P. Osteochondral fractures and their relationship to osteochondritis dissecans of the knee. J Bone Joint Surg 1971;53B:448.
39. Eckstein F, Muller-Gerbl M, Putz R. Distribution of subchondral bone density and cartilage thickness in the human patella. J Anat 1992;180(pt 3):425–433.
40. Emery IH, Meachim G. Surface morphology and topography of patello-femoral cartilage fibrillation in Liverpool necropsies. J Anat 1973;116:103–120.
41. Fujikawa K, Seedhom BB, Wright V. Biomechanics of the patello-femoral joint. Part I: A study of the contact and the congruity of the patello-femoral compartment and movement of the patella. Eng Med 1983;12:3.
42. Hvid I, Andersen LL. The quadriceps angle and its relation to femoral torsion. Acta Orthop Scand 1982;53:577–579.
43. Moller BN, Krebs B, Tidemand Dal C, Aaris K. Isometric contractions in the patellofemoral pain syndrome. An electromyographic study. Arch Orthop Trauma Surg 1986;105:24–27.
44. Stein LA, Endicott AN, Sampalis JS, Kaplow MA, Patel MD, Mitchell NS. Motion of the patella during walking: A video digital-fluoroscopic study in healthy volunteers. AJR Am J Roentgenol 1993;161(3):617–620.
45. Hefzy MS, Yang H. A three-dimensional anatomical model of the human patello-femoral joint, for the determination of patello-femoral motions and contact characteristics. J Biomed Eng 1993;15(4):289–302.
46. Van Eijden TM, De Boer W, Weijs WA. The orientation of the distal part of the quadriceps femoris muscle as a function of the knee flexion-extension angle. J Biomech 1985;18:803–809.
47. Csintalan RP, Schulz MM, Woo J, McMahon PJ, Lee TQ. Gender differences in patellofemoral joint biomechanics. Clin Orthop 2002 Sep;(402):260–269.
48. Abernethy PJ, Townsend PR, Rose RM, Radin EL. Is chondromalacia patellae a separate clinical entity? J Bone Joint Surg 1978;60B:205–210.
49. Ateshian GA, Soslowsky LJ, Mow VC. Quantitation of articular surface topography and cartilage thickness in knee joints using stereophotogrammetry. J Biomech 1991;24(8):761–776.
50. Huiskes R, Kremers J, deLange A, Woltring H, Selvik G, van Rens Th J. Analytical stereophotogrammetric determination of three dimensional knee joint geometry. J Biomech 1985;18:559–570.
51. Sikorski J, Peters J, Watt I. The importance of femoral rotation in chondromalacia patellae as shown by serial radiography. J Bone Joint Surg 1979;61B:435–442.
52. Froimson M, Atheshian G, Soslowsky L, Kelly M, Mow V. Quantification of the surfaces and contact areas of the patellofemoral articulation. Mech Eng 1989;73–78.
53. Fulkerson J. The etiology of patellofemoral pain in young active patients. Clin Orthop 1983;179:129–133.
54. Cohen Z, Roglic H, Grelsamer R, Henry J, Levine W, Mow V, Ateshian G. Patellofemoral stresses during open and closed kinetic chain exercises. Am J Sports Med 2001;29(4):480–487.

55. Heino Brechter J, Powers CM. Patellofemoral stress during walking in persons with and without patellofemoral pain. Med Sci Sports Exerc 2002;34(10):1582–1593.
56. Flatow EL, et al. Computer simulation of glenohumeral and patellofemoral subluxation. Estimating pathological articular contact. Clin Orthop 1994;306:28–33.
57. Hagena F-W, Plitz W, Mühlberger G, Carl C. Retropatellar forces after rupture of the PCL and patello-tibial transfixation: An in vitro study. In Erikson E, ed. Knee Surgery, Sports Traumatology, Arthroscopy. Berlin: Springer-Verlag; 1994, pp. 31–37.

3

History and Physical Examination

William R. Post

"If we could first know where we are, and whither we are
tending, we could then better judge what we do, and
how to do it."

—Abraham Lincoln, from the House Divided
Speech, 1858

Accurate, concise clinical evaluation of patients with patellofemoral disorders is the cornerstone of successful diagnosis and treatment. There are three functions of the history and physical examination: (a) to suggest the diagnosis by eliciting a complete history, (b) to confirm the diagnosis by reproducing symptoms on examination, and (c) to use pertinent physical findings to help direct both nonoperative and operative treatment.

HISTORY

The Complaint

Patients may complain of anterior knee pain and/or patellar instability. Pain related to extensor mechanism (patellofemoral) problems typically is exacerbated by climbing or descending stairs as well as other activities that require strong quadriceps contraction. Descending stairs, which requires a coordinated eccentric contraction to lower one's body weight to the next stair, is particularly painful for many patients with patellofemoral disorders and quadriceps insufficiency. Stair climbing requires more concentric quadriceps contraction to provide knee extension lifting the body up and forward. Strenuous eccentric or concentric extensor mechanism challenge can produce musculotendinous overload and pain in an otherwise "normal" knee if adequate flexibility and strength are not present.

Prolonged periods of knee flexion such as long car rides or watching a movie can also cause pain in the anterior knee area. The reason prolonged flexion causes pain is uncertain but may be related to additional tension in sensitive peripatellar soft tissues and onto deficient patellofemoral cartilage when the knee is held in flexion. As the knee flexes, the iliotibial band (ITB) is drawn posteriorly by normal tibial rollback and its strong connections to the patella exert lateral and posterior force on the lateral patellar border. Such pain is typically relieved if the patient can rest the knee in a more extended position.

Only when there is a history of documented patellar dislocation or when the patient clearly describes the patella shifting during activity should the examiner suspect that patellar instability is present. The ubiquitous "giving way" that patients describe should not be automatically considered a symptom of instability because it is often due to quadriceps insufficiency alone. Such weakness may result from long-term deconditioning or muscular inhibition secondary to pain or effusion (1, 2). Because the vastus medialis has a lower threshold for inhibition than the rest of the quadriceps, unbalanced quadriceps inhibition may contribute to malalignment in the presence of even a small knee effusion (3, 4).

Onset of the Problem

The onset of patellofemoral symptoms provides important clues to the diagnosis. Acute high-energy injuries disrupt normal soft-tissue restraints, musculotendinous units, or cause bony injury. Acute injuries generally fall into two categories: those involving indirect trauma and those involving blunt trauma. High-energy indirect forces can cause acute patellar dislocation/subluxation in athletes during valgus/external rotation injuries. A typical example of high-energy blunt trauma is an automobile accident in which the anterior knee strikes the dashboard. The pathoanatomy of each of these conditions is different. By understanding the differences, the examiner can focus his/her examination appropriately.

The high incidence of osteochondral injury in cases of significant patellar subluxation or dislocation should make the examiner suspicious of loose bodies or articular incongruity on physical and radiographic examinations. Compressive and shearing forces typically cause osteochondral injuries on the distal medial patella or the lateral femoral condyle. Acute lateral instability strains or tears the medial patellofemoral ligaments and medial retinaculum. Often, this tear occurs at the femoral insertion of the medial patellofemoral ligaments, producing tenderness near the medial epicondyle that can lead to misdiagnosis as medial collateral ligament sprain if the clinician does not carefully differentiate these structures on examination (5).

Blunt traumatic injuries often result in chondral injury and bone contusion when the force applied is less than that necessary to produce macroscopic fracture. The knee is usually flexed during such injuries, and therefore the lesions are usually on the proximal patella. Because most knees of the general population do not have preexisting malalignment, most knees that sustain blunt trauma are not malaligned at the time of injury. However, if the injury occurred months or years earlier and pain continues, loss of normal flexibility and strength must be considered in designing a treatment plan. In recent or old blunt anterior knee trauma, one must be aware of potential posterior cruciate ligament (PCL) injury. Chronic PCL deficiency can cause chronic anterior knee pain as a result of relative "posteriorization" of the tibial tubercle that increases patellofemoral joint reaction force.

Just as pathologic fractures occur through weakened and susceptible bone, relatively low-energy "injuries" that cause subluxation or dislocation should suggest the possibility of underlying static or dynamic malalignment. Complaints of a truly insidious nature should raise suspicion of underlying strength/flexibility deficits and/or potential bony malalignment. Patients with insidious onset of symptoms or low-energy injuries should be considered especially likely to have underlying patellar malalignment, and the examination should focus on bony and soft-tissue malalignment factors.

What Is the Nature of the Pain?

Pain secondary to tissue overload from patellofemoral malalignment or to acute musculoskeletal injury is usually activity related. This does not mean that it will not hurt at rest, but it should be exacerbated with periods of increased activity. The pain is achy and sometimes even compared with a toothache. When patients complain of truly constant pain, not related to activity at all, one should be suspicious that the cause of the pain may not be entirely related to musculoskeletal structures. Possible causes of constant pain include post-surgical neuroma, referred neurogenic pain, reflex sympathetic dystrophy (RSD), symptom magnification, or psychologic issues related to secondary gain from pain and perceived disability. In such cases, physical examination should focus on reproducing the patient's symptom and on evaluating the consistency and appropriateness of response to palpation. Exaggerated pain responses and pain with palpation *everywhere* around the knee make diagnosis difficult. Pain out of proportion to physical findings is the most reliable sign of potential RSD. The absence of classic vasomotor findings of RSD such as discoloration and temperature difference does not rule out RSD. O'Brien et al (6) reported a series of 60 patients with RSD of the knee proven by successful sympathetic blockade with no significant vasomotor findings in approximately one-third. In the absence of RSD, exaggerated pain responses may be due to underlying psychosocial issues.

Some patients complain of sharp or burning pain. Constant burning pain indicates possible neuromatous origin. Sharp, intermittent, and unpredictable pains suggest loose bodies in patients with a history of patellar instability because of the high incidence of osteochondral injury. Unstable chondral flaps can also cause similar symptoms. Pathologic hypertrophic synovial plicae classically are thought to cause medial catching and clicking but often seem to cause burning pain when acutely inflamed. Although analysis of the nature of a patient's pain cannot be pathognomonic of his/her disorder, thoughtful critique of the spontaneous complaints and responses to open-ended questioning can help lead to accurate diagnosis.

History of Overuse?

Anterior knee pain frequently results from overuse. Overuse occurs when the type, duration, frequency, and/or intensity of loads applied exceed the body's ability to adapt. Such pain is usually activity related. Tissue overload may occur in peripatellar soft tissues or in the patella itself depending on the type of activity and the areas of relative weakness or inflexibility. Although anatomic malalignment may be present in overuse patients and might even predispose some knees to overload, even normally aligned knees can be plagued by overuse pain syndromes. Although the examiner can rely on physical examination to differentiate involved structures and alignment and make an accurate diagnosis, the history must be probed for correctable instigating causes of overuse injury.

Overuse is relative to the degree of musculoskeletal conditioning present and may occur as a result of activities of daily living, work, or sporting activities. In any of these situations, precipitating causes must be sought. Overuse is common in running athletes and requires evaluation of recent training, taking into account factors such as running surface, mileage increases, excessively worn shoes or orthotics, adequate stretching, and training on hilly terrain or banked tracks. Frequently, training errors will be uncovered and must be corrected to prevent recurrence of symptoms. Job-related overuse demands specific questions to define work activities and positions. Uncovering contributing factors to overuse is an important part of treatment because activity/training adjustments must be made during the healing phase of recovery. Patient education is necessary to prevent recurrence.

History of Surgeries

If a patient has had previous surgery, did the symptoms change postoperatively? If preoperative complaints were related only to pain and postoperative complaints include instability, one should suspect that postoperative instability is the result of unnecessary or excessive realignment surgery. Conversely, if preoperative complaints were primarily instability and constant pain occurs postoperatively, postoperative neuroma, RSD, or inappropriate shifting of articular load onto an articular lesion should be concerns.

Operative notes and, if available, arthroscopic photographs or videotapes provide important information. Particular attention should be paid to the condition of the articular surfaces and the extent of any soft-tissue release or realignment. Patient understanding and recall of information from prior surgeries is sometimes incomplete, and it is the responsibility of the examiner to obtain the most accurate records available. Review of such records can be quite enlightening and is always worth the time invested.

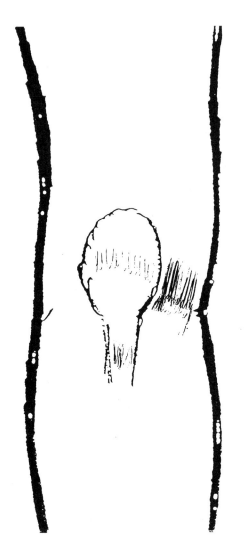

Figure 3.1. Patient-drawn knee pain diagram directs the examiner to areas of tenderness. Reprinted with permission from Post WR, Fulkerson JP. Knee pain diagrams. Correlation with physical exam findings in patients with anterior knee pain. Arthroscopy 1994;10(6): 618–623.

Other Medical History

A complete history should include a review of pertinent medical history including any history of other joint pain or associated systemic diseases. The clinician must be aware of signs and symptoms associated with inflammatory arthritides such as gout, pseudo-gout, rheumatoid arthritis, psoriatic arthritis, Reiter syndrome, and Lyme disease. Metabolic disorders, infections, and neoplasms can also be important causes of myalgias and arthralgias and must not be overlooked.

Patient Goals and Expectations

No history is complete without understanding patient needs and expectations. History taking should include current and desired activity levels and work requirements. An important part of treatment of many patients with patellofemoral disorders is developing realistic goals. Ask the patient to define and discuss specific treatment goals.

Pain Diagrams

Patient-drawn pain diagrams have correlated well with tenderness (Fig. 3.1). In a population of patients with anterior knee pain, 86% of negative patient zones on standardized diagrams correctly predicted a negative examination (7). It has been the author's experience that these diagrams can often correctly direct attention to the heart of the problem in very complex presentations. In addition to predicting areas of tenderness, patient drawings can be useful diagnostically because patients will occasionally draw patterns suggesting radiculopathy. Exaggerations such as stars, arrows, and exclamation points suggest a propensity to symptom magnification, although such correlation has not been clinically proven. Because they accurately predict areas of tenderness, pain diagrams link the history to physical examination of patients with anterior knee pain.

PHYSICAL EXAMINATION

It is not possible to adequately treat patients with patellofemoral disorders without mastering patellofemoral physical examination. The goals of examination in patients suspected of having patellofemoral disorders are (a) to assess factors that affect articular and retinacular forces and alignment and (b) to locate the painful soft tissue or articular structures. The purpose of this discussion is not to present a comprehensive "laundry list" of examination maneuvers but rather to present a logical, focused, and efficient approach to physical examination. Once mastered, an adequate examination will usually take at least 5 minutes and not only confirms the diagnosis of a patellofemoral problem but, as will be seen, helps to focus and direct nonoperative and operative treatment.

Most of the tests to be discussed have not been vigorously studied in normal age-matched populations. Interexaminer/intraexaminer variability is unknown for many tests. The reader must understand and accept these limitations. During the discussion of tests for which background research exists, such data are reviewed. We are unaware of such information for all the other tests. Nonetheless, examination criteria presented have been developed by the careful observation of generations of clinicians and have stood the test of time. Both legs should be examined. Frequently, differences will be found, and, if asymptomatic, a contralateral extremity provides some measure of clinical control. To allow a natural progression through the entire examination, the presentation is as it is practiced in a busy orthopedic surgeon's office.

Evidence of Malalignment

Standing Alignment Examination

Examination begins with the patient standing facing the examiner, barefoot in shorts. Examine for atrophy, extremity alignment including Q angle, pelvic obliquity/limb length, foot type, gait, and the ability to squat and rise smoothly to the standing position.

Atrophy

Observe for evidence of quadriceps atrophy. Measurement of thigh circumference at standard distances from the superior pole of the patella and compare side to side. Do not focus just on the quadriceps, but consider the possibility of atrophy involving the entire extremity as a sign of proximal denervation, extreme disuse, or neuromuscular disease.

Quadriceps weakness implied by atrophy is very important because dynamic muscular control of the patella is so vital to patellar stability. The vastus medialis obliquus (VMO) resists lateral patellar tilt and subluxation. In addition to providing dynamic medial stability, the quadriceps provides shock absorption for the knee joint during weight bearing because it eccentrically resists collapse of the knee into flexion. The function of the quadriceps as a shock absorber is well illustrated by considering the loads imposed by weight acceptance while descending stairs. As weight is transferred to the downstairs foot, the quadriceps must fire while the knee is flexing to prevent the knee from collapsing. Controlled eccentric contraction allows further knee flexion to lower body weight smoothly to the next step. When the quadriceps is weak and fails in its role as a shock absorber, patellofemoral loads may increase. Not only may loads be increased, but if the VMO is relatively deficient, the patella may be somewhat malaligned and the articular surfaces somewhat incongruent while accepting the increased load. Not surprisingly, many quadriceps-deficient patients with patellofemoral disorders have pain while descending stairs. Atrophy indicates a need to make quadriceps strengthening a treatment priority.

Q Angle

The Q angle is the angle formed between a line from the anterior superior iliac spine to the center of the patella and a line from the center of the patella to the tibial tubercle (Fig. 3.2).

Rationale of the Q Angle

The Q angle is frequently discussed as a reflection of the valgus angle of the extensor mechanism. Insall et al (8) initially described examination for the Q angle with the patient supine. Woodland and Francis (9) demonstrated that Q-angle measurements are slightly but significantly greater in standing subjects. Olerud and Berg (10) showed that foot position affects the standing Q-angle measurements. Their study emphasized the need to standardize foot position during Q-angle measurement because internal rotation of the foot and pronation both increased the Q angle. Logically, it seems that standing measurement would reflect weight-bearing function more accurately.

The recommendation of Insall et al of 20 degrees as an upper limit for a normal Q angle has been widely quoted but may not stand up to a review of available literature. This recommendation appears to be based on a personal communication from James and their

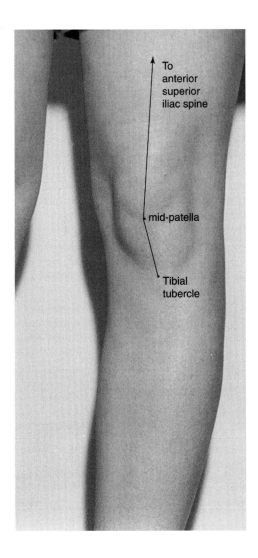

To
anterior
superior
iliac spine

mid-patella

Tibial
tubercle

Figure 3.2. Evaluate the Q angle with the patient standing.

preliminary study of 50 normal knees with an average Q angle of 14 degrees and variation of "no more than a few degrees" (8). Normal populations have been measured, and the results are summarized in Table 3.1 (8, 9, 11–14). Investigators have agreed that female subjects generally have greater Q angles.

The underlying assumption is that the larger the Q angle is, the larger the lateral moment on the patella. Insall et al found that 48% of their patients with chondromalacia had Q angles greater than 20 degrees. Aglietti et al (15) noted that no healthy men had supine Q angles of 20 degrees or greater but 15% of asymptomatic women did. Conversely, 40% of patients who were symptomatic had Q angles of 20 degrees or more. Stated in the opposite way, 60% of the patients of Aglietti et al and 52% of those of Insall et al with patellofemoral pain had Q angles within even their original empiric definition of normal. Among patients with recurrent subluxation in the report of Aglietti et al, the Q angle was not significantly different from that of the control subjects. Fairbank et al (12) demonstrated, however, that there was no significant difference in Q angles between 310 adolescent male and female subjects without knee pain and the 136 who had some

TABLE 3.1. *Normal Population Q-Angle Review*

	Supine			Standing	
Author	Q angle (deg)	No. of knees/ age (y)	Author	Q angle (deg)	No. of knees/ age (y)
Insall et al (20)	14	50/NS	Woodland et al (9)	17.0 ± .072 (F) 13.6 ± .072 (M)	57/20.0 69/22.3
Aglietti et al (15)	17 ± 3 (F) 14 ± 3 (M)	75/23 75/23	Fairbank et al (12)	23 ± 1.2 (F) 20 ± 1.2 (M)	150/14.8 ± 0.1 160/14.6 ± 0.1
Hsu et al (14)	18.8 ± 4.7 (F) 15.6 ± 3.5 (M)	60/NS 60/NS	Horton and Hall (13)	15.8 ± 4.5 (F) 11.2 ± 3.0 (M)	50/22.6 50/22.6
Woodland et al (9)	15.8 ± .072 (F) 12.7 ± .072 (M)	57/20.0 69/22.3			

F, female; M, male; NS, not specified.

knee pain within the previous year. *The Q angle has not been shown to predict patellofemoral symptoms.*

One of the theoretical concerns with using the Q angle as an estimate of the lateral moment of the extensor force is that as the patella subluxates laterally, the Q angle decreases. In other words, lateral subluxation masks the measurement that is designed to evaluate it. Fithian et al (16) attempted to address this concern by measuring the Q angle with the knee in 30 degrees of flexion with the patella manually reduced into the trochlea. Using this technique, they did find higher angles in 22 patients with a history of patellar dislocation. It is interesting that contralateral uninvolved knees also had higher Q angles compared with their normal population of 94 control subjects. This modified Q-angle measurement may not accurately represent a dynamic vector because reduction of the patella into the trochlea depends on adequate patellar mobility. Kujala et al (17) compared Q angles measured at 0 and 30 degrees and found a change of −6 degrees as the knee was flexed. Although it has been said that derotation of the tibia is less than normal in patients with patellofemoral pain (18), the decrease in Q angle in the study of Kujala et al was identical for 34 asymptomatic army recruits and 28 with exertional anterior knee pain. Although interesting, further studies are necessary before endorsing the evaluation of the Q angle in 30 degrees of flexion.

In summary, Q-angle measurements are widely discussed, but no direct correlation with the incidence of patellofemoral disorders is well established by scientific criteria. The range of normal values established by multiple studies is wide. Although some authors have used Q angles as part of the criteria to determine realignment strategies, such approaches are empiric (19, 20). Should the Q angle even be measured? Understanding the theoretical importance of the degree of valgus extensor moment is important. The Q angle is presumably one method of estimating the lateral moment acting on the patella, but one must remember that no solid data link specific Q-angle measurements to diagnosis or results of treatment. *Although a traditional part of patellofemoral discussion, actual clinical utility of the Q angle is uncertain despite extensive study.*

Leg-Length Measurement

Screen for leg-length equality by palpating the top of the iliac crest and comparing sides (Fig. 3.3). If inequality exists and measurement is desired, level the pelvis by having the patient stand on an object of known height such as standardized blocks.

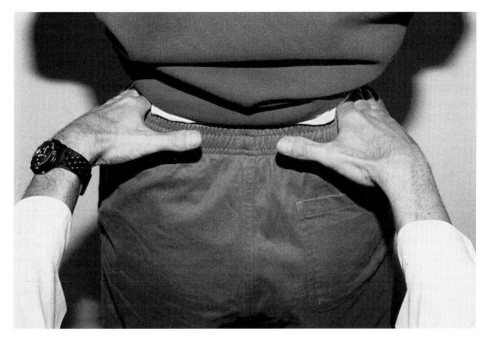

Figure 3.3. Standing estimation of pelvic obliquity/leg-length discrepancy.

Leg-length difference results in abnormal gait and may be associated with patellofemoral pain in the short leg. A short limb results in ipsilateral pelvic drop in terminal swing phase, causing an increased valgus moment at the knee (21). Length difference greater than 0.5 in. (12.5 mm) occurs in 4% to 8% of normal controls and has been correlated with an increased incidence of low back pain (22, 23). Although no studies link leg-length inequality with anterior knee pain, it is logical to correct length differences in symptomatic extremities with heel lifts in the hope of reducing or eliminating aggravating stress.

Foot Type, Alignment, Gait

Ask the patient to turn around and observe both feet for excessive pronation and associated hindfoot valgus (Fig. 3.4). If the patient has excessive pronation, ask him/her to stand on his/her toes and see whether pronation is flexible. Ask the patient to walk. Watch for excessive and prolonged pronation and abnormal valgus or varus moments at the knee.

Why to Do It

Judge pronation during weight bearing. Evaluation of standing heel position has been shown to be reproducible and is a good screening tool for pronation (24). Valgus hindfoot position generally indicates hindfoot pronation, and simply having the patient stand on his/her toes quickly defines whether the flatfoot is rigid or supple. If the pronation is flexible, it will reverse when the patient stands on his/her toes. Observation of the hind-

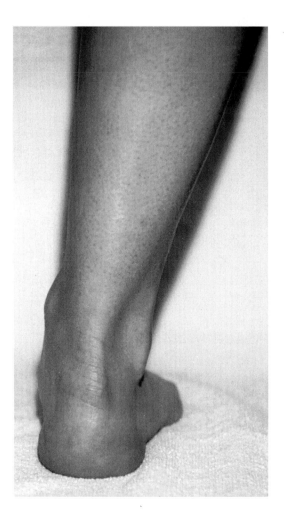

Figure 3.4. Evaluate weight-bearing hindfoot alignment.

foot and arch during standing and walking seems adequate for clinical estimation of the degree of pronation.

Excessive and prolonged hindfoot pronation produces obligatory internal tibial rotation (25). The hindfoot normally pronates from heelstrike until footflat, causing obligatory internal tibial rotation (26, 27). External rotation of the tibia, femur, and pelvis normally occurs from the beginning of the stance phase until the beginning of the swing phase. Excessive pronation may prolong internal rotation of the tibia into the stance phase until supination and hindfoot eversion begin as the foot begins to push off. This relative internal rotation is translated up the lower extremity and causes internal femoral rotation that effectively forces the lateral portion of the trochlea anteromedially against the lateral patellar facet during weight bearing. If pronation continues through the footflat phase and if the involved extremity pronates more than the patient's "normal" contralateral leg, the examiner should be suspicious that pronation is excessive and potentially aggravating to patellofemoral function. Prescription orthotics or shoes with good arch support and hindfoot control may help to control tibial rotation and patellofemoral forces and facilitate rehabilitation (28, 29).

Squatting

Ask the patient to squat, and observe the mechanics and ease of squatting. The ease with which the patient can squat and rise to a standing position gives the examiner instant information regarding the severity of the condition. Correlate the intensity of patient complaints with observations of this simple provocative activity. If the patient can do this without using manual support, evaluation of dynamic closed chain patellar tracking is possible. Occasionally, one will observe a sudden medial shift of the patella as it enters the trochlea in early flexion. This finding is a positive J sign, so-named because the patellar path resembles that of an upside down J. This indicates abnormal lateral tracking in early flexion secondary to multiple factors including relative VMO weakness and/or lateral retinacular tightness in most cases.

Seated Alignment Examination

Tubercle Sulcus Angle

The patient sits on the edge of the examination table. Measure the 90-degree tubercle sulcus angle by observing the position of the tibial tubercle relative to the center of the patella (Fig. 3.5).

When the knee is flexed to 90 degrees, the patella is generally captured within the trochlea. Measurement of this angle is therefore a reflection of lateral displacement of the tubercle with reference to the femoral sulcus. Hughston et al (30) considered the normal 90-degree tubercle sulcus angle to be 0 degrees. Kolowich et al (31) consider that the

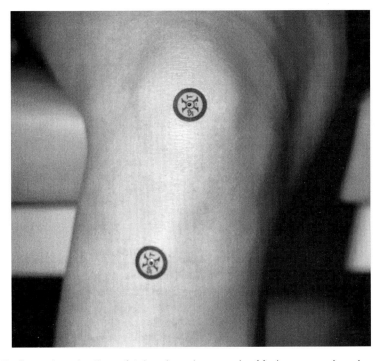

Figure 3.5. Seated evaluation of tubercle sulcus angle. Markers are placed on center of patella and tibial tubercle for the purpose of illustration only.

upper limit of normal is 10 degrees lateral displacement, although data have not been presented to substantiate this range. Compared with analysis of tubercle position by measurement of the Q angle, observation of lateral displacement of the tubercle relative to the patella in flexion more accurately portrays lateralization of the tubercle relative to the trochlea. Although the normal population values for the tubercle sulcus angle have not been well defined, lateralization of the tibial tubercle correlates with anterior knee pain (32), and examination of this relationship is helpful in understanding the contribution of tubercle position to the valgus alignment of the extremity.

Passive Patellar Tracking

Passively extend each knee, watching patellar tracking and considering any difference with previously observed dynamic tracking.

Observation of tracking without quadriceps contraction allows the examiner to understand the contribution of the passive restraints (lateral retinaculum, ITB, medial patellofemoral ligaments) to observed alignment. Observe particularly the entrance of the patella into the trochlea. The patella normally enters the trochlea by approximately 10 degrees of flexion. It should enter the trochlea smoothly without catches or sudden shifts. The J sign, which occurs when the patella shifts suddenly medially to enter the trochlea, is observed more often in passive tracking when the VMO is not actively guiding the patella into the trochlea. Comparison with the contralateral side is important.

Supine Patellar Mobility

Patellar Tilt Test

Test the patella for resistance to correction of lateral patellar tilt (rotation) by pushing posteriorly on the medial border of the patella while palpating the lateral margin of the patella to assess whether the patella corrects to at least neutral (Fig. 3.6). If the patellar tilt does not correct to neutral (parallel to the table) or beyond, one should be suspicious that mobility is significantly restricted. A patellar tilt test should be done in full extension with the quadriceps relaxed because this allows evaluation of the lateral soft-tissue restraints in their most relaxed position. As with other supine tests for patellar mobility, walk around the table to examine the patient's opposite knee.

The lateral retinaculum includes contributions from the lateral patellofemoral and patellotibial ligaments and the ITB (33). The ITB is drawn posteriorly as the knee flexes, causing tension to increase in the iliopatellar band, the portion of the ITB that inserts into the lateral retinaculum (34). Patellar mobility tests should therefore be done in full extension because it is in this position that there is normally the greatest mobility.

Lateral retinacular tightness is very common in patients with patellofemoral pain and is the hallmark of excessive lateral pressure syndrome as described by Ficat and Hungerford (35). The direction of the lateral retinaculum is posterior and lateral, but primarily posterior. Because the vector of the lateral retinaculum is principally posterior, excessive tension produces relatively more tilt (lateral rotation) than subluxation (lateral translation). Excessive tension can produce pain from soft-tissue overload or secondarily from lateral patellar facet overload. The examiner should expect to be able to correct patellar tilt to neutral, but contralateral comparison is important because normal population data are lacking. Limited lateral retinacular flexibility is a very important finding, and, if present, nonoperative treatment must include stretching of tight structures.

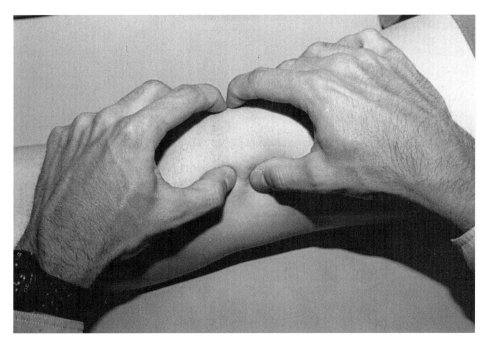

Figure 3.6. Patellar tilt test with knee extended. Tilt should correct to neutral.

Medial-Lateral Glide Test

Medial to lateral mobility should be tested by judging the amount of translation in each direction when firm pressure is applied (Fig. 3.7). Be careful to keep the patellar tilt constant during medial-lateral glide testing. Watch for evidence of apprehension during medial-lateral translation. If the patella is pushed medially and tilt is not controlled, the patella rotates externally. The examiner gets the false impression that the patella is displacing medially when much of the perceived displacement is rotational.

Static and dynamic factors affect patellar alignment. Normal tracking is the result of balance in the static peripatellar soft-tissue restraints and good dynamic quadriceps strength and coordination. Medial-lateral glide testing is useful to assess the static aspect of patellar alignment. Anatomically, Conlan et al (36) showed that the medial patellofemoral ligament is the major static restraint to lateral displacement at full extension, conferring 53% of the medial restraining force. Although the amount of restraining force due to the medial patellofemoral ligament was somewhat variable (23%–80%), when it was anatomically distinct, it was the primary medial restraint. The second most important medial static restraint was the medial patellomeniscal ligament that contributed 22% of restraining force. These laboratory data correlate well with the clinical findings of Sallay et al (37) who noted that 15 of 16 patients who had undergone surgical exploration had tears of the medial patellofemoral ligament from the adductor tubercle after acute dislocation. Thus, when increased unilateral lateral translation is observed in full extension, the deficient tissues likely include the medial patellofemoral and patellomeniscal ligaments.

Medial-lateral glide testing has been described in full extension (18, 38) and also with the knee in 30 degrees of flexion (16, 39). When this test is done in full extension, it is

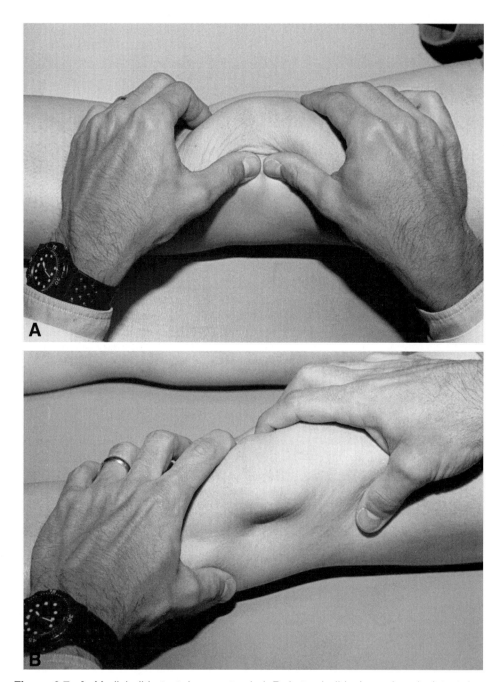

Figure 3.7. A, Medial glide test, knee extended. **B,** Lateral glide (apprehension) test, knee extended.

more purely a test of peripatellar soft-tissue compliance because there is less resistance from engagement of the patella in the trochlea. Estimation of the amount of translation may be accomplished by dividing the patella into longitudinal quadrants and estimating the degree of number of quadrants worth of translation that can be induced on examination. Kolowich et al (31) measured mobility in 20 to 30 degrees of flexion and suggested that three quadrants of lateral glide suggested an incompetent medial restraint. Conversely, their opinion regarding medial glide was that one quadrant or less indicated an abnormally tight lateral retinaculum, whereas medial glide of three to four quadrants implied hypermobility.

Actual measurement of patellar mobility may become a welcome addition to patellofemoral examination because intertester reliability of more subjective evaluation has been shown to be poor among experienced physical therapists (40). Fithian et al (16) reported that patellar mobility measurements were reproducible between examiners and between repeated examinations by the same person. They suggested patellar "balance" be analyzed by calculating the difference between measured medial and lateral translations. Using this calculation, they found a difference between asymptomatic knees and knees with a history of patellar dislocation. As might be expected, contralateral knees of the patients with instability were abnormal compared with asymptomatic controls but more normal than knees with symptomatic instability. Skalley et al (39) measured medial translation in full extension and found average translations to be 9.5 mm medially and 5.4 mm laterally. Standard deviations were not given, but the ranges cited for each direction were large (4–15 mm) and again emphasize the importance of searching for contralateral asymmetry.

The apprehension sign occurs when the patient recognizes the sensation of impending dislocation during lateral glide testing. It is important to differentiate between pain and impending instability symptoms during the apprehension test. If the patient is truly apprehensive because of perceived instability, this strongly suggests that lateral patellar instability is an important part of that patient's diagnosis.

Special Tests for Medial Subluxation

Although lateral instability is much more commonly encountered, medial instability should be suspected if medial glide testing duplicates symptoms in a patient with a history of patellar realignment surgery. This can be considered a "reverse" apprehension test. In fact, physical examination is the primary method for diagnosis of medial subluxation (41–44). Fulkerson's relocation test for symptomatic medial subluxation involves holding the symptomatic patella medially with the patient supine and the knee extended. On active or passive knee flexion, the patella falls into the trochlea and, when positive, reproduces the patient's pain or feeling of instability. The gravity subluxation test, as described by Nonweiler and DeLee (44), can also be helpful to confirm medial instability. They reported five symptomatic hypermobile patients in whom the vastus lateralis had been transected at the time of lateral release. When the patella is subluxed medially by the examiner with the patient in the lateral decubitus position, none of these patients could actively reduce their patella. Because medial subluxation occurs rarely, the gravity subluxation test need not be performed on all patients unless clinical suspicion exists for medial subluxation.

Superior-Inferior Glide Test. Test superior and inferior patellar mobility in full extension by passive displacement of the patella (Fig. 3.8). Compare with the contralateral knee. Correlate with radiographic findings. Decreased superior glide is a hallmark of infrapatellar contracture syndrome. This syndrome can result in debilitating anterior knee pain in the aftermath of knee surgery or blunt trauma. In florid cases, a knee flexion contracture is present, and the peripatellar soft tissues, including the infrapatellar fat pad, become fibrosed and firm. In less advanced cases, decreased superior glide may be one of the first signs of a developing infrapatellar contracture syndrome. If diagnosed

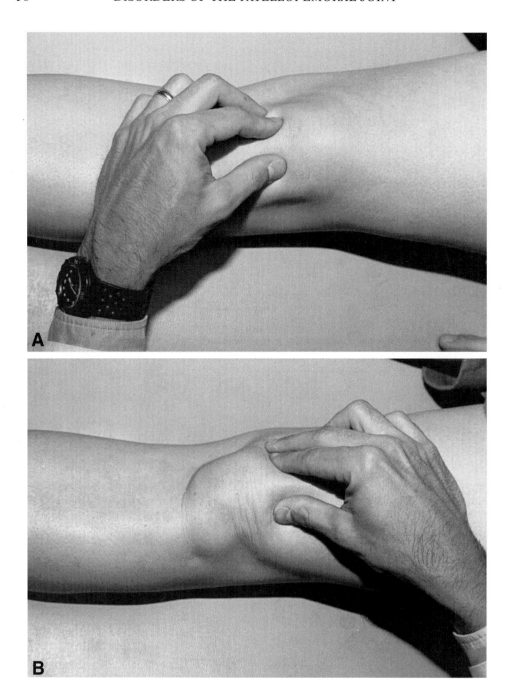

Figure 3.8. A, Superior glide test, knee extended. **B,** Inferior glide test, knee extended.

promptly, this problem can be treated by physical therapy, particularly gentle persistent mobilization of the patella and peripatellar tissues. Surgical treatment of advanced cases can be difficult, and results are not uniformly good (45).

Reproducing the Patient's Pain

Supine Palpation

Soft-Tissue Palpation

Systematic palpation of peripatellar soft tissues should focus on soft-tissue static restraints and the tendinous insertions of each portion of the quadriceps muscle. Place the soft-tissue structures under tension before palpation. This will help to limit the pressure transmitted to underlying structures and help the examiner to know that the painful structure is most likely the one under tension (Fig. 3.9). Palpate the medial and lateral retinacular tissues, the medial femoral condyle in the region of the medial parapatellar plica, each of the quadriceps tendon insertions, and the patellar tendon in each patient. Palpate deep to the patellar tendon for evidence of increased density and/or reproduction of the patient's pain. Palpation of the quadriceps muscle bellies can occasionally reveal tenderness. Palpate all scars for neuromata, especially if the history suggests this diagnosis. Reproducing symptoms by palpation of the adductor hiatus suggests saphenous nerve entrapment. In patients with suspected acute lateral dislocation, palpate the adductor tubercle for tenderness at the origin of the medial patellofemoral ligament. *Medial and lateral joint lines should also be examined for tenderness, which may suggest meniscal problems or tibiofemoral arthrosis.*

Remember that a primary goal of examination is to reproduce and localize the patient's pain. Innervated tissues of the patellofemoral joint, which could generate anterior knee pain, include the subchondral bone of the patella and trochlea, synovium (including plicae), patellar and quadriceps tendons, and retinacular soft-tissue restraints medially and laterally. Tenderness is very common in the medial and lateral patellar retinacula and the patellar tendon, all of which rank high among the most densely innervated soft tissues in the knee (46). Tenderness is common in the peripatellar tissues that are overly tight and have been chronically overloaded. This tenderness may result from the neuromatous degeneration found in such retinacular tissues excised at the time of lateral release (47, 48).

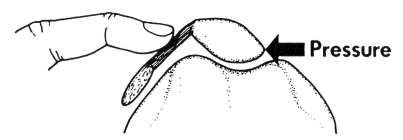

Figure 3.9. Place soft tissues under tension before palpation. Reprinted with permission from Fulkerson JP. Awareness of the retinaculum in evaluating patellofemoral pain. Am J Sports Med 1982;10:147–149.

Precise diagnoses in acute injuries and chronic pain are often made by careful mental visualization of the specific structures that are most tender. Particular attention should be paid to the medial femoral condyle area where the medial parapatellar plica can often be readily palpated. Tenderness as the plica is rolled underneath a finger is diagnostic of medial plica irritation and medial plica syndrome. Patients with soft-tissue pain secondary to excessive lateral patellar tilt commonly have tenderness in the vastus lateralis insertion, the lateral retinacular insertion, and the inferior portion of the medial retinaculum just above the patellar tendon origin. Quadriceps muscle belly tenderness occurs in severe overuse syndromes and more unusual situations such as peripatellar hemangioma. Patellar tendon tenderness diagnoses patellar tendinitis/tendinosis.

Postsurgical neuroma is a physical examination diagnosis. Discovery of a hypersensitive scar, which reproduces patient complaints, is not rare and should be sought in patients with previous surgery. Characteristic patterns of numbness or hypesthesia are often present in patients with symptomatic neuromata or nerve entrapment (Fig. 3.10). Postsurgical, posttraumatic, or idiopathic saphenous nerve entrapment near the adductor canal is an unusual cause of anterior knee pain. If palpation over the adductor canal replicates the patient's complaint, injection of local anesthetic can confirm the diagnosis. Effective treatment by decompression or neurectomy is possible, but only if persistent palpation leads to the correct diagnosis (49–51).

In acutely injured knees, palpation of the medial parapatellar structures helps to differentiate acute lateral patellar instability and medial collateral ligament sprain. Sallay et al (37) reported 70% of their patients were maximally tender over the adductor tubercle after acute lateral dislocation. Acute evaluation of possible extensor injuries must also include palpation for defects in the quadriceps and patellar tendons.

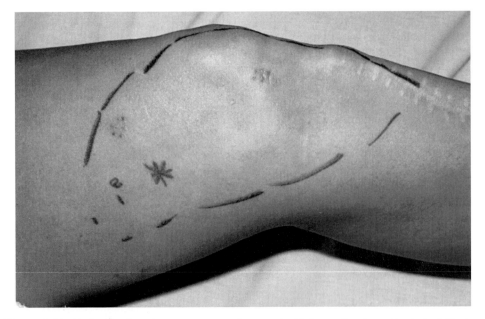

Figure 3.10. Patient had saphenous nerve entrapment with hypesthesia as illustrated. Saphenous decompression relieved her pain. Reprinted with permission from Post WR. Surgical decision making in patellar pain and instability 1994;2(4):273–284.

Supine Articular Examination

Evaluate the knee joint for effusion by milking the suprapatellar pouch with one hand and checking to see whether the patella is ballotable with the other. Compress the patella directly into the trochlea with your thenar eminence (Fig. 3.11). Be careful to not touch any peripatellar tissues during compression. Compress the patella at various angles of flexion from full extension to full flexion. Beware of patients who have prepatellar bursitis that may cause pain with this test. Hold your hand over each patella during active and passive knee flexion observing for crepitus and pain. Note carefully which knee flexion angles are associated with pain or crepitus.

Effusion signifies serious intraarticular pathology. A full discussion of the possible causes of knee effusion is beyond the scope of this chapter, but causes include meniscal, ligamentous, degenerative, and inflammatory pathology. In patients with patellofemoral pathology, effusion suggests moderate to severe patellofemoral arthrosis, osteochondral or chondral loose bodies, and severe plical inflammation. Joint effusion causes reflex quadriceps inhibition. As little as 15 mL of fluid injected into normal knees has been shown to produce marked reflex inhibition (1–4). The threshold for VMO inhibition is approximately 20 to 30 mL of intraarticular fluid compared with the 50 to 60 mL required to inhibit the rectus femoris and the vastus lateralis (3). Thus, asymmetric inhibition may result in some dynamic malalignment even with a small joint effusion. This might help to explain the patellofemoral pain so common during rehabilitation after many types of knee surgery.

Compression of the patella into the trochlea often produces pain when significant articular lesions exist on the portion of the patella or trochlea being compressed. The pain produced from articular compression must originate from irritation of the subchondral bone because articular cartilage is devoid of nerve endings. By meticulously avoiding the peripatellar tissues when compressing the patella, you can be certain that any pain produced originates from bony pathology. If the anterior knee appears very swollen, but the patella is not ballotable, suspect that prepatellar bursal swelling is present. When present, such bursitis is generally self-evident and not easily confused with intraarticular effusion by experienced examiners.

Worthwhile palpation of "facet tenderness" through the medial retinaculum (52) seems anatomically dubious given the interposition of the densely innervated retinaculum and synovium. Because the patella is not drawn into the trochlea until approximately 10 degrees of flexion, pain on compression of the patella with the knee in full extension is not truly evidence of articular pain. Because the distal patella first contacts the proximal trochlea, compression in early flexion suggests distal patellar pathology. As flexion proceeds, the articular surfaces compressed become progressively proximal on the patella and distal in the trochlea.

Although crepitus suggests the possibility of significant articular changes, crepitus is very common in asymptomatic knees and is a more serious discovery when absent or asymmetric in the contralateral knee. Pain with patellar compression when the knee is moving is not an accurate test for articular pain because peripatellar soft tissues stretch as the knee is moving and can contribute to pain during motion. Occasionally, a discrete catch can be produced on examination, reproducing the symptom that the patient recognizes as their primary complaint. This is important diagnostically and can correspond to a traumatic chondral flap or a pathologic hypertrophic plica.

McCoy et al (53) quantified crepitus by measuring joint sounds detected by vibration arthrography and found that these correlate with specific intraarticular pathology. Jiang

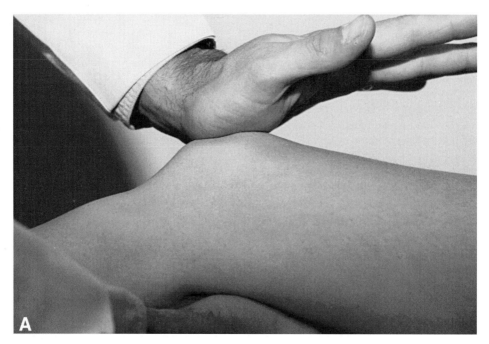

Figure 3.11. Perform direct articular compression at various angles of flexion. Be careful to avoid compressing the peripatellar soft tissues. Articular compression at various angles of flexion helps to localize articular lesions.

et al (54) also found the degree of patellar crepitus measured by vibration arthrometry correlated well with operative findings of patellar arthrosis. Neely et al (55) used laser optic technology to document the "sticking and slipping of the patella" and resultant microvibrations (20–180 mm) of physiologic patellofemoral crepitus in normal knees. Although vibration arthrography and related technologies are still research tools, they have potential to quantify crepitus and related "joint noise" in a way that may eventually be clinically useful (56). Because crepitus is frequently found in normal knees, remember that it is clinically important only when it is asymmetric or reproduces symptoms.

Supine Examination for Flexibility

Lift each leg independently and measure the popliteal angle as a measure of hamstring tightness (Fig. 3.12). This is also essentially a straight-leg raising test and serves as a screening test for lumbar radiculopathy. Measure gastrocsoleus flexibility by ankle dorsiflexion with the knee extended and with the knee flexed 90 degrees (Fig. 3.13). Evaluate hip flexion contracture by flexing the contralateral hip completely and checking to be sure that the ipsilateral thigh can remain flat on the examination table (Fig. 3.14). If the ipsilateral hip cannot lie flat on the table, hip flexion contracture is present.

Patellofemoral pain is often associated with flexibility deficits in the lower extremity. Muscle affects patellar alignment actively through contraction and statically through muscular compliance or flexibility. The static effects of antagonist muscles are important because they represent a portion of the force that must be overcome to complete agonist activity. For example, hamstring tightness causes a relative knee flexion contracture that

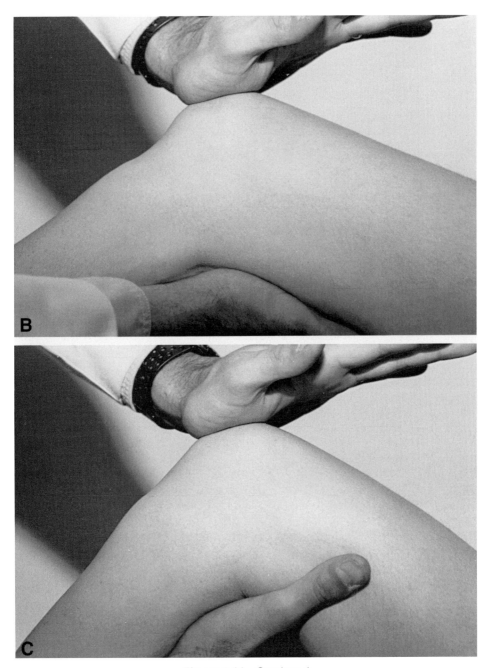

Figure 3.11. *Continued.*

increases the quadriceps force required to extend the knee. Because more quadriceps force is necessary, patellofemoral joint reaction force is also increased. Although "normal" values for hamstring flexibility are unavailable, most young athletic individuals have popliteal angles in the 160- to 180-degree range. As always, contralateral examination is helpful.

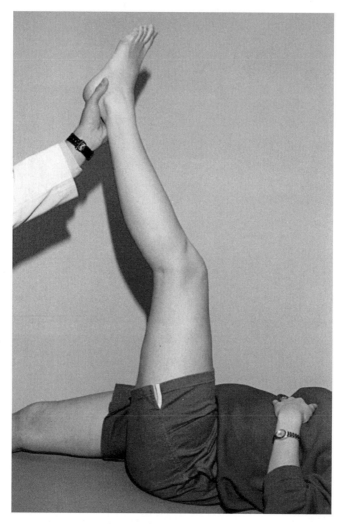

Figure 3.12. Evaluate hamstring tightness while the patient is supine.

Hip flexion contracture results in increased knee flexion through stance. As an extreme example, consider the crouched gait of patients with spastic diplegia and hip flexion contractures. In the presence of increased hip flexion during stance, the knee is flexed more to keep the foot underneath the center of gravity. Increased knee flexion results in increased patellofemoral joint reaction force.

Tightness of the gastrocsoleus complex limits ankle dorsiflexion. Because the gastrocnemius muscles cross the knee joint, evaluation of dorsiflexion with the knee extended is necessary. Clinically, ankle dorsiflexion is more often limited with the knee extended. If dorsiflexion is limited, the subtalar joint compensates by increased pronation. Increased subtalar pronation causes increased tibial internal rotation, which, as previously discussed, has detrimental effects on patellofemoral mechanics.

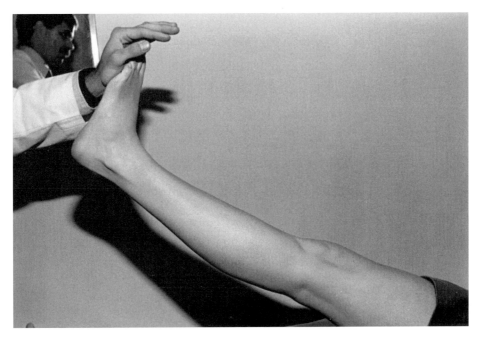

Figure 3.13. Check for gastrocnemius tightness.

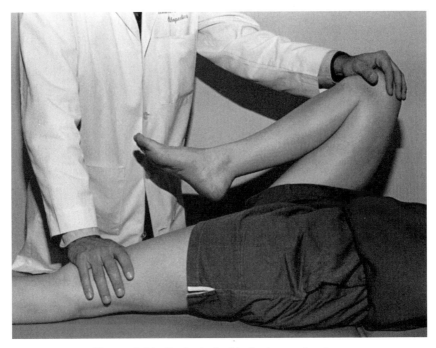

Figure 3.14. Evaluate for hip flexion contracture.

Prone Examination

Prone Quadriceps Flexibility

With the patient prone, flex each knee with one hand while stabilizing the pelvis (Fig. 3.15). Bring the heel as close as possible to the buttock. Record the distance from the heel to the buttock and any side-to-side asymmetry. If the patient has discomfort during this test, ask whether the pain is in the knee or thigh.

Treating quadriceps inflexibility is a critical part of restoring efficient extensor function. When flexibility is lacking, a muscle is less able to absorb energy eccentrically. Because the energy must be absorbed somewhere in the extremity, overload elsewhere becomes a possibility. Clinically, it seems that the sites most often subject to secondary overload are the patellar and quadriceps tendons. Active knee flexion also must overcome greater resistance when the quadriceps is relatively tight. Again, joint reaction forces may be increased. Patients with patellar tendinitis and "failed" postoperative patellar pain patients often have large quadriceps flexibility deficits that become obvious when measuring prone knee flexion.

Prone measurement is important because the rectus femoris crosses the hip and the prone position keeps the hip extended. When this test is performed, stabilize the pelvis to prevent compensatory hip flexion that a patient attempts in order to move his/her heel closer to the buttock. A patient also tries to abduct his/her hip to shorten the distance from the patella to the rectus origin at the anterior inferior iliac spine. A convenient method of measuring the heel-to-buttock distance is by fingerbreadths of the examiner's hand. Although somewhat inexact, this allows adequate data to assess relative improvements between patient visits. Many young active patients can bring their heels to their buttock or at least within a few fingerbreadths. It is not rare to find patients with prone flexion

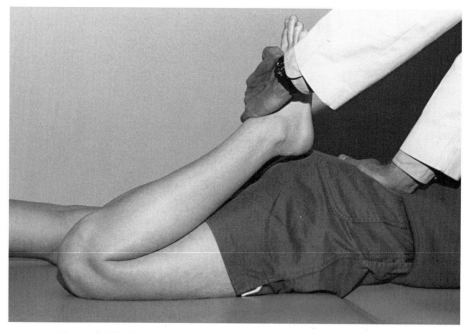

Figure 3.15. Test for quadriceps flexibility while the patient is prone.

limited to 110 degrees or less. When the heel comes less than eight fingerbreadths from the buttock, it is more convenient to record quadriceps flexibility as degrees of prone knee flexion.

Prone Hip Rotation

Because the patient is prone for evaluation of quadriceps flexibility, it is a convenient time to assess femoral anteversion. With the knee flexed 90 degrees, rotate the leg internally until the greater trochanter is maximally prominent laterally. At this degree of rotation, the femoral neck is parallel to the table and the angle between the vertical femur and the tibia is the angle of hip anteversion (Fig. 3.16). After noting the anteversion angle, screen for limitations in hip motion by looking at entire range of internal and external rotation bilaterally.

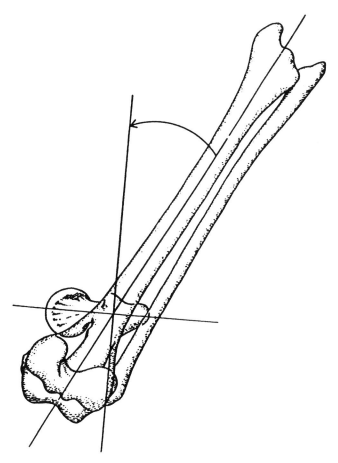

Figure 3.16. Drawing demonstrating the lateral prominence of the greater trochanter and the measurement of femoral anteversion in the prone position. Reprinted with permission from Ruwe PA, Gage JR, Ozonoff MB, DeLuca PA. Clinical determination of femoral aversion. J Bone Joint Surg 1992;74A(6):821.

Why to Do It

Examination of anteversion is important to understand its potential influence on patellar mechanics in each patient. Physical examination, as described, is as sensitive as radiographic measurement for femoral anteversion (57). Although femoral anteversion is the most variable component of femoral anatomy (58), normal values are well established. Anteversion is greatest in childhood and decreases during skeletal maturation (59, 60). According to Kingsley and Olmstead (59), who studied 630 cadaver femurs, anteversion averaged 8.02 degrees. Sixty-six percent of cadavers had anteversion angles between 0 and 15 degrees. Large variations occur between subjects, and side-to-side differences of 13 to 15 degrees occur in normal subjects (61, 62).

Although increased anteversion has been classically associated with patellofemoral pain and instability, no studies prove an association. Excessive anteversion causes relative internal rotation of the femur during gait. As discussed in the section on hindfoot pronation, internal rotation moves the trochlea medially and the lateral trochlea anteriorly. Because the quadriceps origin on the pelvis does not rotate internally, the Q angle increases. Careful evaluation of the range of motion is also an important screening tool for hip pathology, especially in the child or adolescent whose complaints of anterior knee pain occasionally represent referred pain from Perthes disease or other hip pathology. Adults may also present with referred anterior knee pain, most commonly from osteoarthrosis of the hip. Prone hip rotation will usually be limited and painful in such patients.

ITB Flexibility

Ober Test (Fig. 3.17)

To evaluate ITB flexibility, have the patient lie on his/her side. For examination of the right leg, stand behind the patient who lies with his/her left hip down and fully flexed to eliminate lumbar lordosis and stabilize the pelvis. Flex the right knee and hip 90 degrees each. Then abduct the hip and extend it to neutral.

If the hip cannot extend to neutral, consider the possibility of hip flexion contracture. Do not allow the pelvis to rotate externally during this maneuver. During positioning of the tested hip into full extension, stabilize the pelvis with your left hand to maintain neutral femoral rotation. When the upper leg is maximally abducted and extended, allow it to drop (adduct) by gravity while gently maintaining the knee flexion and femoral rotation. This position places the ITB on stretch, and flexibility is assessed by observing how much adduction is possible. Comparison with the asymptomatic side is important, but, generally, the thigh should adduct to a position at least parallel to the examination table. *Palpation of the ITB just lateral to the patella during maximal stretch usually reproduces pain in patients with excessive ITB/lateral retinacular tightness.*

Excessive tension in the ITB can result in malalignment and also in soft-tissue pain. *The importance of the ITB in patients with lateral retinacular tightness cannot be overemphasized.* Melchione and Sullivan (63) showed excellent intratester and good intertester reliability of Ober test in patients with anterior knee pain using a fluid filled inclinometer to quantify thigh adduction. ITB inflexibility as documented by the Ober test was correlated with lateral knee pain and anterior hip pain in ballet dancers (64). Although Ober (65) initially described this test as part of an investigation into low back pain, tightness is very common in patients with patellofemoral pain. The ITB links the pelvis and the tibia. When ipsilateral hip abductor weakness allows the contralateral ilium

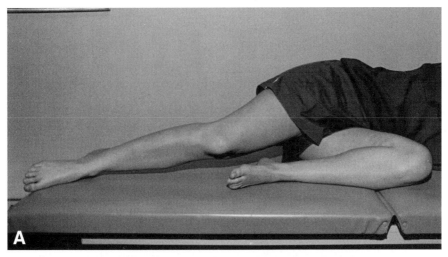

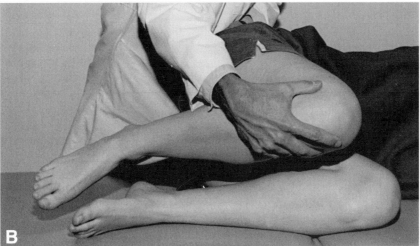

Figure 3.17. A, The contralateral hip is maximally flexed to eliminate lumbar lordosis. **B,** Flex the hip of the leg to be tested. *Continued on next page.*

to drop during weight bearing, tension is also increased in the ITB. When examining the ITB, remember that hip pathology, including hip abductor weakness, flexion contracture, and rotational limitations can affect patellofemoral forces. Such problems, if detected, should be addressed in the rehabilitation plan.

Evaluation of Systemic Hypermobility

Screen for knee and elbow hyperextension greater than 10 degrees. If fifth finger metacarpophalangeal hyperextension and thumb-forearm apposition are also present, the patient fits the criteria for hypermobility as described by Beighton and Horan (66).

Rünow (67) showed that patellar dislocation was six times more frequent in hypermobile patients compared with age-matched controls. Both Rünow (67) and Stanitski (68) found that hypermobile patients are less than half as likely to sustain articular injury dur-

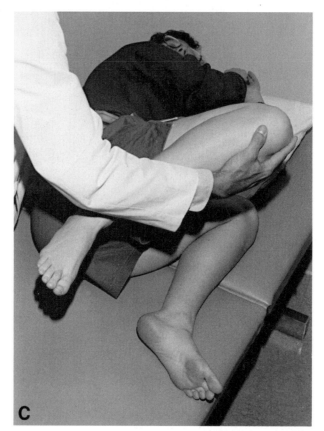

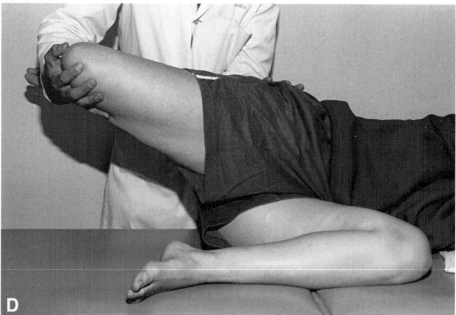

Figure 3.17. *Continued.* **C,** While the hip is flexed, abduct the hip maximally. **D,** Extend the hip while stabilizing the pelvis to keep it perpendicular to the examination table.

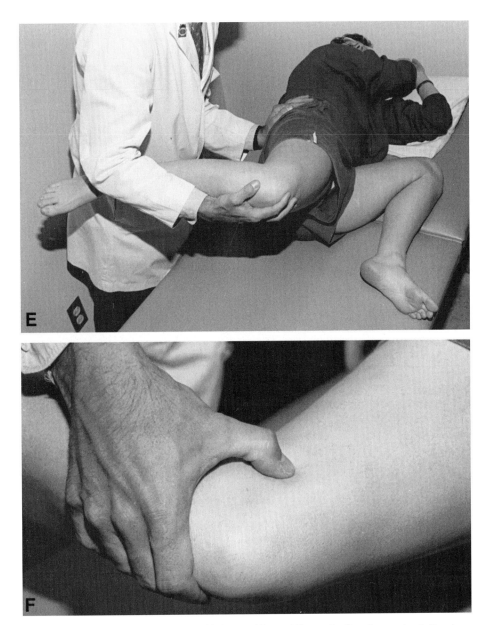

Figure 3.17. *Continued.* **E,** Allow the thigh to adduct while controlling femoral rotation in neutral. Note continued control of the pelvis with the examiner's left hand. **F,** At the position of maximal adduction, palpation over the distal iliotibial band often reproduces the patient's pain.

ing patellar dislocation. Stanitski also found that none of his patients with hypermobile patellar dislocation had medial patellar avulsions compared with one-third of patients without hypermobility. Because the pathoanatomy of patellar instability is different in patients with hypermobility, a screening examination is important. Ehlers-Danlos or Marfan syndromes should be suspected in patients with marked hypermobility and appropriate referrals should be considered when serious systemic manifestations are suspected.

Knee Ligament Stability

Check each knee for evidence of anterior cruciate ligament, PCL, and rotatory instability. Include the Lachman test and posterior drawer and pivot shift maneuvers (Fig. 3.18).

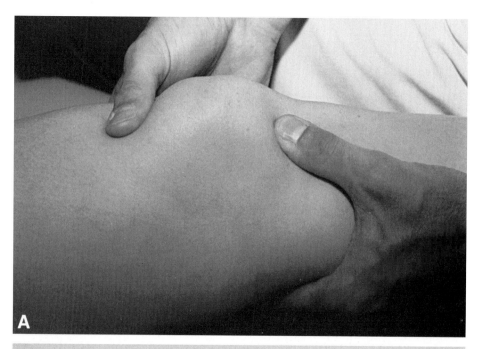

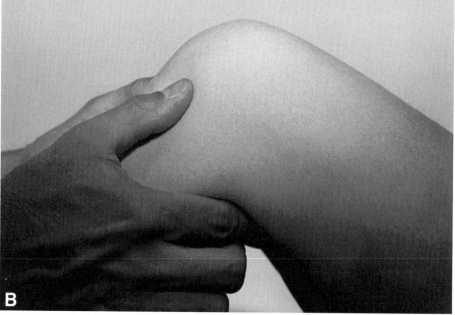

Figure 3.18. A, Lachman test for excessive anterior tibial translation. **B,** Posterior drawer test: Palpate normal position of tibia anterior to femoral condyle with the knee flexed 90 degrees.

Patients with ligament insufficiency often describe pain and giving way, which can be confused with patellofemoral pain and instability. Chronic anterior cruciate ligament deficiency is associated with a 20% to 27% incidence of anterior knee pain (69, 70). As many as 90% of patients with PCL tears report knee pain with activity (71). Parolie and Bergfeld (72) reported that 48% of their chronic PCL-deficient patients had stiffness after prolonged sitting (i.e., the classic patellofemoral "movie-theater sign"). PCL tears increase patellofemoral joint reaction forces by posterior displacement of the tibial tuberosity. This effect is exactly the opposite of the beneficial unloading accomplished by tubercle anteriorization. Because cruciate ligament injuries occur commonly, a knee ligament stability examination is important to identify factors that may contribute to knee pain in each patient. If cruciate ligament deficiency is discovered, treatment must be modified accordingly.

Putting It All Together

After history and physical examination define patellofemoral malalignment and/or patellofemoral soft-tissue pain as the diagnosis, examination findings direct treatment. So, even if the history is diagnostic, careful examination is important. Put together the "whole picture" of extremity alignment, soft-tissue mobility, and dynamic control when making treatment decisions. Remember to include evaluation of the entire extremity. When flexibility is asymmetric in patients with anterior knee pain, stretching should be focused on all tight muscle groups. Consider not only quadriceps atrophy and weakness but also the timing of VMO contraction. Avoid the painful ranges of motion identified by articular compression during initial strengthening. Treat painful foci of tendinitis or retinacular inflammation with antiinflammatory modalities, massage, and ice. Address static factors contributing to malalignment such as excessive hindfoot pronation and leg-length discrepancy by orthotic and heel lift prescriptions. Patients with soft-tissue tightness and resultant malalignment may benefit from patellar taping and stabilizing braces. The importance of an accurate examination and precise diagnosis to successful treatment should be clear.

If surgery becomes necessary, examination findings also affect surgical selection. For example, hypermobile patients are less likely to benefit from lateral release. Significant signs of pain on articular compression and crepitus suggest advanced articular injury and the need for pressure-relieving anteriorization, patellectomy, or arthroplasty instead of isolated realignment. Observing the degree of flexion that provokes the most pain on articular compression probably helps to predict the site of patellofemoral arthrosis. Because some cadaver models of tubercle anteriorization have shown better unloading of distal lesions (73, 74), more articular pain near extension may prove to be prognostic for superior results after anteriorization.

In summary, history and physical examination form the cornerstones of accurate diagnosis and treatment in patients with patellofemoral disorders. *There is no substitute for a thorough history and physical examination.* Radiographic studies usually corroborate the clinical impression and must not be relied on in the absence of confirmatory clinical data. Combining knowledge of the mechanics and natural history of patellofemoral problems with information from the history and physical examination, logical treatment can begin.

REFERENCES

1. de Andrade JR, Grant C, Dixon A St J. Joint distension and reflex muscle inhibition in the knee. J Bone Joint Surg 1965;47A:313–322.
2. Kennedy JC, Alexander IJ, Hayes KC. Nerve supply of the human knee and its functional importance. Am J Sports Med 1982;10:329–335.

3. Spencer JD, Hayes KC, Alexander IJ. Knee joint effusion and quadriceps inhibition in man. Arch Phys Med Rehabil 1984;65:171–177.
4. Wood L, Ferrell WR, Baxendale RH. Pressures in normal and acutely distended human knee joints and effects on quadriceps maximal voluntary contractions. Q J Exp Physiol 1988;73:305–314.
5. Bassett FH. Acute dislocation of the patella, osteochondral fractures and injuries to the extensor mechanism of the knee. Instr Course Lect 1976;25:40–49.
6. O'Brien SJ, Ngeow J, Gibney MA, Warren RF, Fealy S. Reflex sympathetic dystrophy of the knee: Causes, diagnosis and treatment. Am J Sports Med 1995;23(6):655–659.
7. Post WR, Fulkerson JP. Knee pain diagrams: Correlation with physical examination findings in patients with anterior knee pain. Arthroscopy 1994;10(6):618–623.
8. Insall J, Falvo KA, Wise DW. Chondromalacia patellae: A prospective study. J Bone Joint Surg 1976;58A:1–8.
9. Woodland LH, Francis RS. Parameters and comparisons of the quadriceps angle of college-aged men and women in the supine and standing positions. Am J Sports Med 1992;20(2):208–211.
10. Olerud C, Berg P. The variation of the Q angle with different positions of the foot. Clin Orthop 1984;191:162–165.
11. Aglietti P, Insall JN, Cerulli G. Patellar pain and incongruence. Clin Orthop 1983;176:217–224.
12. Fairbank JCT, Pynsent PB, van Poortvliet JA, Phillips H. Mechanical factors in the incidence of knee pain in adolescents and young adults. J Bone Joint Surg 1984;66B:685–693.
13. Horton MG, Hall TL. Quadriceps femoris muscle angle: Normal values and relationships with gender and selected skeletal measures. Phys Therapy 1989;69(11):897–901.
14. Hsu RWW, Himeno S, Coventry MB, Chao EYS. Normal axial alignment of the lower extremity and load-bearing distribution at the knee. Clin Orthop 1990;255:215–227.
15. Aglietti P, Insall JH, Cerulli G. Patellar pain and incongruence. Clin Orthop 1983;122:217–224.
16. Fithian DC, Mishra DK, Balen PF, Stone ML, Daniel DM. Instrumented measurement of patellar mobility. Am J Sports Med 1995;23(5):607–615.
17. Kujala UM, Dvist M, Osterman K, Friberg O, Aalto T. Factors predisposing army conscripts to knee exertion injuries incurred in a physical training program. Clin Orthop 1986;210:203–212.
18. Fulkerson JP, Hungerford DS. Disorders of the Patellofemoral Joint, 2nd ed. Baltimore: Williams & Wilkins; 1990.
19. Hughston JC, Walsh WM. Proximal and distal reconstruction of the extensor mechanism for patellar subluxation. Clin Orthop 1979;144:36–42.
20. Insall J, Falvo KA, Wise DW. Chondromalacia patellae, a prospective study. J Bone Joint Surg 1976;58A:1–8.
21. Perry J. Gait Analysis, Normal and Pathological Gait. Thorofare, NJ: Slack; 1992.
22. Nichols PJR. Short-leg syndrome. BMJ 1960;1:1863–1865.
23. Rush WA, Steiner HA. A study of lower extremity length inequality. AJR Am J Roentgenol 1946;56:616–623.
24. Sell KE, Verity TM, Worrell TW, Pease BJ, Wiglesworth J. Two measurements for assessing subtalar joint position: A reliability study. J Orthop Sports Phys Ther 1994;19:162–176.
25. Inman VT, Ralston HJ, Todd F. Human Walking. Baltimore: Williams & Wilkins; 1981.
26. Levens AS, Inman VT, Blosser JA. Transverse rotation of the segments of the lower extremity in locomotion. J Bone Joint Surg 1948;30A:859–872.
27. Tiberio D. The effect of excessive subtalar joint pronation on patellofemoral mechanics: A theoretical model. J Orthop Sports Phys Ther 1987;(Oct):160–165.
28. Eng JJ, Pierrynowski MR. Evaluation of soft foot orthotics in the treatment of patellofemoral pain syndrome. Phys Ther 1993;73(2):62–70.
29. Gross MT. Lower quarter screening for skeletal malalignment-suggestions for orthotics and shoewear. J Orthop Sports Phys Ther 1995;21(6):389–405.
30. Hughston JC, Walsh WM, Puddu G. Patellar Subluxation and Dislocation. Philadelphia: WB Saunders; 1984.
31. Kolowich PA, Paulos LE, Rosenberg TD, Farnsworth S. Lateral release of the patella: Indications and contraindications. Am J Sports Med 1990;18(4):359–365.
32. Muneta T, Yamamoto H, Ishibashi T, Asahina S, Furuya K. Computerized tomographic analysis of tibial tubercle position in the painful female patellofemoral joint. Am J Sports Med 1994;22(1):67–71.
33. Fulkerson JP, Gossling HR. Anatomy of the knee joint lateral retinaculum. Clin Orthop 1980;153:183–188.
34. Terry GC, Hughston JC, Norwood LA. The anatomy of the iliopatellar band and the iliotibial track. Am J Sports Med 1986;14(1):39–45.
35. Ficat P, Hungerford D. Disorders of the Patellofemoral Joint. Baltimore: Williams & Wilkins; 1977.
36. Conlan T, Garth WP, Lemons JE. Evaluation of the medial soft-tissue restraints of the extensor mechanism of the knee. J Bone Joint Surg 1993;75A:682–693.
37. Sallay PI, Poggi J, Speer KP, Garrett WE. Acute dislocation of the patella, a correlative pathoanatomic study. Am J Sports Med 1996;24(1):52–60.
38. Kujala UM, Kvist M, Osterman K, et al. Factors predisposing army conscripts to knee exertion injuries incurred in a physical training program. Clin Orthop 1986;210:203–212.
39. Skalley TC, Terry GC, Teitge RA. The quantitative measurement of normal passive medial and lateral patellar motion limits. Am J Sports Med 1993;21:728–732.
40. Fitzgerald GK, McClure PW. Reliability of measurements obtained with four tests for patellofemoral alignment. Physical Therapy 1995;75(2):84–89.

41. Hughston JC, Deese M. Medial subluxation of the patella as a complication of lateral retinacular release. Am J Sports Med 1988;16:383–388.
42. Miller PR, Klein RM, Teitge RA. Medial dislocation of the patella. Skeletal Radiol 1991;20:429–431.
43. Teitge RA. Iatrogenic Medial Patellar Dislocation. In: Proceedings of the 1991 AAOS Meeting, Anaheim, CA. Rosemont, IL: AAOS Publications; 1991.
44. Nonweiler DE, DeLee JC. The diagnosis and treatment of medial subluxation of the patella after lateral retinacular release. Am J Sports Med 1994;22(5):680–686.
45. Paulos LE, Wnorowski DC, Greenwald AE. Infrapatellar contracture syndrome. Diagnosis, treatment and long-term follow-up. Am J Sports Med 1994;22(4):440–449.
46. Riedert RM, Stauffer E, NF Friederich. Occurrence of free nerve endings in the soft tissue of the knee joint. Am J Sports Med 1992;20:430–433.
47. Fulkerson JP, Tennant R, Jaivin JS, et al. Histologic evidence of retinacular nerve injury associated with patellofemoral malalignment. Clin Orthop 1985;187:196–205.
48. Mori Y, Fujimoto A, Okumo H, Kuroki Y. Lateral retinaculum release in adolescent patellofemoral disorders: Its relationship to peripheral nerve injury in the lateral retinaculum. Bull Hosp Joint Dis 1991;51:218–229.
49. House JH, Ahmed K. Entrapment neuropathy of the infrapatellar branch of the saphenous nerve. Am J Sports Med 1977;5(5):217–224.
50. Luerssen TG, Campbell RL, Defalque RJ, Worth RM. Spontaneous saphenous neuralgia. Neurosurgery 1983;13(3):238–241.
51. Worth RM, Ketteldamp DB, Defalque RJ, Duane KU. Saphenous nerve entrapment: A cause of medial knee pain. Am J Sports Med 1984;12(1):80–81.
52. Carson WG, James SL, Larson RL, Singer KM, Winternitz WW. Patellofemoral disorders: Physical and radiographical examination. Clin Orthop 1984;185:165–177.
53. McCoy GF, McCrea JD, Beverland DE, Kernohan WG, Mollan RAB. Vibration arthrography as a diagnostic aid in diseases of the knee. J Bone Joint Surg 1987;69B:288–293.
54. Jiang CC, Liu YJ, Yip KM, Wu E. Physiological patellofemoral crepitus in knee joint disorders. Bull Hosp Joint Dis 1993;53(4):22–26.
55. Neely LA, Kernohan WG, Barr DA, Mee CHB, Mollan RAB. Optical measurements of physiological patellofemoral crepitus. Clin Phys Physiol Meas 1991;12(3):219–226.
56. Kernohan WG, Reverland DE, McCoy GF, et al: The diagnostic potential of vibration arthrography. Clin Ortho 1986;210:106–112.
57. Ruwe PA, Gage JR, Ozonoff MB, DeLuca PA. Clinical determination of femoral anteversion. J Bone Joint Surg 1992;74(A):820–830.
58. Yoshioka Y, Sin D, Cooke DV. The anatomy and functional axes of the femur. J Bone Joint Surg 1987;69(A):873–880.
59. Kingsley PC, Olmsted KL. A study to determine the angle of anteversion of the neck of the femur. J Bone Joint Surg 1948;30A:745–751.
60. Staheli LT, Corbett M, Wyss C, King H. Lower-extremity rotational problems in children. J Bone Joint Surg 1985;67A:39–47.
61. Brouwer KJ, Molenaar JC, van Linge B. Rotational deformities after femoral shaft fractures in childhood-a retrospective study. Acta Orthop Scand 1981;52(1):81–89.
62. Briten M, Terjesen T, Rossvoll I. Femoral anteversion in normal adults. Acta Orthop Scand 1992;63(7):29–32.
63. Melchione WE, Sullivan S. Reliability of measurements obtained by use of an instrument designed to indirectly measure iliotibial band length. J Orthop Sports Phys Ther 1993;18(3):511–515.
64. Reid DC, Burnham RS, Saboe LA, Kushner SF. Lower extremity flexibility patterns in classical ballet dancers and their correlation to lateral hip and knee injuries. Am J Sports Med 1987;15(4):347–352.
65. Ober FR. The role of the iliotibial band and fascia lata as a factor in the causation of low-back disability and sciatica. J Bone Joint Surg 1936;18A:105–110.
66. Beighton P, Horan F. Orthopaedic aspects of the Ehlers Danlos syndrome. J Bone Joint Surg 1969;51B:444–453.
67. Rünow A. The dislocating patella: etiology and prognosis in relation to generalized joint laxity and anatomy of the patellar articulation. Acta Orthop Scand 1983;54(suppl):201.
68. Stanitski CL. Articular hypermobility and chondral injury in patients with acute patellar dislocation. Am J Sports Med 1995;23(2):146–150.
69. Bonamo JJ, Fay C, Firestone T. The conservative treatment of the anterior cruciate deficient knee. Am J Sports Med 1990;18(6):618–623.
70. Buss DD, Min R, Skyhar MJ, et al. Conservatively treated anterior cruciate ligament injuries. Orthop Trans 1990;14:561.
71. Keller PM, Shelbourne KD, McCarroll JR, Rettig AC. Nonoperatively treated isolated posterior cruciate ligament injuries. Am J Sports Med 1993;21(1):132–136.
72. Parolie JM, Bergfeld JA. Long-term results of nonoperative treatment of isolated posterior cruciate ligament injuries in the athlete. Am J Sports Med 1986;14:35–38.
73. Lewallen DG, Riegger CL, Myers ER, Hayes WC. Effects of retinacular release and tibial tubercle elevation in patellofemoral degenerative joint disease. J Ortho Res 1990;8:856–862.
74. Fulkerson JP, Becker GJ, Meaney JA, et al. Anteromedial tibial tubercle transfer without bone graft. Am J Sports Med 1990;18:490–497.

4

Imaging the Patellofemoral Joint

*"The value of experience is not in seeing much but in
seeing wisely."*

—*Sir William Osler*

Standard radiography is sufficient in the evaluation of most patients with patellofemoral pain. Imaging the patellofemoral joint with techniques such as computed tomography (CT), magnetic resonance imaging (MRI), and radionuclide scan (bone scan), however, may be very helpful in understanding more complex and resistant patellofemoral disorders. There are significant limitations of standard radiographs, and the student of patellofemoral disorders should be ready to request other appropriate diagnostic studies when necessary.

STANDARD VIEWS

Anteroposterior View

With a patient supine on the radiograph table, there is a natural tendency for the legs to roll into external rotation. This must be controlled if the examiner wishes to obtain consistent and reproducible radiographs. In general, a standing anteroposterior (AP) view is most appropriate so that medial or lateral articular cartilage loss ("joint space narrowing") may be detected.

Turning the feet to straight AP alignment may introduce internal rotation and distort the patellar alignment. Fick (1) has shown that there is an average 12-degree change of rotation by aligning the feet in this manner. By obtaining standing AP views of the knees in normal alignment for the patient, the relationship of the patella to the femur will be shown as it exists under normal standing conditions. Nonetheless, because there is some lateralization of the patella normally with the knees in full extension, the standing AP radiograph does not really provide much meaningful information except when there is more extreme malalignment or a lesion in the patella. Standing posteroanterior (PA) views are most helpful in determining whether there is medial or lateral compartment narrowing or evidence of arthrosis. These should be taken in full extension and at 30 degrees of knee flexion (10 degrees caudal). Also, evidence of other problems in the knee, which may be confused with a patellofemoral disorder, might be discovered on the PA radiograph. Finally, the examiner can determine whether there is an unusually high- or low-riding patella by carefully evaluating the AP (or PA) radiograph (Fig. 4.1). Patellar and condylar measurements may be taken also, if desired, from an accurate AP (or PA) radiograph.

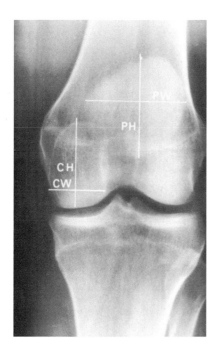

Figure 4.1. Anteroposterior radiograph of the knee. The patella is well seen, but its functional relationship to the remainder of the knee cannot be assessed. Rotation can introduce considerable artifact. Tension on the quadriceps will also change its position compared with the resting position. Factors concerning patellofemoral function such as varus or valgus can be assessed. *PW*, patella width; *PH*, patella height; *CW*, condylar width; *CH*, condylar height. Tibial plateau dimensions and tibial spine dimensions and relationships can also be assessed.

In cases of anterior knee trauma, one may wish to obtain oblique radiographs (2), angling the radiograph tube 45 degrees both medially and laterally. These projections can reveal details about patellar fractures that are not detectable on standard AP or lateral radiographs.

Lateral View

The lateral radiograph may be taken in the lateral decubitus position or standing with the knee extended and flexed (30 degrees) (Fig. 4.2). This places the patellar tendon under tension and demonstrates the functional relationship of the patella to the tibia and, more important, of the patellar facets to the femur. The beam is centered on the tibiofemoral joint line. This degree of flexion should correspond to that of the tangential view.

The lateral view adds considerably to our knowledge of the patella. Patellar height and thickness can be measured. One can observe the general morphology and determine whether there is subchondral sclerosis, evidence of arthrosis, or calcification in the quadriceps or patellar tendon. Lund and Nilsson (3) noted a shallow excavation in the patella of most patients with proven "chondromalacia patellae," which may be noted on the lateral radiograph. One can also determine the vertical distance of the patella from the tibia.

Maldague and Malghem (4–6) described the interpretation of a precise lateral radiograph of the knee with regard to patellar alignment. This interpretation, however, depends on an exact lateral of the knee in which the posterior and distal femoral condyles are overlapped. Consistent reproduction of the precise lateral requires fluoroscopy. An experienced radiology technician, however, can obtain precise laterals in the majority of

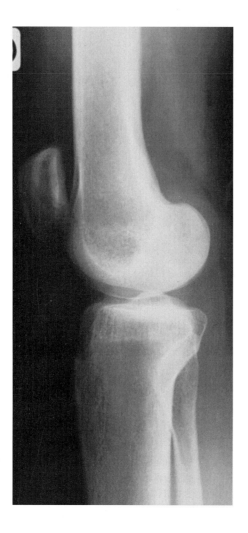

Figure 4.2. Lateral radiograph of the knee.

patients. This requires palpation of the posterior condyles and experience in lining up the posterior femoral condyles on the radiograph cassette.

One major advantage of the lateral view is that it provides information regarding patellar rotation (tilt) with the patient in a weightbearing position. The lateral view may be taken in full extension and again at the desired degree of knee flexion. In most patients, this will be 30 degrees of knee flexion or, to correlate with a standard Merchant view, at 45 degrees of knee flexion. Thus, the clinician is able to get a more functional view of patellar rotation in weightbearing. Murray and Dupont (7) established the sensitivity of the lateral view compared to routine axial radiographs.

Figure 4.3, A to C show what can be seen with a precise lateral. Note that the normally aligned patella demonstrates a central ridge that is posterior to the lateral facet line (Fig. 4.3, A). When the patella is rotated (tilted), one may notice overlap of the central ridge and lateral facet lines (Fig. 4.3, B). With more extreme rotation of the patella, usually associated with some subluxation (lateral translation), the central ridge may actually rotate anterior to the lateral facet, giving a picture as seen in Figure 4.3, C. The precise lateral view, therefore, becomes an excellent image for determining rotation of the patella. Unfortunately, the lateral view really does not help much in evaluating transla-

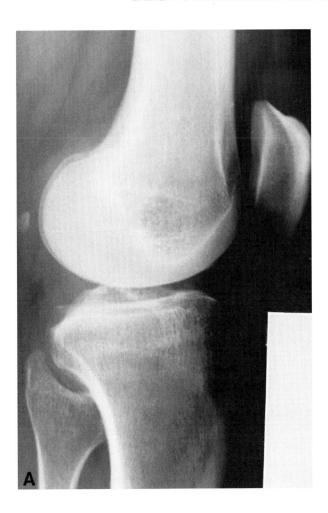

Figure 4.3. A, Normal alignment; **B,** lateral facet line and central ridge overlap; **C,** gross subluxation of patella. (Courtesy of J. Y. Dupont, Quimper, France.) *Continued on next page.*

tion of the patella (as considered separately from tilt). Translation (subluxation) will be better evaluated on the axial view.

The lateral view is also very helpful in evaluating trochlear morphology (8). The center of the trochlea will be seen as the most posterior line (small arrow), whereas the medial (large arrow) and lateral (open arrow) condyles may be seen separately (Fig. 4.4). Normally, the lateral trochlear line should terminate well proximal to the medial trochlear line without crossing the central trochlear line. With experience, the clinician will learn to appreciate morphology of the trochlea better on the lateral view than is possible on any other view, including the axial. This is because the axial view only gives one portion of the trochlea, whereas the entire trochlea may be seen on the lateral view with full excursion of the medial and lateral condyles and the center of the trochlea. Thus, it is possible on the lateral view to obtain an impression of the entire trochlea with regard to its depth and proximal configuration. This information is extremely important because it relates directly to patellofemoral stability.

Blumensaat (9) has described the normal relationship of the patella to an anterior prolongation of a dense line that marks the ventral border of the intercondylar fossa (Blumensaat's line) (Fig. 4.5). Elevation of the distal pole of the patella above this line with

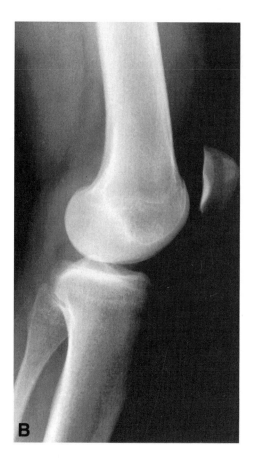
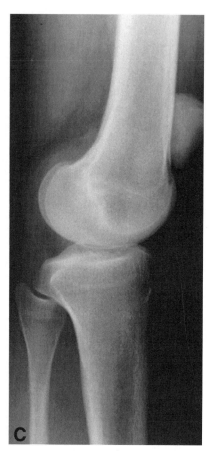

Figure 4.3. *Continued.*

the knee flexed 30 degrees has been widely accepted as indicative of patella alta. Insall and Salvati (10) demonstrated that Blumensaat's line is not an accurate measurement for the position of the normal patella at 30 degrees of flexion. This was confirmed by Jacobsen and Berthensen (11) on bilateral knee radiographs in 50 asymptomatic volunteers. Their method is simple and does not depend on exact positioning of the degree of flexion. It consists of determining the ratio of patellar tendon length to greatest diagonal length of the patella. Both series (10, 11) indicate an upper limit of normal of 1.2 (at the 90% level). Grelsamer and Meadows (12), however, showed that the Insall-Salvati ratio lacks sensitivity because of variations in patella morphology. A long, distal, nonarticulating portion in a patella with a short articular area will give an inaccurate impression in some patients when the Insall-Salvati ratio is used (Fig. 4.5, A to D). Grelsamer and Meadows described a "morphology ratio" relating the patellar articular length to the overall patellar length (Fig. 4.6). Blackburne and Peel (13) proposed another modification of this technique using the tibial articular surface as the reference level for patellar height (Fig. 4.7). These researchers measured the patellar articular length and determined its ratio to the distance between the tibial articular surface and the patellar articular surface. This ratio is 0.8 in normal knees flexed at 30 degrees. Caton et al (14) described a similar method.

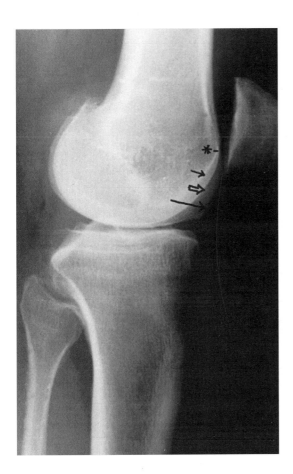

Figure 4.4. Lateral view of the patellofemoral joint, posterior condyles overlapped. *Small arrow* denotes central trochlea, *large arrow* shows medial condyle, and *open arrow* shows a shallow dysplastic lateral condyle (note that the proximal edge of the lateral condyle line crosses the central trochlea (*asterisk*), as described by Dejour et al (8)). (Courtesy of J. Y. Dupont, Quimper, France.)

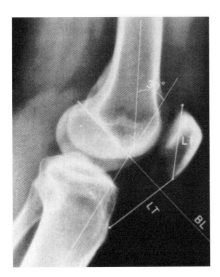

Figure 4.5. Lateral radiograph of the knee in 30 degrees of flexion. Blumensaat's line (*BL*) is marked. The method of Insall and Salvati comparing patellar length (*LP*) and patellar tendon (*LT*) is perhaps less accurate than other alternative measurements when evaluating the patellofemoral articular relationship.

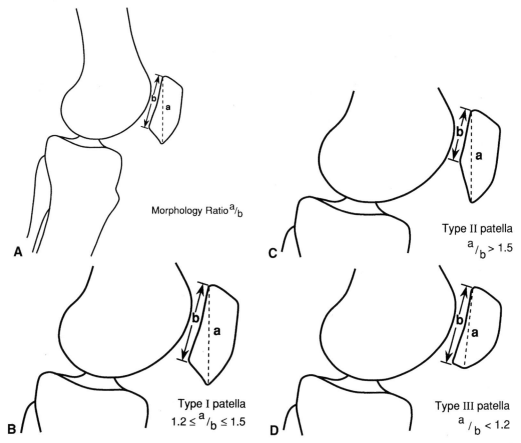

Morphology Ratio $^a/_b$

A

C

Type II patella
$^a/_b > 1.5$

B

Type I patella
$1.2 \leq {}^a/_b \leq 1.5$

D

Type III patella
$^a/_b < 1.2$

Figure 4.6. A, The morphology ratio described by Grelsamer et al relates the length of patella articular surface to the overall patella length. **B** to **D,** patella types as determined using Grelsamer's morphology ratio. Reprinted with permission from Grelsamer RP, Proctor CS, Bazos AN. Evaluation of patellar shape in the sagittal plane. A clinical analysis. Am J Sports Med 1994;22(1):61–66.

Bernageau and Goutallier (15) emphasized the proximal trochlea and its relationship to the patella (Fig. 4.8). Ultimately, the clinician must identify whether the patella is correctly aligned and whether there is smooth entry of the patella into the trochlea. The Bernageau-Goutallier technique makes a lot of sense in this regard and is currently the author's preference.

Tangential (Axial) View

Standard tangential ("axial" or "sunrise") views of the patellofemoral joint provide good, basic information regarding the condition of this joint (16–19). There are several techniques for taking a tangential patellar radiograph, but those of Laurin et al (18) and Merchant et al (19) have been most helpful in the author's experience. The Merchant view requires a special cassette holder and frame. This view is widely used in the United States.

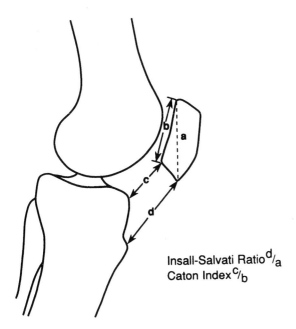

Insall-Salvati Ratio $^d/_a$
Caton Index $^c/_b$

Figure 4.7. The Blackburne and Peel index has also been described by Caton et al. This illustration demonstrates the importance of considering articular length in evaluating patellar height. Reprinted with permission from Caton J, Deschamps G, Chambat P, Lerat JL, Dejour H. Les rotules basses. A propos de 128 observations. Rev Chir Orthop 1982;68:317–325.

Variable anatomy of the femoral trochlea, however, can make interpretation of tangential radiographs difficult. The tangential radiograph also has image distortion and overlapping shadows that may affect interpretation. Most tangential radiographs are taken of both patellae simultaneously, such that the radiograph beam is directed in a slightly oblique direction across the patellofemoral joints, thereby introducing further possibility of error. Furthermore, subtle patellar tracking abnormalities in the first 20 to 30 degrees of knee flexion are difficult or impossible to detect with tangential radiographs of the patella because it is technically difficult to capture the patella on a radiograph cassette in this range of minimal knee flexion. Nonetheless, tangential radiography of the patella is helpful in the basic evaluation and understanding of patellofemoral disorders. A well-controlled, standard tangential radiograph emphasizing early (20–45 degrees) knee flexion can provide important baseline information for the examining physician.

Historical Review

Settegast (20), in 1921, recognized the axial/tangential view of the patellofemoral joint. He described a method in which the patient lies prone with the knee acutely flexed. The beam passes parallel to the posterior surface of the patella and perpendicular to the plate on which the knee rests. The disadvantages of this approach include distortion of the patella with the patient prone and lack of adequate visualization of the proximal trochlea.

In 1924, Jaroschy (21) described a different technique with the patient lying supine. The beam passes parallel to the tibia, and the cassette rests on the distal thigh. He later modified the technique to the prone position with the knee flexed 50 to 60 degrees and the plate lying under the patient's distal thigh. Here, the disadvantage is distortion produced by the beam striking the plate at a 45-degree angle. Also, the high knee flexion angle diminishes sensitivity. Independently in 1941, Wiberg (22) and Knutson (23)

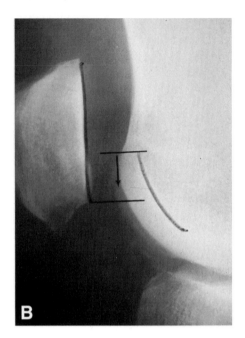

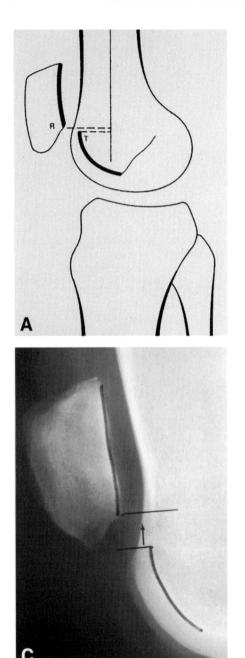

Figure 4.8. A, Bernageau and Goutallier pointed out the importance of describing the patella articular surface as it relates to the proximal, central trochlea. **B,** Patella infera. **C,** Patella alta.

described techniques that reversed the direction of the beam. The cassette rests on the anterior tibia and is perpendicular to the beam, which is horizontal. Furmaier and Breit (24), in 1952, improved this technique by elevating the legs to include both knees, placing one foot against the other, thereby controlling rotation and reducing one source of error. Projecting both knees simultaneously allowed useful comparison. This technique gives a good view but because the plate is resting on the tibia, views of less than 45 degrees of flexion are difficult if not impossible. Positioning with all these views is often difficult. Brattstrom (25), in studying dysplasia of the trochlea in relationship to recurrent dislocation of the patella, put forth an accurate but complicated technique with which we have no clinical experience.

Merchant et al (19) described a technique similar to those of Wiberg (22) and Knutson (23) by flexing the leg 45 degrees over the end of the table and angling the tube 30 degrees from the horizontal, thus overcoming some of the positioning problems of the tube. Merchant et al (19) found difficulty, however, in obtaining satisfactory films at low knee flexion angles. This technique, nonetheless, has been well accepted, is reproducible, and provides an excellent overview of patellofemoral congruence. The methods are summarized in Figure 4.9.

Ficat et al (26) described a technique in which both knees are taken simultaneously, thus controlling rotation and offering comparison on a single film. This technique was recommended for obtaining tangential views at 30 to 90 degrees of knee flexion. Because the cassette is placed on the thigh, it can be close to the joint and, thus, will minimize dis-

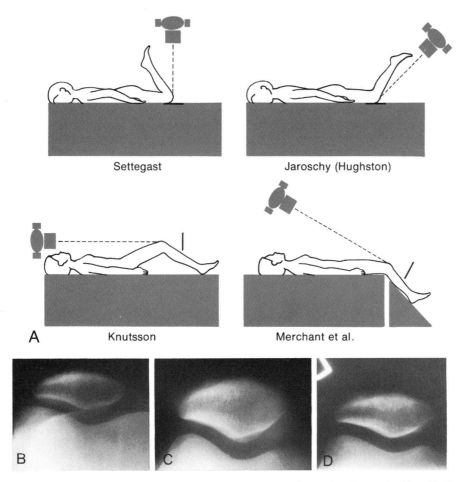

Settegast

Jaroschy (Hughston)

A   Knutsson

Merchant et al.

B   C   D

Figure 4.9. A, Some techniques for obtaining axial patellofemoral radiographs. **B** to **D,** Comparison of three techniques on the same knee shows the variation of images caused by position (**B** and **D**) and distortion (**C**).

tortion. Unfortunately, however, this also increases radiation delivery to the patient. This technique consists of directing the radiograph beam from the subject's feet toward the patellae, with the beam passing through the contact area to project it onto the cassette.

When only one tangential (axial) view is desired, a Laurin 20-degree knee flexion tangential view (18) or a Merchant view (19) provides valuable information. The Laurin view (Fig. 4.10) is difficult to obtain and requires careful instruction of the radiology technician but is helpful in detecting patients with more subtle tracking abnormalities as well as those with more severe patellar tilt, subluxation, or dislocation. When patellar articulation up to 45 degrees of knee flexion is desired, the Merchant view is satisfactory. This view is widely accepted, reproducible, and clinically helpful. Because contact pressure on the patella becomes maximal around 60 degrees of knee flexion and because some patients exhibit progressive patellar tilt, a tangential view at 45 to 60 degrees of knee flexion will provide some useful information. Occasionally, because of obesity or a very prominent tibial tubercle, it will not be possible to obtain a 20- or 30-degree view or even an adequate Merchant view.

Laurin et al (18) showed that the patella is well into the trochlea in 97% of normal individuals by 20 degrees of knee flexion. Further flexion will bring some abnormally aligned patellae back into the trochlear sulcus, which deepens as flexion proceeds, and the desired documentation of abnormal alignment in early flexion may be missed. Using CT, we have found that many young patients with patellofemoral pain will show subtle tracking abnormalities with early knee flexion as compared with asymptomatic control volunteers. With increasing knee flexion, significant patellar malalignment will improve in some patients, which suggests that there are patients with patellofemoral pain related to mild tilt or subluxation (as compared with normal controls) but without detectable abnormality of patellar tracking further into knee flexion.

Malghem and Maldague (27) have introduced the axial (30-degree) radiograph with lateral rotation of the leg. This may be useful in the assessment of patellar subluxability. Toft (28) recommended axial radiographs of the patellofemoral joint with the patient weight bearing. Egund (29) described another patellofemoral axial view using a standard 15-degree inclination of the lower leg with the patient erect. Turner and Burns (30) also recommended the erect position for obtaining tangential views.

Despite attention to detail, tangential radiographs have certain limitations that must be recognized. It is difficult to center the beam perfectly tangential to the contact zone in a way that does not separate the superior and inferior borders of the patella. Image distortion, therefore, is common on tangential radiographs. Knee asymmetry or leg-length dis-

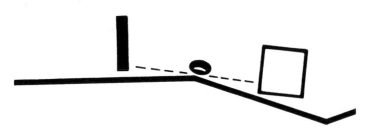

Figure 4.10. The Laurin 20-degree tangential view is difficult to obtain but will provide useful information.

crepancy may make absolute comparative views impossible. Some radiograph units do not permit lowering of the tube and collimator below the level of the table. This requires some modification of the actual technique of taking radiographs but does not invalidate the basic method. Finally, an accurate reference line for determining patellar tilt is not possible with tangential radiographs because of variable anatomy of the femoral trochlea. Nonetheless, the tangential radiograph is useful for the general evaluation of patients with patellofemoral disorders.

Interpretation

If the beam has been centered well, the joint line is revealed without overlapping bony structures and is examined for height and degree of parallelism of the opposing subchondral plates. The quality of orientation of trabecular and subchondral bone in both the patella and trochlea should be observed and compared. In the clinical evaluation of patients, we have found two measurements to be most helpful: the Laurin lateral patellofemoral angle (patellar tilt angle) (18) and the Merchant congruence angle (19).

Lateral Patellofemoral Angle and the Patellar Tilt Angle

Laurin et al (18) described their criteria for patellar tilt based on lines drawn along the lateral patellar facet and the anterior margins of the femoral trochlea. As shown in Figure 4.11, the lateral patellofemoral angle should be open laterally. Laurin et al found that 97% of their controls demonstrated a lateral patellofemoral angle open laterally, whereas 60% of patients with patellar subluxation showed parallel lines, and 40% had a medial facing patellofemoral angle. This simple measurement is a good indicator, for screening purposes, of abnormal patellar tilt. Although the lateral patellofemoral angle has been used to assess subluxation, it is more appropriate to use this measurement to assess tilt and to use other criteria, such as Merchant's congruence angle, to assess subluxation. The patellar tilt angle (as distinct from the lateral patellofemoral angle determined on an axial radiograph) determined by CT or MRI is particularly useful in differentiating tilt from subluxation because the posterior femoral condyles provide a much more consistent reference line for determining tilt (31). This will become clearer in the section on CT. The term patellar tilt angle will define this relationship of the lateral facet to the posterior condylar line.

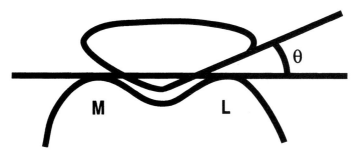

Figure 4.11. The lateral patellofemoral angle of Laurin should open laterally (*L*). This measurement is helpful in screening patients for patellar tilt.

Merchant's Congruence Angle

We have used Merchant's technique (19) for measuring the congruence angle and have applied it to views of the patellofemoral articulation using CT. The patella normally becomes centralized in the trochlea by 10 to 20 degrees of knee flexion. The trochlea cannot be defined well enough at full knee extension to permit accurate appraisal of congruence with the knee extended. Schutzer et al (32) noted that a congruence angle greater than 0 degrees at 10-degree knee flexion should be considered abnormal. Merchant et al (19) had noted in their study that normal congruence is −6 ± 11 degrees at 45-degree knee flexion. In the study by Schutzer et al (32), there were patients with patellofemoral pain who had abnormal congruence at 10-degree knee flexion, with correction of this subtle abnormality on further flexion of the knee. Imai et al (33) pointed out that this is most likely caused by progressive tightening of the medial retinaculum with increasing knee flexion. These distinct but subtle differences (determined by CT) from an asymptomatic control population may not be detected on standard tangential radiographs in all patients.

The congruence angle described by Merchant et al (19) is a good indicator of patella centralization and/or subluxation (as opposed to tilt). Merchant's congruence angle may be applied to tangential radiographs at any degree of knee flexion as well as at the 45-degree knee flexion angle originally described by Merchant. We believe that abnormal congruence should be sustained at 10 and 20 degrees of knee flexion to be considered

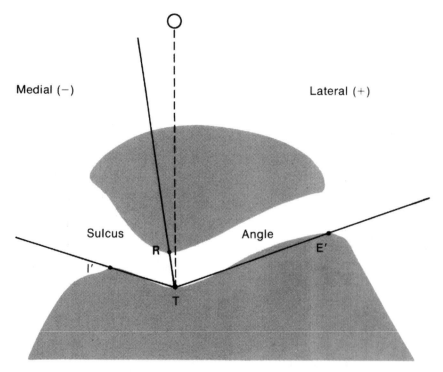

Figure 4.12. Functional relationship. *TO*, neutral reference line bisecting angle *E'TI'*. *RT*, line connecting median ridge to trochlear depth. Adapted from Merchant AC, Mercer R L, Jacobsen RH, Cool, CR. Roentgenographic analysis of patello-femoral congruence. J Bone Joint Surg 1974;56A:1391-1396.

truly abnormal in determining treatment. Certainly, those patients who exhibit abnormal congruence only at 10- and 20-degree knee flexion with normal congruence at 45-degree knee flexion must be considered less severely afflicted, although their congruence angles are certainly not quite consistent with those of the normal population.

To determine the congruence angle, the sulcus angle, E′TI′, as shown in Figure 4.12, is bisected by a neutral reference line, TO. The apex of the median patellar ridge is connected to the lowest point on the sulcus. When this line, RT, is medial to the neutral reference line, the angle is given a negative value; when lateral, a positive value is assigned.

Other Patellofemoral Indices

Several other measurements may be used on occasion but are not often helpful in the analysis of most clinical conditions. These normal patellofemoral indices are based on a 60-degree knee flexion tangential view and are summarized in Figure 4.13. Of these indices, the sulcus angle may be most helpful in gaining insight into reasons for patellar instability. Serial evaluation of the sulcus at increasing angles of knee flexion using CT has been most helpful in understanding trochlear morphology.

COMPUTED TOMOGRAPHY

To define patellar tracking accurately, CT offers sequential images at any degree of knee flexion using the midtransverse patella as a stable plane of reference. Unlike tangential radiographs, CT images through specific segments of the femoral trochlea, omitting image overlap and distortion. Consequently, one can define accurately the relationship between a specific reference plane (midtransverse patella) and its exact counterpart on the femur, the femoral trochlea (Fig. 4.14). Particularly helpful also is the possibility of tomographic sectioning into the posterior femoral condyles where the anatomy is quite symmetric (31), providing a reliable reference plane (Fig. 4.15) for determining patellar tilt as compared with a line drawn across the variable anterior femoral trochlear (Fig.

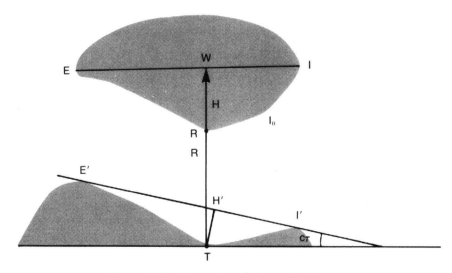

Figure 4.13. Normal patellofemoral indices.

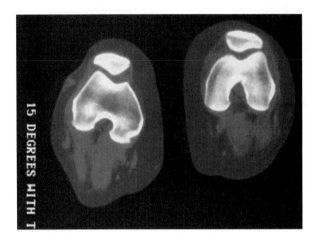

Figure 4.14. This computed tomography image demonstrates the precision possible with tomographic slices centered on the midtransverse patella. Because there is no image overlap, a true picture of patellofemoral congruity is possible.

4.16) margins. With sequential tomographic images from 0 to 60 degrees of knee flexion, one can appreciate early engagement of the patella into the trochlea by 10 to 20 degrees of knee flexion in normal patellofemoral function (32–34). Under normal circumstances, the patella should not exhibit tilt or subluxation through the subsequent range of knee motion. Using CT criteria, it is possible to note a variety of different tracking patterns that are not as well defined using standard radiographs. In addition, CT with contrast has proven helpful in the appraisal of patellar articular cartilage (35). With its more sensitive reference planes for determining tilt, CT has revealed three basic tracking

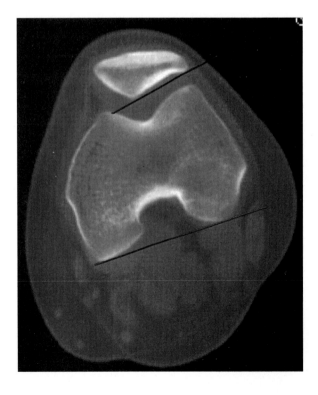

Figure 4.15. The posterior femoral condyles of this computed tomography image are anatomically very consistent and provide a reliable reference plane for evaluating patellar tilt. The angle formed by the lateral facet and posterior condyle lines is the patellar tilt angle.

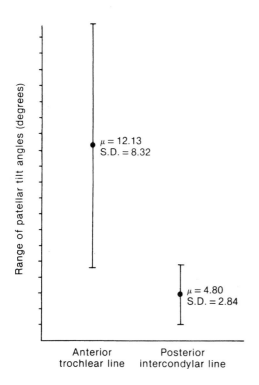

Range of patellar tilt angles (degrees)

$\mu = 12.13$
S.D. = 8.32

$\mu = 4.80$
S.D. = 2.84

Anterior trochlear line   Posterior intercondylar line

Figure 4.16. When the anterior trochlear line is used to determine tilt, there is a much greater chance of inaccuracy when compared to the posterior intercondylar line (see Fig. 4.15). S.D., standard deviation. Reprinted with permission from Fulkerson JP, Schutzer SF, Ramsby GR, Bernstein RA. Computerized tomography of the patellofemoral joint before and after lateral release or realignment. Arthroscopy 1987;3 (1):19–24.

abnormalities (Fig. 4.17). Stanciu et al (36) confirmed the improved sensitivity of CT of the patellofemoral joint compared with standard radiographs.

Within each of these categories, there is additional variability as to degree and correctability. Studies have shown that normal patellae engage the trochlea and are centered, without tilt, by 10 to 20 degrees of knee flexion (32). The patella normally sits lateral to the trochlea with the knee extended. One study has suggested evaluation of subluxation

MALALIGNMENT PATTERNS

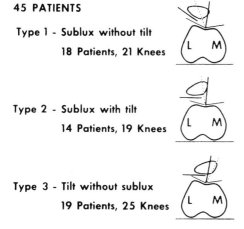

45 PATIENTS

Type 1 - Sublux without tilt

　18 Patients, 21 Knees

Type 2 - Sublux with tilt

　14 Patients, 19 Knees

Type 3 - Tilt without sublux

　19 Patients, 25 Knees

Figure 4.17. Malalignment patterns determined by computed tomography. It is most important to recognize that tilt may occur with or without subluxation. Reprinted with permission from Schutzer S F, Ramsby G R, Fulkerson JP. Computed tomographic classification of patellofemoral pain patients. Orthop Clin North Am 1986;17(2):235–248.

using CT with the knee extended (37), but the patella is mostly above the trochlea, at this point making accurate evaluation of patellar alignment less reliable until 10 to 20 degrees of knee flexion. Using CT, a patella that is still significantly tilted or subluxated by 20 degrees of knee flexion is malaligned. Using the sensitive CT criteria, some subtle abnormalities may be detected even at 10 degrees of knee flexion, but in our experience these changes should be sustained to 15 to 20 degrees of knee flexion to control for variability in technique. On further flexion of the knee, subluxation or tilt may improve or worsen. By examining a technically well-done CT study of patellofemoral tracking, one can gain clear insight into the tracking pattern of each individual patient, leaving little to the imagination. It is extremely important, however, that these studies be performed in a standardized, accurate, and reproducible manner, centered on the midtransverse patella. Classification of tilt and/or subluxation becomes particularly important in developing a prognosis and appropriate treatment plan. Also, CT is extremely helpful in the evaluation of patellofemoral realignment or lateral release (31). Figures 4.18 and 4.19 show the patterns of subluxation and tilt exhibited by patients. Evaluation of patellofemoral congruence with the quadriceps both contracted and relaxed may improve sensitivity selectively (38). At 30 to 40 degrees of knee flexion, quadriceps contraction causes slight medialization of the patella and a relative decrease of the congruence angle. Dynamic CT of the patellofemoral joint is also possible (39).

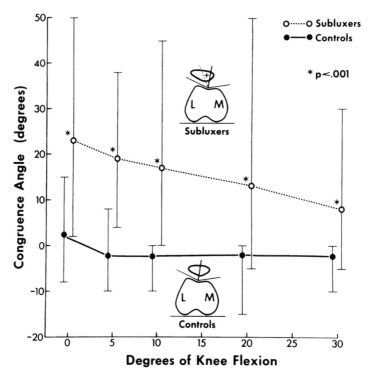

Figure 4.18. There are many patients with patellofemoral pain whose patellae are relatively subluxated when compared with controls. Reprinted with permission from Schutzer SF, Ramsby GR, Fulkerson JP. Computed tomographic classification of patellofemoral pain patients. Orthop Clin North Am 1986;17(2):235–248.

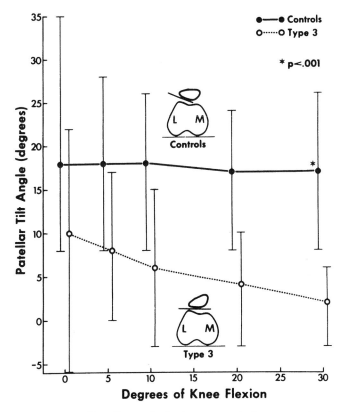

Figure 4.19. Note that patellar tilt tends to be somewhat progressive in patients with patellofemoral pain. Reprinted with permission from Schutzer SF, Ramsby GR, Fulkerson JP. Computed tomographic classification of patellofemoral pain patients. Orthop Clin North Am 1986;17(2):235–248.

Performing Patellofemoral CT

The patient is examined in a comfortable standing position to evaluate distances between the medial malleoli and femoral condyles. Rotation of the feet is also noted. The patient is then placed in the scanner gantry, reproducing this normal standing alignment as closely as possible using bolsters. Beginning at neutral knee flexion/extension (not full extension because some patients may hyperextend), sequential CT slices are taken, centering the beam on the midtransverse patella (which is labeled with a marking pen) of both knees simultaneously. This is best accomplished with the patient in a lateral decubitus position. It is important to use the same reference plane for sequential tomographic slices, and it is extremely important to define the midtransverse patella because tomographic cuts at different levels will give less accurate indications of tilt. Tomographic cuts may be taken as desired, but it is currently our preference to obtain tomographic slices at 0, 15, 30, 45, and 60 degrees of knee flexion. By so doing, one can accurately assess the patella as it enters the trochlea and progresses to a point of maximal contact stress. Progression and/or correction of tilt or subluxation can then be determined. When this technique is mastered, the entire study can be obtained in approximately 20 minutes at a cost that is approximately the same as a full set of four knee radiographs. Biedert and Gruhl (40) noted that CT with the quadriceps muscle relaxed is preferable.

Our approach to analyzing a CT study is described in some detail, emphasizing the differentiation between subluxation and tilt.

DETERMINING SUBLUXATION AND TILT USING TOMOGRAPHIC IMAGES

Measurements of the patellar tilt angles or congruence angles are routinely taken from midpatellar transverse tomographic images. The purpose is to assess patellar alignment just after the patella has engaged the femoral sulcus (15 degrees), in the midrange of knee flexion (30 and 45 degrees), and at flexion consistent with maximal or near-maximal patellar contact stress (60 degrees).

First, suitable images are obtained that are consistent with excellent technique, emphasizing reproduction of normal standing alignment, midpatellar transverse cuts, and straight through the femur so that the femoral sulcus and posterior condyles are well visualized (Fig. 4.20).

Next, lines are drawn with a fine grease pencil along the lateral patellar facet and posterior femoral condyles (Fig. 4.21).

The angle formed by these two lines is the patellar tilt angle (Fig. 4.22).

This angle should always be greater than 7 degrees even in full extension and has been 12 to 14 degrees or more on the 15- to 20-degree knee flexion tomographic slice in the knees of asymptomatic controls.

After measuring the tilt angles, the congruence angles are determined. In our modification of Merchant's technique (19), the femoral sulcus angles are drawn (lines C and D) (Fig. 4.23) on the same images for which patellar tilt was just determined (if necessary, the previous lines are removed). The sulcus angle is measured on each image and bisected (line E) (Fig. 4.23).

One then forms the congruence angle by drawing a line F from the deepest point in the femoral trochlea (where lines C and D meet) to point R at the tip of the patella (Fig. 4.24).

The congruence angle (Fig. 4.25, angle a) is created by lines E and F and is our preferred index of subluxation [as recommended earlier by Merchant et al (19)].

Using CT, we (32) noted that the congruence angle consistently became 0 or negative by 10 degrees of knee flexion in the knees of ten age-matched asymptomatic volunteers. We consider a patella to be congruent when it centers in the trochlea (as determined by CT) by 15 to 20 degrees of knee flexion.

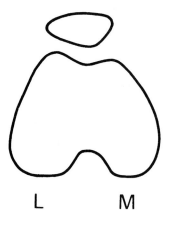

L   M

Figure 4.20. A high-quality tomographic study of the patellofemoral joint should include adequate delineation of the femoral sulcus and posterior condyles and must be centered on the midtransverse patella.

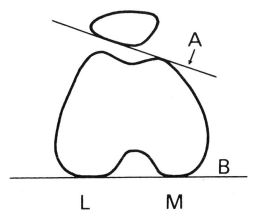

Figure 4.21. A and **B,** The posterior femoral condyles provide a reliable reference plane for evaluating patellar tilt.

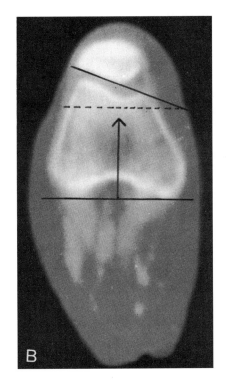

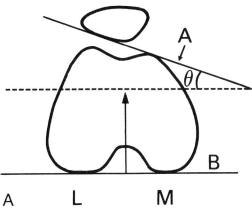

Figure 4.22. A, The patellar tilt angle is more reliable when determined in this manner. The anatomy of the anterior femoral trochlea changes considerably as the patella moves through flexion, but the posterior condyles provide a stable reference line. **B,** This computed tomography image demonstrates a normal patellar tilt angle (*PTA*) at 20 degrees of knee flexion (PTA = 18 degrees).

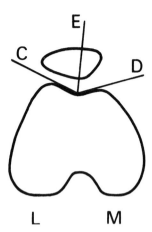

L   M

Figure 4.23. Bisecting the femoral sulcus angle.

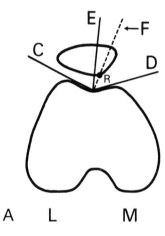

A   L   M

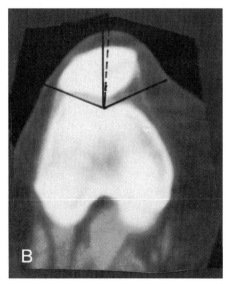

Figure 4.24. A, A line drawn to the tip of the patella (point R) forms line *F.* **B,** This computed tomography image (CT) demonstrates a normal (≤0) CT congruence angle at 20 degrees of knee flexion.

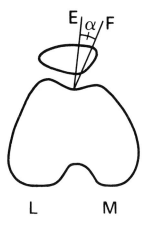

Figure 4.25. The congruence angle (α) is used to evaluate subluxation of the patella. If α is medial to line E, it is negative. If α is lateral to line E, it is positive.

ARTHROGRAPHY

Evaluation of the patellofemoral joint with contrast material is rarely necessary if MRI is available. A small amount of contrast material may be injected, however, and radiographs are taken to evaluate congruence (Fig. 4.26). Tomographic imaging is most desirable. Imai et al (33) found arthrography helpful in evaluating the space between the medial facet and the trochlea and graded patellofemoral alignment based on reduction of this space with increasing knee flexion.

Ficat et al (41) found single-contrast arthrography very helpful in the evaluation of patients with patellofemoral pain, and Horns (42) noted an accuracy of 90% in localizing chondromalacia of the patella using arthrography.

Today, however, there are very few reasons to perform patellofemoral joint arthrography. When MRI is not available or is contraindicated and nonoperative evaluation of patellar or trochlear articular cartilage is indicated, patellofemoral joint arthrography may be an alternative. CT with contrast may be particularly helpful in difficult cases.

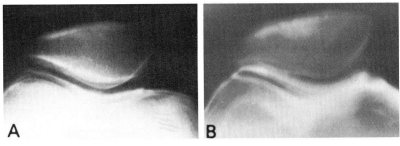

Figure 4.26. A, Good quality arthrogram shows the joint line well delineated. **B,** The radiograph beam has been angled 5 degrees differently from **A** (same knee), showing that precision is necessary to have an interpretable arthrogram.

PATELLOFEMORAL RADIOGRAPHIC EVALUATION IN CHILDREN

This subject is special enough to require a small separate section. Until the individual is 4 or 5 years of age, the patella remains wholly cartilaginous and thus radiographically invisible. This is important in diagnosing some of the early disorders affecting this joint. The action of abnormal stress on a patella is particularly difficult to evaluate, unlike many joints, until approximately age 11 years. The normal patellofemoral joint passes through three radiographic stages.

Birth to 5 Years

The patellar ossification center has not yet appeared, and the patella is radiographically invisible. The trochlea will, however, show the sulcus but usually less markedly than it actually is (Fig. 4.27).

Five to Eleven Years

The ossific nucleus appears (Fig. 4.28) and gradually increases in size, attaining more or less final adult appearance by the end of this time. The trochlea likewise reveals more and more of its form as the cartilage anlage ossifies. During this period, little can be appreciated of the relationship between the two bones because of the large volume that remains radiographically invisible. The shape and orientation of the ossific nucleus are directed by the forces applied to the patella. Equilibrated forces result in the ossific nucleus appearing in the center of the patella. Eccentric forces may result in displacement (usually laterally) of the ossific nucleus. We do not know yet whether most dysplastic forms are present at birth or formed during the course of development. Based on experience with the hip, one could surmise that it is a little of the former and a lot of the latter.

After 11 Years

The adult form is now recognizable (Fig. 4.29), but in the earlier part of this period, the joint line is thicker than it will be later because not all the cartilaginous anlage has

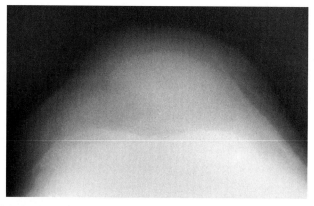

Figure 4.27. Axial view of a 3-year-old child. The patella is not visible, but the trochlear sulcus is seen in the femoral ossific nucleus.

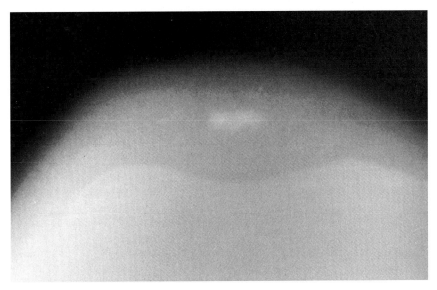

Figure 4.28. Axial view of a 6-year-old child in whom the patella ossific nucleus is seen to be well centered in the cartilaginous anlage.

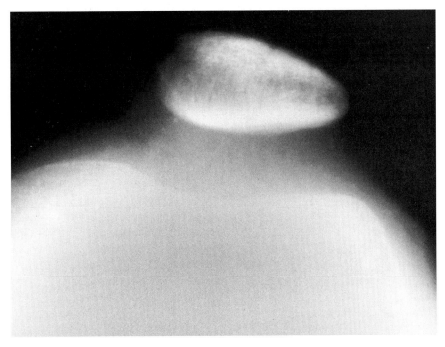

Figure 4.29. Axial view of an 11-year-old in whom the adult patella form is evident, although the joint line is still considerably thicker than it eventually will be.

ossified. By the end of puberty (14–18 years), the joint line will have assumed its permanent adult form, which now will be changed only by disease.

MAGNETIC RESONANCE IMAGING

MRI has been used extensively to evaluate the patellofemoral joint (43–46). Because it gives a direct picture of hydrated structures, it is the most effective noninvasive modality currently available to view patellar articular cartilage (Fig. 4.30). Ghelman and Hodge (47) reviewed the role of MRI for the patellofemoral joint. Nakanishi et al (48) noted that MRI is very useful in the evaluation of cartilage injury. These researchers noted also, however, that early changes observed by arthroscopy were "underestimated" on MRI. Therefore, MRI was more useful for evaluating moderate to advanced patellar cartilage damage. Conway (49) made similar observations. McCauley et al (50) noted that patients with chondromalacia patellae have focal defects in patellar cartilage on T2-weighted MRI. Many previous studies on detection of chondromalacia have used T1-weighted images. Brown and Quinn (51) further emphasized the value of T2-weighted images for detecting chondromalacia, and these authors reiterated the lack of MRI sensitivity in detecting soft, but unbroken, articular cartilage. Nonetheless, as imaging techniques improve and computer software packages improve, sensitivity for detecting articular cartilage lesions may also continue to improve. At the present, however, arthroscopic (or open) evaluation of patellar articular cartilage remains superior to MRI.

MRI of the patella for intraarticular fractures and neoplasms, however, may be very helpful. Figure 4.31 shows a hemangioma of the quadriceps muscle immediately above the patella in a patient with anterior knee pain. Whenever there is a need specifically for soft-tissue imaging, MRI is the method of choice.

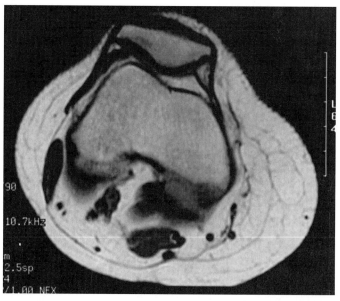

Figure 4.30. Magnetic resonance provides the advantage of soft tissue and cartilage imaging. This is particularly beneficial when evaluating articular cartilage of the patella or trochlea.

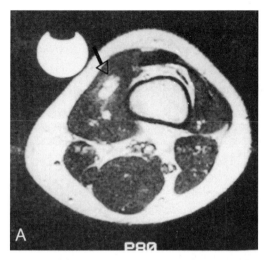

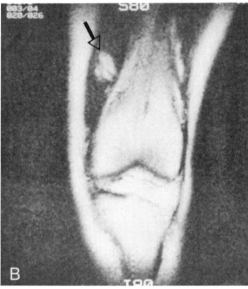

Figure 4.31. These magnetic resonance images of the peripatellar quadriceps muscle demonstrate a hemangioma (later removed) that had caused resistant anterior knee pain. (Courtesy of John Elliott, Westerly, RI.)

MRI with progressive knee flexion is possible, and kinematic MRI (52), even in this range, is interesting. From a practical point of view, however, static tomographic images are more useful for accurately measuring tilt and subluxation. Some clinicians and radiologists believe that a more subjective interpretation of images is equally valid, but one cannot deny the benefits of objective criteria of abnormal alignment using carefully established normal limits.

CT is less expensive, although this may change. CT currently offers greater ability to obtain tomographic slices at varying knee flexion angles. I continue to recommend CT for evaluation of patellar alignment when history, physical examination, and well-done plain radiographs yield insufficient information. I have found that more sophisticated imaging techniques are less necessary with improved clinical examination skills and precise radiographs. Nonetheless, in selected patients, MRI can be extremely helpful. Shellock et al (53) introduced a "positioning device" that permits loading of the knee and normalized stress to the patellofemoral joint during imaging. This load-bearing platform, together with kinematic MRI, may provide some interesting insight into functional behavior of the patellofemoral joint. Using this positioning system, they later demonstrated the effect of bracing on patellar position (54).

RADIONUCLIDE IMAGING

Dye and Boll (55) pointed out that radionuclide imaging may be helpful in the evaluation of patients with patellar pain (Fig. 4.32). As with arthrosis in other areas, one might expect that significant articular breakdown might result in a subchondral bone remodeling response in the patellofemoral joint. Also, if there is significant trauma to the patella, one might expect an osseous remodeling response, as suggested by Dye and Boll (55) and Dye and Chew (56). Subsequently, and particularly if articular cartilage is disrupted, excessive stress on the patella may aggravate or perpetuate bone remodeling in the patella. This process could result in increased activity in the patella as determined by radionuclide scan.

Brill (57) noted that bone scans are usually not positive in young athletes who have complaints of anterior knee pain. In our opinion, this is not surprising because we believe that many anterior knee pain problems, particularly in young athletes, are localized to the peripatellar retinacular structures and patellar tendon.

In the evaluation of patients with resistant anterior knee pain that has not responded to the usual nonoperative treatment, radionuclide scanning may be very helpful (58). Spotty tracer uptake in the central patella appears pathognomonic of chondromalacia patellae in older patients (59). Certainly, if one is contemplating a major decompression procedure with anteriorization of the tibial tubercle, it would be reasonable to determine that there

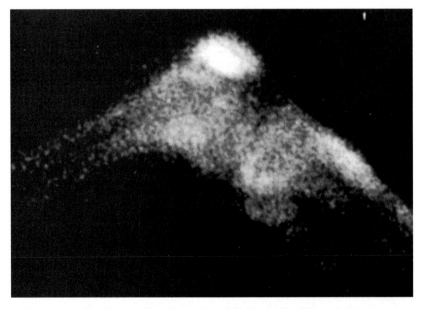

Figure 4.32. Technetium 99m radionuclide scan will detect significant intraosseous remodeling of patellar or trochlear bone in response to injury, excessive pressure, or arthrosis. (Courtesy of Scott Dye, San Francisco, CA.)

is a significant articular and subchondral osseous remodeling problem in the patella. Also, in those patients who do not have other objective findings regarding the patellofemoral joint, one may wish to obtain a bone scan to rule out the possibility of significant patellar disease. After trauma, one may need to wait 18 to 24 months, as suggested by Dye and Boll (55), for equilibrium and homeostatic restoration of normal bone function. In short, the radionuclide scan may be helpful in a variety of patellofemoral pain problems that are resistant to accurate diagnosis.

OTHER IMAGING TECHNIQUES

A sensitivity rate of 92% has been reported by Derks et al (60) who used ultrasound for delineation of plica synovialis. Brussaard et al (61), however, found that 22% of patellar cartilage defects were missed using ultrasound.

Intraosseous venography (62) has been reported also to be used in patients with chondromalacia and patellofemoral arthritis, demonstrating venous engorgement of the patella in both disorders.

Single-photon emission computed tomography (SPECT) bone scintigraphy has been useful in evaluating the extent of knee osteoarthritis. This technique was created by Waisbrod and Treiman (62) and Collier et al (63) to be useful for distinguishing synovitis and articular cartilage damage in the patellofemoral joint. SPECT was also useful in detecting meniscus tears, but this function has now mostly been replaced by MRI.

Minkoff and Fein (64) pointed out that SPECT may be uniquely helpful in some difficult diagnostic problems. They describe SPECT as "a CT scan of a bone scan."

Disler et al (65) reported the use of fat-suppressed, three-dimensional, spoiled gradient-recalled acquisition in the steady state in maximizing contrast between articular cartilage and fluid, fat, or muscle. This technique may be useful to enhance articular cartilage images of the patella.

Three-dimensional reconstructions of the patellofemoral joint may provide unique insights into patellofemoral structure in some special cases. Fractures, dysplasias, and some malalignments may be clarified using this technique (Fig. 4.33).

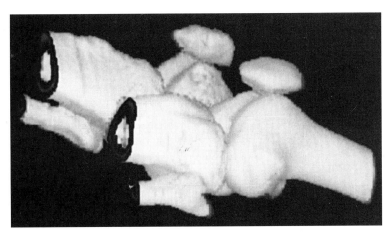

Figure 4.33. Three-dimensional reconstruction of the patellofemoral joint using computed tomography may be particularly helpful in difficult cases involving fracture, dysplasia, or deformity.

Optical coherence tomography offers a very detailed view of articular cartilage, and, although not available except in a very few major academic facilities, it offers a new and exciting way to view articular cartilage and the cellular level. Perhaps this technology will provide insight into reasons why some patients with so little actual cartilage damage have so much pain.

PRACTICAL ALGORITHM FOR IMAGING THE PATELLOFEMORAL JOINT

In the initial evaluation of patients with patellofemoral pain, one should obtain a standard AP; a precise standing lateral (posterior condyles superimposed), preferably weight bearing at 0 and 30 degrees of knee flexion; and axial radiographs of the patellofemoral joints (at 30 and/or 45 degrees of knee flexion). The majority of patients will require nothing more. Even when surgery becomes necessary, detailed physical examination and precise radiography may provide all that is needed in most patients.

When diagnosis and treatment become more difficult, tomographic imaging will give considerable insight into the intricacies of patellofemoral function. In particular, tomography centered on the midpatella and obtained at 0, 15, 30, 45, and 60 degrees of knee flexion will determine whether there is significant subluxation or tilt of the patella. CT and MRI may be very helpful in uncovering suspected interosseous, subchondral, and peripatellar lesions.

Of the other available studies, radionuclide scanning may be helpful in selected patients when there is concern about the presence, location, or severity of patella arthrosis. The radionuclide scan may be most helpful when other studies are normal or if there is a history of anterior knee trauma and chronic patellofemoral pain. This is particularly true when the clinician wishes to establish objective findings in cases that involve compensation or litigation.

REFERENCES

1. Fick R. Handbuch der Anatomic and Mechanik der Gelenke. Jena, East Germany: G. Fischer; 1910.
2. Daffner RH, Tabas JJ. Trauma oblique radiographs of the knee. J Bone Joint Surg 1987;69A(4):568–572.
3. Lund F, Nilsson BE. Radiologic evaluation of chondromalacia patellae. Acta Radiol (Diagn) (Stockholm) 1980; 21(3):413–416.
4. Maldague B, Malghem J. Apport du cliché de profil du genou dans le dépistage des instabilités rotuliennes. Rapport préliminaire. Rev Chir Orthop 1985;71(suppl II):5–13.
5. Maldague B, Malghem J. Imagerie du genou en 1987. In: Cahiers d'Enseignement de la S.O.F.C.O.T. Expansion Scientifique Française. Paris; 1987, pp 347–370.
6. Malghem J, Maldague B. Le profil du genou. Anatomic radiologique différentielle des surfaces articulaires. Radiology 1986;67:725–735.
7. Murray T, Dupont J-Y, Fulkerson J. Axial and lateral radiographs in evaluating patellofemoral malalignment. Am J Sports Med 1999;27:580–584.
8. Dejour H, Walch G, Neyret P, Adeleine P. Dysplasia of the intercondylar groove. Rev Chir Orthop 1990;76: 45–54.
9. Blumensaat C. Die lageabweichungen and verrunkungen der kniescheibe. Ergeb Chir Orthop 1938;31:149–223.
10. Insall J, Salvati E. Patella position in the normal knee joint. Radiology 1971;101:101–104.
11. Jacobsen K, Berthensen K. The vertical location of the patella. Acta Orthop Scand 1974;45:436–145.
12. Grelsamer RP, Meadows S. The modified Insall-Salvati ratio for assessment of patellar height. Clin Orthop 1992;282:170–176.
13. Blackburne J, Peel T. A new method of measuring patellar height. J Bone Joint Surg 1977;58B:241.
14. Caton J, Deschamps G, Chambat P, Lerat JL, Dejour H. Les rotules basses. A propos de 128 observations. Rev Chir Orthop 1982;68:317–325.
15. Bernageau J, Goutallier D. Affections fémoro-patellaires. Encyclopedic Med. Chir, Radiodiagnostic II 1977;31: 312 (C-10).

16. Carson WG Jr, James SL, Larson RL, Singer KM, Winternitz WW. Patellofemoral disorders: Physical and radiographic evaluation. Part II. Radiographic examination. Clin Orthop 1984;185(May):178–186.
17. Hughston J. Subluxation of the patella. J Bone Joint Surg 1968;50A:1003.
18. Laurin CA, Dussault R, Levesque HP. The tangential x-ray investigation of the patellofemoral joint: X-ray technique, diagnostic criteria and their interpretation. Clin Orthop 1979;144(Oct):16–26
19. Merchant AC, Mercer RL, Jacobsen RH, Cool CR. Roentgenographic analysis of patello-femoral congruence. J Bone Joint Surg 1974;56A:1391–1396.
20. Settegast J. Typische roentgenbilder von normalen menschen. Lehmanns med. Atlanten 1921;5:211.
21. Jaroschy W. Die diagnostiche verwertbarkeit der patellaraufnahmen. Fortschr Roentgenstr 1924;31:781.
22. Wiberg G. Roentgenographic and anatomic studies on the femoro-patellar joint. Acta Orthop Scand 1941;2:319–410.
23. Knutson F. Uber die rontgenologie des femoropatellargelenkes sowie eine gute projecktion fur das kniegelenk. Acta Radiol 1941;22:371.
24. Furmaier A, Breit A. Uber die roentgenologie des femoro-patellargelenkes. Arch Orthop Unfallchir 1952;45:126–138.
25. Brattstrom H. Shape of the intercondylar groove normally and in recurrent dislocation of the patella. Acta Orthop Scand 1964;68(suppl):134–148.
26. Ficat P, Phillipe J, Bizou H. Le defile femoro-patellaire. Rev Med Toulouse 1970;6:247–244.
27. Malghem J, Maldague B. Patellofemoral joint 30 degrees axial radiograph with lateral rotation of the leg. Radiology 1989;170:566–567.
28. Toft J. Stress radiography of the patello-femoral joint. Ital J Orthop Traumatol 1981;7(3):365–369.
29. Egund J. The axial view of the patello-femoral joint. Description of a new radiographic method for routine use. Acta Radiol (Stockholm) 1986;27(1):101–104.
30. Turner GW, Burns CB. Erect position/tangential projection of the patello-femoral joint. Radiol Technol 1982;54(1):11–14.
31. Fulkerson JP, Schutzer SF, Ramsby GR, Bernstein RA. Computerized tomography of the patellofemoral joint before and after lateral release or realignment. Arthroscopy 1987;3(1):19–24.
32. Schutzer SF, Ramsby GR, Fulkerson JP. Computed tomographic classification of patellofemoral pain patients. Orthop Clin North Am 1986;17(2):235–248.
33. Imai N, Tomatsu T, Nakaseko J, Terada H. Clinical and roentgenological studies on malalignment disorders of the patello-femoral joint. Part II: Relationship between predisposing factors and malalignment of the patello-femoral joint. Nippon Seikeigeka Gakkai Zasshi 1987;61(11):1191–1202.
34. Fujikawa K, Seedham B, Wright V. Biomechanics of the patellofemoral joint. Eng Med 1983;12(1):3.
35. Boven F, Bellemans MA, Geurts J, Potvliege R. A comparative study of the patello-femoral joint on axial roentgenogram, axial arthrogram, and computed tomography following arthrography. Skeletal Radiol 1982;8(3):179–181.
36. Stanciu C, LaBelle HB, Morin B, Fassier F, Marton D. The value of computed tomography for the diagnosis of recurrent patellar subluxation in adolescents. Can J Surg 1994;37(4):319–323.
37. Inoue M, Shino K, Hirose H, Horibe S, Ono K. Subluxation of the patella: Computed tomography analysis of patellofemoral congruence. J Bone Joint Surg 1988;70A:1331.
38. Guzzanti V, Gigante A, Di Lazzaro A, Fabbriciani C. Patellofemoral malalignment in adolescents. Computerized tomographic assessment with or without quadriceps contraction. Am J Sports Med 1994;22(1):55–60.
39. Pinar H, Akseki D, Gent I Karaoglan O. Kinematic and dynamic axial computerized tomography of the normal patellofemoral joint. Knee Surg Sports Traumatol Arthroscopy 1994;2:27–30.
40. Biedert R, Gruhl C. Axial CT of the patellofemoral joint with and without quadriceps contraction. Arch Orthop Trauma Surg 1997;116:77–82.
41. Ficat RP, Phillipe J, Hungerford DS. Chondromalacia patellae: A system of classification. Clin Orthop 1979;144(Oct):55–62.
42. Horns JW. The diagnosis of chondromalacia by double contrast arthrography of the knee. J Bone Joint Surg 1977;59A(1):119–120.
43. Soudry M, Lanir A, Angel D, Roffman M, Kaplan N, Mendes DG. Anatomy of the normal knee as seen by magnetic resonance imaging. J Bone Joint Surg 1986;68B(1):117–120.
44. Wojtys E, Wilson M, Buckwalter K, Braunstein E, Martel W. Magnetic resonance imaging of knee hyaline cartilage and intraarticular pathology. Am J Sports Med 1987;15(5):455–463.
45. Yulish BS, Montanez J, Goodfellow DB, Bryan PJ, Mulopulos GP, Modic MT. Chondromalacia patellae: assessment with MR imaging. Radiology 1987;164(3):763–766.
46. Kujala U, Osterman K, Kormano M, Nelimarkka O, Hurme M, Taimela S. Patellofemoral relationships in recurrent patellar dislocation. J Bone Joint Surg 1989;71B(5):788–792.
47. Ghelman B, Hodge JC. Imaging of the patellofemoral joint (review). Orthop Clin North Am 1992;23(4):523–543.
48. Nakanishi K, et al. Subluxation of the patella: Evaluation of patellar articular cartilage with MR imaging. Br J Radiol 1992;65(776):662–667.
49. Conway WF. Cross-sectional imaging of the patellofemoral joint and surrounding structures. Radiographics 1991;11(2):195–217.

50. McCauley TR, Kier R, Lynch KJ, Jokl P. Chondromalacia patellae: Diagnosis with MR imaging. AJR Am J Roentgenol 1992;158(1):101–105.

51. Brown TR, Quinn SF. Evaluation of chondromalacia of the patellofemoral compartment with axial magnetic resonance imaging. Skeletal Radiol 1993;22(5):325–328.

52. Shellock RG, Mink JH, Fox JM. Patellofemoral joint: Kinematic MR imaging to assess tracking abnormalities. Radiology 1988;168(2):551–553.

53. Shellock FG, Mink JH, Deutsch AL, Foo TK, Sullenberger P. Patellofemoral joint: Identification of abnormalities with active-movement, "unloaded" versus "loaded" kinematic MR imaging techniques. Radiology 1993;188(2):575–578.

54. Shellock F, Mullin M, Stone K, Coleman M, Crues J. Kinematic MRI of the effect of bracing on patellar position. J Athletic Training 2000;35(1):44–49.

55. Dye S, Boll D. Radionuclide imaging of the patellofemoral joint in young adults with anterior knee pain. Orthop Clin North Am 1986;17(2):249–262.

56. Dye SF, Chew MH. The use of scintigraphy to detect increased osseous metabolic activity about the knee. J Bone Joint Surg 1993;75A:1388–1406.

57. Brill D. Sports nuclear medicine. Bone imaging for lower extremity pain in athletes. Clin Nucl Med 1984;8: 101–116.

58. Hejgard N, Diemer H. Bone scan in the patellofemoral pain syndrome. Int Orthop 1987;11(1):29–33.

59. Bakh YW, Park YH, Chung SK, Kim SH, Shinn KS. Pinhole scintigraphic sign of chondromalacia patellae in older subjects: A prospective assessment with differential diagnosis. J Nucl Med 1994;35(5):855–862.

60. Derks WH, de Hooge P, van Linge B. Ultrasonographic detection of the patellar plica in the knee. J Clin Ultrasound 1986;14(5):355–360.

61. Brussaard C, Naudts P, De Schepper A. Ultrasonographic diagnosis of chondromalacia of the femoropatellar joint. J Belge Radiol 1991;74(4):303–306.

62. Waisbrod H, Treiman N. Intra-osseous venography in patellofemoral disorders. A preliminary report. J Bone Joint Surg 1980;62B(4):454–456.

63. Collier BD, et al. Chronic knee pain assessed by SPECT: Comparison with other modalities. Radiology 1985;157(3):795–802.

64. Minkoff J, Fein L. The role of radiography in the evaluation and treatment of common anarthrotic disorders of the patellofemoral joint. Clin Sports Med 1989;8(2):203.

65. Disler DG, et al. Fat-suppressed spoiled GRASS imaging of knee hyaline cartilage: Technique optimization and comparison with conventional MR imaging. AJR Am J Roentgenol 1994;163(4):887–892.

5

Arthroscopy of the Patellofemoral Joint

David A. Buuck and John P. Fulkerson

"Eventually all things merge into one. And the river runs through it."

Arthroscopy is an extremely important adjunct in the diagnosis and treatment of patellofemoral joint disorders Many authors have reported their results (1–7).

The key to success in each patient depends on a good preoperative history/physical examination as well as accurate interpretation of imaging data before the operation itself. Many complications have arisen from inappropriate arthroscopic procedures on patients who had had an inadequate preoperative examination. Accurate diagnosis will help to avoid the dreaded multiply operated on knee. It seems each additional surgery becomes more involved in an attempt to overcome the initial inappropriate procedure. This builds to a crescendo in an unhappy patient with a painful knee that makes the orthopedist ask him/herself, "What went wrong?" This chapter deals with the indications, techniques, and results of patellofemoral arthroscopy, with the hope that well-done arthroscopy will help to establish accurate decision making and thereby avoid complications.

Patellofemoral arthroscopy must be regarded as only one part of a thorough examination of the knee joint and not as an isolated procedure. Surgical applications in this chapter include

1. Diagnostic viewing of all anterior knee articular structures and observation of patellar tracking and trochlear dysplasia,
2. Description of size, depth, and location of articular lesions,
3. Debridement of the patella and trochlea,
4. Arthroscopic lateral release,
5. Arthroscopic proximal realignment,
6. Arthroscopic arthroplasty,
7. Resection of symptomatic plica and synovium.

BASIC SETUP AND TECHNIQUE

When the primary area of interest is the patellofemoral joint, the patient is in the supine position, with the end of the operating table flat. After the anesthetic is administered, a tourniquet is placed high around the proximal thigh and covered distally with an adhesive drape to prevent sliding during the surgery. If the tourniquet is placed too distal on the femur, the proximal patellar portals will be difficult to use because the arthroscope will lever on the tourniquet and prevent adequate mobility. The standard arthroscopy leg holder that fits around the tourniquet is too bulky and is not used.

The patient's knee is prepped and draped, and a post is placed next to the knee in the down position for later use if needed. This basic setup allows the surgeon to do the patellofemoral arthroscopy with the knee extended, yet allows the knee to be flexed off the table later for examination of the notch and other compartments. When the time arises to examine the rest of the knee joint, a circulatory nurse or assistant in the room will raise the post on the side of the table that allows the surgeon to apply a valgus force to look medially. The standard "figure 4" position can be used to look laterally. The unaffected leg is padded and secured to the table.

We routinely begin our diagnostic arthroscopy of the patellofemoral joint with the superomedial portal described by Schreiber (8). This portal may be more comfortable to use if the surgeon stands on the opposite side of the table for this part of the procedure. The monitor is at the head of the table on the affected side. If the primary area of interest is going to be the patellofemoral joint, we start with the end of the table flat. The portal is made two to three fingerbreadths above the patella just medial to the midline. The larger the leg, the more proximal the starting point (it is unusual to need to start more than three fingerbreadths proximal to the patella). This keeps the scope out of the thick quadriceps tendon and will allow a good view of the patellofemoral joint (Fig. 5.1). A no. 11 scalpel blade is used to make a longitudinal incision at the angle that you want the can-

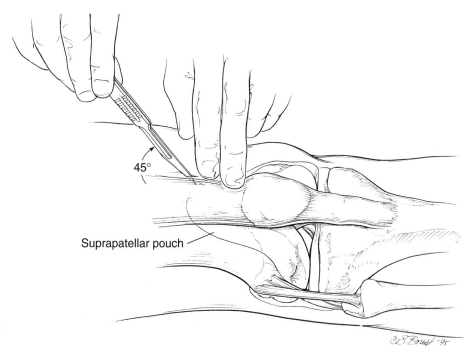

Figure 5.1. From the superomedial portal, the skin incision is made just medial to the midline. It is two fingerbreadths proximal to the superior pole of the patella, angled 45 to 60 degrees off the horizontal. (Illustration by Susan Brust.)

nula to enter the suprapatellar pouch and is carried down through the skin only. We find that angling the arthroscope 60 degrees off the horizontal works well, entering the suprapatellar pouch 2 cm above the patella, and then the scope may be flattened once the cannula is in place (Fig. 5.2). This makes a shorter distance from skin to joint and still allows a flatter angle to be obtained when the scope is inserted. If you allow the arthroscope to enter the suprapatellar pouch too close to the proximal border of the patella, this area is difficult to visualize.

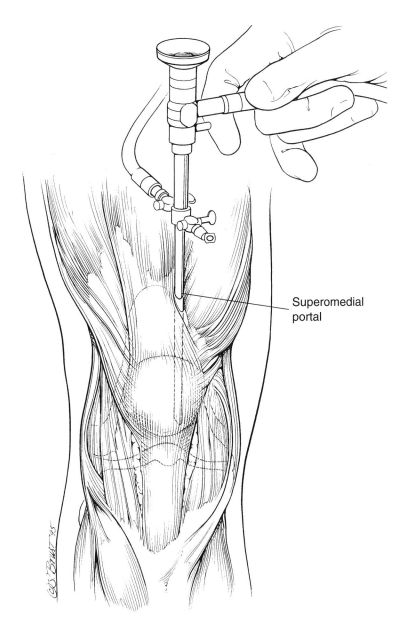

Superomedial portal

Figure 5.2. The arthroscope enters the joint approximately 2 cm proximal to the patella for the superomedial portal. (Illustration by Susan Brust.)

After the incision is made, follow the same course with your blunt trocar. The supero-medial aspect of the trochlea may be more prominent from the anterior view than from the lateral (9), and you will often feel your trocar contact this area, preventing you from entering the joint. By redirecting your hand slightly laterally (thus, the tip of the trochar medially), you may enter the joint by getting the trochar to slide down the medial gutter. Another option is to slightly raise the tip of the trocar to get up over the lip and gently advance into the joint. Care must be taken not to score the articular cartilage with the trochar.

When the cannula and arthroscope are in the knee joint, the fluid may be attached to the cannula or a separate portal may be made for inflow. Inferolateral or inferomedial portals are established under direct vision. Keep in mind when making these working portals that they will be used later for the arthroscope to view the remainder of the joint, so place them in an appropriate position, usually approximately 5 to 10 mm distal to the patella. The easiest way to establish working portals is to use a spinal needle as a guide and make sure that the needle can reach the area of interest before making your incision.

From the superomedial portal, you are able to visualize the patella, trochlea, fat pad, anterior horns of the menisci, plicae, medial and lateral gutters, a portion of the anterior cruciate ligament, and ligamentum mucosum. From this proximal view, you may easily watch the patella track in varying degrees of flexion. The patella will begin to engage the trochlea at 10 to 20 degrees of flexion and should be centered in the trochlea without tilt by 45 degrees (Figs. 5.3 and 5.4). The pump should be at no more than 60 mm Hg pressure during this maneuver to allow the patella to engage and center in the trochlea more physiologically. As you watch the patella enter the trochlea, try to identify causes of articular lesions. For example, chronic lateral tilt viewed arthroscopically may reveal "kissing lesions" on the far *lateral trochlea* and the *central ridge* or *lateral facet* of the patella because these two areas may be receiving the most contact (10). Patients with a history of patellar dislocation, however, may have *lateral trochlea* and *medial facet* lesions (Fig. 5.5) because the medial patella facet is frequently damaged at the time of patella relocation after the dislocation. Patients who have a history of a dashboard-type injury in which the patellofemoral joint takes the brunt of injury may be seen with specific lesions. Proximal pole lesions of the patella are common in these types of patients (Fig. 5.6). There may also be concomitant damage of the trochlea from these injuries; a Merchant view is sometimes helpful in delineating these lesions (Fig. 5.7) (11). Place a hook probe through the inferolateral portal and palpate the articular surfaces of the patella and trochlea. Record the size, depth, and loca-

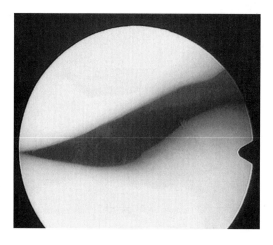

Figure 5.3. Lateral patellar tilt looking from the anterolateral view. Note how far lateral the central ridge appears at 45 degrees of flexion.

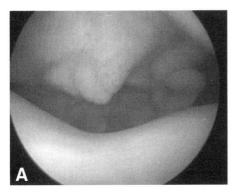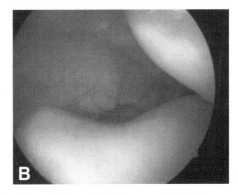

Figure 5.4. A and **B,** Lateral patellar subluxation at 30 and 45 degrees of flexion.

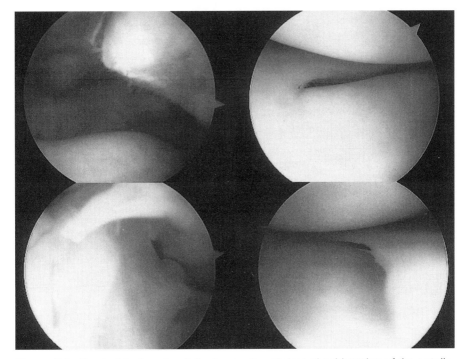

Figure 5.5. Grade 4 lesion of patella due to chronic lateral subluxation of the patella.

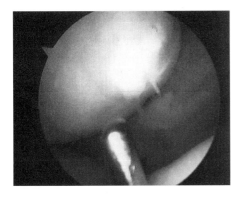

Figure 5.6. Proximal patellar pole crush injury from the superomedial portal view.

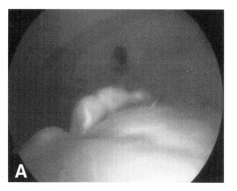 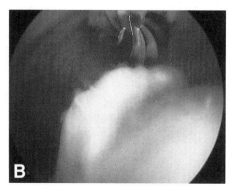

Figure 5.7. A, Traumatic medial trochlear osteophyte from dashboard injury in a 26-year-old patient. Initially seen on Merchant view, this lesion was resected with a burr, and subsequently symptoms abated **(B)**.

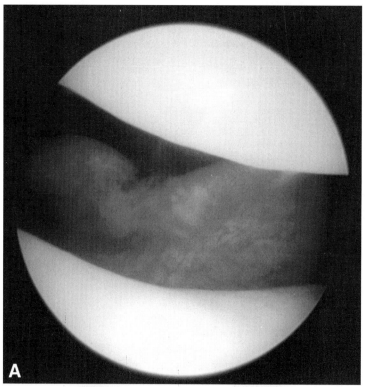

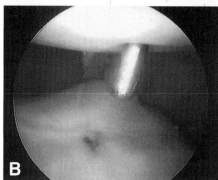

Figure 5.8. A, Pristine patello-femoral joint. **B,** Minimal dimpling of articular cartilage of patella.

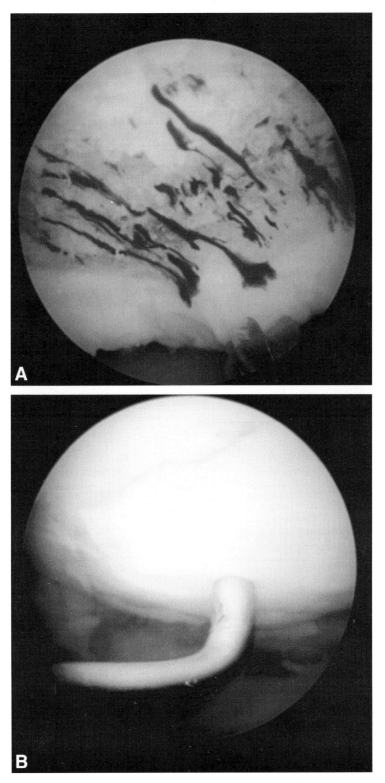

Figure 5.9. A, Abrasion arthroplasty of Grade 4 patellar lesion. **B,** Second-look arthroscopy 1 year later; fibrocartilage has been laid down. (Courtesy of J. Y. DuPont, Quimper, France.)

tion of any lesion(s). Articular cartilage is usually firm on palpation. Your probe should not do more than slightly dimple the cartilage with mild pressure (Fig. 5.8).

After the diagnostic portion of the arthroscopy, one may then debride loose articular lesions using a curved shaver through one of the working portals. Remove only loose cartilage and do not bevel the edges because you will be damaging normal articular cartilage. You may also drill or abrade exposed bone (Fig. 5.9). Recently, straight and angled picks have been available to arthroscopically create small holes in the exposed subchondral bone to create bleeding that will allow fibrocartilage to form in the defect. These are technically easier to use than a drill and do not cause the significant increase in local tissue temperature when a drill is used.

After this is accomplished, move your arthroscope into the inferolateral portal and complete the arthroscopy. *More information may be obtained about the patellofemoral joint if it is viewed from two directions.* From this inferior portal, the proximal one-third of the patella and suprapatellar pouch are better visualized. You may use the inferomedial portal as your working portal if additional debridement is necessary. You may also work through your superomedial portal, but you need to keep a cannula in the portal because it is difficult to get in and out due to the thickness of soft tissue. Also, repeated trauma to the quadriceps by repeated entry is not advisable. The remainder of the knee joint should be inspected at this time to rule out concomitant diagnoses. The post at the side of the table should be raised to aid in applying a valgus force to look medially. Although the central approach is excellent (12) for visualizing other areas of the knee, this central portal is not ideal for viewing the patellofemoral joint.

CLASSIFICATION OF ARTICULAR LESIONS

Chondromalacia has been a term misused over the years to represent everything from softened cartilage to a wastebasket phrase for "I don't know why your knee hurts." Taken literally, chondromalacia means "softened cartilage," which leaves us with the task of defining new language for the rest of the articular lesions that we encounter at arthroscopy.

The Outerbridge classification (9) has been widely used to describe articular lesions. Grade 1 represents softening or swelling of the cartilage (Fig. 5.10), Grade 2 is cartilage fibrillation of 0.5-in. diameter or less, Grade 3 is breakdown of greater than 0.5 in. (Fig. 5.11), and Grade 4 is erosion of cartilage down to bone (9).

It is easy to see why confusion arises in this classification. The surgeon is able to classify each lesion regarding character and depth or its size but not both with this classification. This makes classification of certain lesions difficult when there are characteristics of more than one grade. A good example of this would be a lesion 5 to 10 mm in diameter. Whether it consists of mild superficial fibrillation or deep fissures down to subchondral bone, the lesion is classified as Grade 2 purely based on size. Other classification systems have been implemented to correct this inconsistency. Insall's (13) classification is based on depth and character of the lesion.

This system's major difference from the Outerbridge system is that it does not take size directly into account. Insall's grading describes character and depth only. Grade 1 is softening or blistering of the cartilage without disruption of the surface, Grade 2 has superficial fibrillation or mild fissuring in the softened area, Grade 3 is deeper fibrillation and breakdown of the lesion involving greater than half the thickness of the articular cartilage ("crab meat"), and Grade 4 represents erosion to bone. Location and size are then described in addition to the Grade (13). A grading system reported by Beguin and Locker (14) is very similar to the one that Insall introduced.

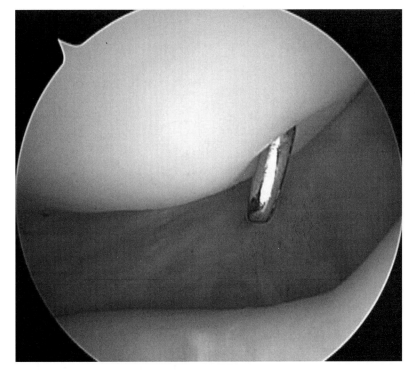

Figure 5.10. Grade 1 soft patella cartilage.

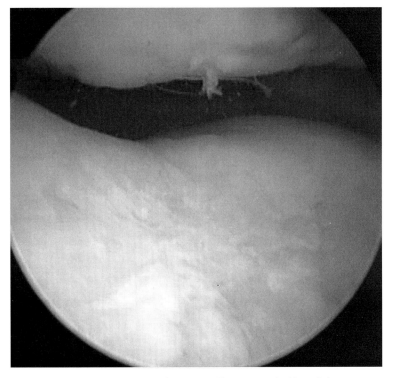

Figure 5.11. Trochlear Grade 3 diffuse chondral breakdown.

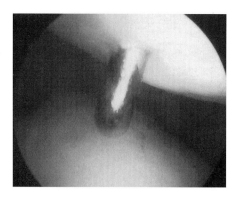

Figure 5.12. Grade 1 lesion on patella: note softening of cartilage without frank breakdown.

Noyes and Stabler (15) introduced an ambitious system for grading all articular lesions in the knee. Their system was based on depth, character, size, and location. The criticism with this system was that these authors reported the lesions on their diagrams as circles. Because many lesions are not circular, this created problems with classification (16).

The Noyes classification system combines elements of Insall's system with location. The patella or trochlea lesion location gives insight into the potential outcome of surgery and must, therefore, be recorded (17). The patella is divided into nine zones. Three vertical areas are subdivided by three horizontal areas. The width of the three vertical areas will vary depending on location of the central ridge. The medial vertical area corresponds to the medial facet, the central vertical area contains the central ridge, and the lateral vertical area contains the lateral facet. The odd facet is described separately, if involved. The horizontal areas remain constant with a proximal, middle, and distal area, all of equal widths. The trochlea is then divided into nine equal zones similar to those on the patella.

Grading of the lesions is similar to that of Insall's system. Grade 1 is a softening or blister of the cartilage with no frank disruption of the cartilage (Fig. 5.12). Grade 2 is superficial breakdown of the cartilage. Fissuring or scuffing of the cartilage is representative of this type of lesion (Figs. 5.13 and 5.14). Grade 3 is deep fissuring or disruption of cartilage that goes down to subchondral bone, but the bone is not exposed (Figs. 5.15 and 5.16). Grade 4 is exposed bone due to a traumatic event such as a patellar dislocation or crush injury without the associated degenerative changes previously listed (Fig. 5.17). Grade 5 is exposed bone with associated degenerative changes such as osteophytes along the patellar or trochlear edges (Fig. 5.18). It is important to differentiate between

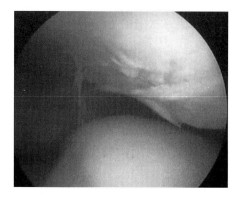

Figure 5.13. Grade 2 lesion on lateral facet of patella secondary to chronic lateral tilt.

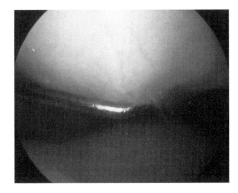

Figure 5.14. Grade 2 lesion on central ridge of patella: note fissuring and depth of probe.

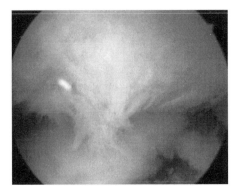

Figure 5.15. Grade 3 lesion on central ridge of patella with a "crab meat" appearance.

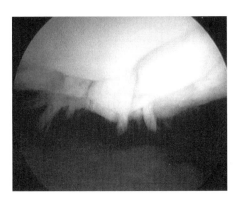

Figure 5.16. Grade 3 deep central ridge patellar lesion.

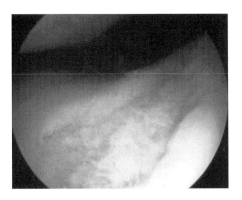

Figure 5.17. Grade 4 trochlear lesion from crush injury in central portion (patella had reciprocal Grade 2 lesion).

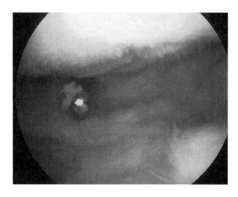

Figure 5.18. Noyes Grade 5 degenerative patellar lesion, eroded down to bone, with surrounding arthritic changes.

the Grade 4 and 5 lesions because their outcomes may be different. Additionally, you should characterize lesions when possible as distal central (Ficat critical zone), lateral facet (excessive lateral pressure), medial patella lesion caused by dislocation (Fig. 5.5), or a proximal crush injury (18).

ARTHROSCOPIC DEBRIDEMENT

Lesions of the patella and trochlea can be debrided readily using arthroscopic technique. Federico and Reider (19) noted 58% relief in patients with traumatic chondromalacia. This is particularly important because this can be an extremely difficult patient to treat. Arthroscopy is usually easiest with the patient supine, knee extended. A curved tip arthroscopic rotary shaving tool is often helpful. Care must be exercised to remove all loose flaps and mobile fragments. If exposed bone is left, drilling or picking the bone is usually advisable. Although debridement alone may be palliative if the flap(s) alone is symptomatic, realignment or release to relieve pressure on the deficient area may be necessary. Treatment must be adapted to the specific degenerative findings (20–22). When there is advanced arthritis, arthroscopy is unlikely to help (23, 24). This study by Moseley et al (23) was widely cited in 2002 but did not really demonstrate anything new to the experienced arthroscopic surgeon. In the patellofemoral joint, as in the knee generally, arthroscopic care is most effective when there are *specific lesions to treat, with or without arthritis.*

Arthroscopic debridement of small osteochondral fragments from osteochondritis dissecans or dislocation is appropriate, but large fragments with bone attached (usually more than 1 to 1.5 cm in diameter) should be replaced and fixed securely. Arthroscopic technique may also be used judiciously for the treatment of infrapatellar tendonitis (25).

Radiofrequency ablation and laser have been used for cartilage debridement in some centers, but we have been happy with sharp removal of loose cartilage fragments. Depth of penetration is a major issue in the use of thermal ablation, and any risk of cartilage damage beyond what is removed should be avoided. There are reports of subchondral bone necrosis after laser ablation of cartilage. Newer radiofrequency techniques, particularly monopolar ablation, carry less risk of inadvertent damage to healthy cartilage and subchondral bone. In general, however, the authors have not found these thermal methods necessary in the treatment of patellofemoral articular lesions but have found thermal ablation extremely beneficial in synovectomy and hemostasis.

ARTHROSCOPIC LATERAL RELEASE

Isolated release of the lateral retinaculum was described by Merchant and Mercer (26) in 1974. This was an open procedure, indicated at the time for patients with recurrent subluxation or dislocation. The indications have changed. Today, the primary indication for lateral release is *clinical and radiographic* tilt (or lateral rotation) of the patella (27) without subluxation (translation). We know now that lateral release can actually make subluxation worse in some cases! The release may be done open or arthroscopically, depending on the surgeon's preference and experience. An open lateral release has the advantages of easier hemostasis and is technically easier. In addition, looking at the patella under direct visualization is the most accurate way to determine the actual location and size of the lesion. It gives one the ability to stand back and look compared with an arthroscopic view that is from just millimeters away (Fig. 5.19). An arthroscopic release may give a subjectively better cosmetic result but may lead to a higher rate of hemarthrosis, even with electrocautery. In either case, strict hemostasis after tourniquet and pressure release is imperative.

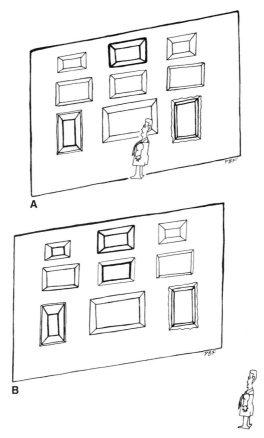

Figure 5.19. A, When looking at the patella through the arthroscope, the surgeon is so close to the patellar surface that his/her view is somewhat distorted, and he/she may not appreciate other important areas. **B,** During an open procedure or viewing from a second portal, the surgeon may gain a better perspective of the patellar surface. (Illustration by Phoebe Fulkerson.)

The decision to do a lateral release is made preoperatively, not intraoperatively. One of the major reasons for failure of lateral release is a poor indication for the procedure. Patients with vague knee pain and no definitive diagnosis of tilt are poor candidates. Patients with moderate-to-severe subluxation are not optimal candidates. The purpose of the lateral release is to transect the posterolateral tethers of the patella. This will correct tilt (lateral rotation) but not subluxation (lateral tracking) (27).

Many techniques for arthroscopic lateral release have been described (1, 2, 5, 26, 28). The following technique is the authors' preference. The patient is supine on the operating table, a tourniquet around the proximal thigh, but is not usually inflated. The end of the table remains up with the knee extended. A standard examination under anesthesia is performed as well as a systematic arthroscopic inspection of the entire knee joint. A superomedial or inferomedial portal is used for visualization. The advantage of the superomedial portal is that you may look all the way down the lateral gutter from the suprapatellar pouch to the insertion of your electrocautery unit or knife inferolaterally.

A spinal needle may be placed at the most superior point of your proposed release (Fig. 5.20, A). This area is just superior and lateral to the most superolateral portion of the patella. This gives you an arthroscopic "key" for your release. You need to stay out of the vastus lateralis tendon because cutting this may lead to quadriceps weakness and medial subluxation of the patella, a well-described and potentially devastating complication (29).

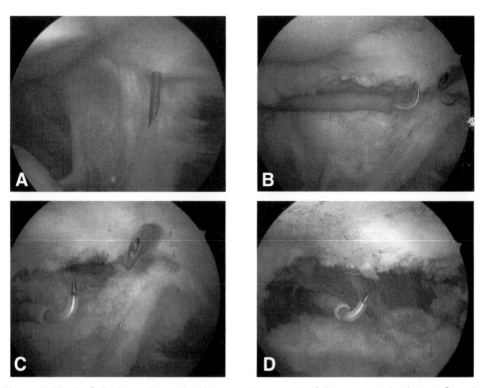

Figure 5.20. A, Spinal needle marks the superior aspect of the proposed release. Care is taken to stay out of the vastus lateralis tendon. **B,** The initial cautery is through the synovium, a few millimeters lateral to the patella. **C,** The cautery starts through the lateral retinaculum. Note the insulated tip on the cautery. **D,** Completed arthroscopic lateral release.

It is safer to stay more posterior proximally to stay out of the vastus lateralis. The release is started proximally and carried distally, staying a few millimeters lateral to the patella (Fig. 5.20, B). The release is carried through the synovium and lateral retinaculum only (Fig. 5.20, C). The release finishes distally at the inferolateral portal (Fig. 5.20, D). With the knee drained of fluid, one should be able to manually elevate the patella perpendicular to the trochlea. If you cannot obtain this amount of tilt, the release is inadequate and needs to be improved.

Areas frequently not released are the proximal epicondylopatellar band and the distal patellotibial band. The distal band may be reached by switching your electrocautery or knife to the superomedial portal and reaching distally while looking from below. *In some patients with tilt, the fat pad has become somewhat fibrotic and helps tether the patella distally.* If you have completed your release and still are unable to elevate the lateral patella satisfactorily, this may be the problem. Releasing the fat pad is difficult arthroscopically. At this point, you need to extend your inferolateral portal for better visualization. The fat pad should be dissected off the patellar tendon posteriorly, and then you may cut across it laterally to medially. Cutting across the fat pad approximately 50% to 75% of its diameter will usually free up the patella satisfactorily. This area is very vascular and will bleed when you let the tourniquet down. Hemostasis can be difficult to obtain with arthroscopic technique, and specific attention also needs to be paid to the geniculate arteries. If an adequate release cannot be obtained arthroscopically or hemostasis is difficult to obtain, convert to an open procedure for better visualization and direct palpation.

When appropriate passive elevation of the lateral patella and hemostasis are obtained, the portals are closed and local anesthetic instilled. A compressive dressing is applied to aid in tamponade, and some form of cold therapy is applied. The surgery is done on an outpatient basis, and the patient is discharged weight bearing as tolerated on crutches. The patient is encouraged to get motion back quickly, and no brace is used. Crutches may be discontinued when the patient is ambulating safely. Formal postoperative rehabilitation is covered elsewhere in this book. The most common reasons for failure of lateral release are poor indications, inadequate release, overzealous release (vastus lateralis), inadequate rehabilitation, and the surgeon missing concomitant pathology (e.g., meniscus tear). Most of these can be prevented with attention to detail preoperatively, intraoperatively, and postoperatively. Numerous complications from arthroscopic lateral release have been reported. These include hemarthrosis, deep vein thrombosis, infection, loss of range of motion, weakness, transection of the vastus lateralis, persistent or worse pain, reflex sympathetic dystrophy, excessive release causing medial patellar instability, and thermal injury (30). Small (7) reported a 7% complication rate with lateral release. Hemarthrosis, the most common complication, is avoidable in the vast majority of patients.

Results of arthroscopic lateral release vary in the literature. Fabbriciani et al (2) reported on 50 patients who underwent arthroscopic lateral release, with a 36-month average follow-up. Seventy-one percent of patients who underwent lateral release for patellar pain alone had satisfactory results. Seventy-six percent satisfactory results were reported in patients who had the release done for complaints of instability. Incomplete release, severe articular changes, and inadequate rehabilitation were reasons that the authors cited for unsatisfactory results (2). Henry et al (28) reported 88% good results at 3-year average follow-up. Their primary indication was patellofemoral subluxation. The release was completed through the inferolateral portal under arthroscopy control with a Smillie meniscotome. These authors had a 13% complication rate (mostly hemarthrosis) and emphasized that arthroscopic lateral release is not an innocuous procedure (28).

Lankenner et al (31) reported 62% good/excellent results from arthroscopic lateral release for a diagnosis of patellofemoral stress syndrome. The release was done under arthroscopic control with a Mayo scissors. The average follow-up was 25.6 months. Aderinto and Cobb (32) noted 59% satisfaction after lateral release for patellofemoral arthritis.

Much of the confusion in the literature about results of lateral release arises from the different indications and criteria of success. Whether open or arthroscopic, success of the lateral release depends more on proper patient selection than on technique.

ARTHROSCOPIC MEDIAL IMBRICATION

Availability of arthroscopic tools that facilitate suture passage inside a joint has made arthroscopic medial imbrication quite feasible. Radiofrequency thermal shrinkage has been tried by some surgeons after lateral release, but it is unlikely that medial capsule will "pull" a patella medially as a result of tissue shrinkage. In fact, thermal techniques inevitably damage tissue in the short run and could lead inadvertently to weakening of the medial capsule or medial patellofemoral ligament.

When there is lateral patella subluxation, medial capsule imbrication may be necessary to reduce a patella into the trochlea and restore normal tracking mechanics. Using an 18-gauge needle and a penetrating (bird-beak) grasper, several sutures (preferably no. 2 non-absorbable) may be placed into the deficient medial capsule/patellofemoral ligament such that the tissue is gathered and tightened on tying the suture ends (Fig. 5.21). This may be accomplished tying knots inside (Holbrecht) or outside (Pienovi). The surgeon must be certain that there is adequate tissue gathering to ensure a true realignment (Fig. 5.22). We believe that these patients must be protected for 5 to 6 weeks, but with limited, single-cycle flexion of the knee daily after the first 2 to 3 weeks, depending on the quality of the imbrication and tissue.

ARTHROSCOPIC ARTHROPLASTY

When a larger articular lesion requires resurfacing in the patellofemoral joint, there are several options. The surgeon may harvest articular cartilage for culture and plan a later articular cartilage implantation. Another option is to perform an osteochondral autograft. At the time of arthroscopy, however, the surgeon may also abrade or penetrate the subchondral bone in the defect to accomplish resurfacing by bone marrow stimulation. In general, we favor this last option, whenever possible, as described by Steadman (personal communication).

Particularly for smaller (<1.5 cm) lesions, arthroscopic microfracture arthroplasty (Steadman) has been effective in our experience (Fig. 5.23). Under arthroscopic control, the Steadman arthroscopic microfracture picks are used in a circumferential fashion to penetrate the subchondral bone of the articular defect with 3 to 4 mm between the penetrations. Of course this can be done with a drill or wire, but we find the picks extremely easy to use and effective. After this procedure, motion is desirable, but loading of the treated area should be very limited for approximately 6 weeks. When there is more extensive damage (Fig. 5.24), an unloading procedure or alternative procedure will be needed and microfracture alone is unlikely to help.

In our experience to date, osteochondral transfer arthroplasty and articular cartilage cell implantation are best performed as open procedures.

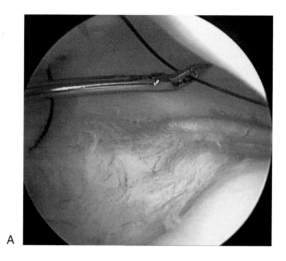

A

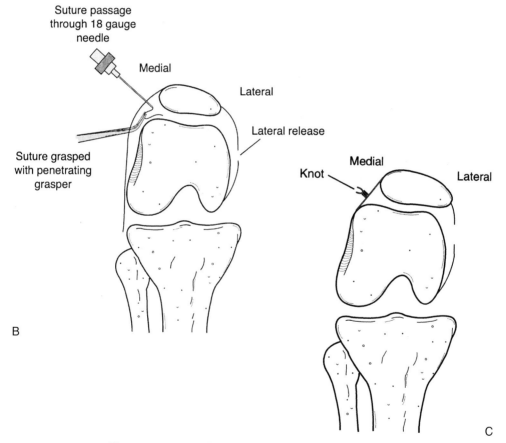

B

C

Figure 5.21. A to **C,** Arthroscopic proximal imbrication.

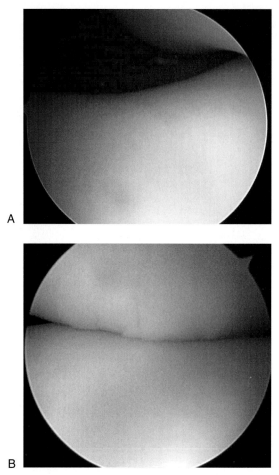

Figure 5.22. A, Tilt and subluxation of patella before proximal realignment. **B,** Patella centralization after arthroscopic proximal realignment.

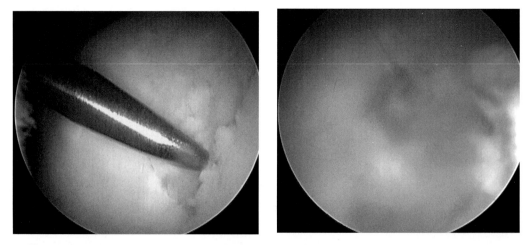

Figure 5.23. A, Microfracture arthroplasty of the trochlea. **B,** Bleeding after trochlear microfracture.

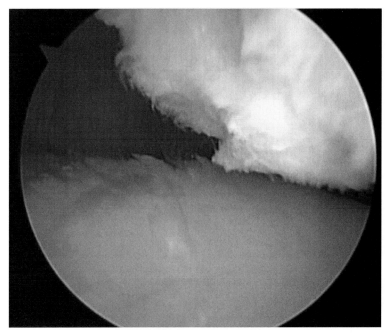

Figure 5.24. Extensive medial facet damage from dislocations.

SYMPTOMATIC PLICA AND SYNOVIAL RESECTION

Plicae are naturally occurring synovial folds in the knee. They are present in various locations in the knee with medial, superior, and inferior plicae being the most common (33–36). Inferior plicae (ligamentum mucosum) are the most common but have not been reported to cause symptoms. Superior plicae are rarely a problem. Medial plicae most frequently become symptomatic. A medial plica has been reported to be present in approximately 25% of all knees; 87% of these lesions are bilateral (33). These may become painful with overuse or blunt trauma (Fig. 5.25). The medial plica runs from the synovium just medial to the patella to the synovium of the anterior fat pad. A patient with

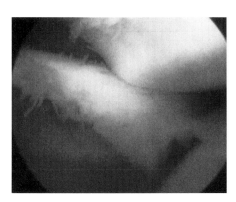

Figure 5.25. Inferomedial plica looking from superomedial portal view. The plica is thicker and more inflamed at point of contact on the medial femoral condyle.

a symptomatic medial plica will often complain of pain, grating, or even "catching" at the edge of the medial femoral condyle. This may rarely be accompanied by an effusion. A good physical examination will usually differentiate between the location of a symptomatic medial plica and a medial meniscus tear (most commonly confused with a medial plica), as the meniscus pain will be located along the tibiofemoral line. Not all medial plicae noted at arthroscopy are symptomatic, making the *meticulous* preoperative physical examination imperative. The confidence level of relieving symptoms by removing the plicae at arthroscopy rises with positive preoperative findings. Palpate for a snapping, *painful* band over the medial femoral condyle near the edge of the trochlea as you flex and extend the patient's knee between 30 and 90 degrees. Other common causes of pain in this area can be an osteophyte or synovitis along the medial aspect of the trochlea. These can often be palpated, and an osteophyte may be noted on a Merchant radiograph or other knee radiographs. Removing these symptomatic synovia or osteophytes will often give pain relief.

Conservative treatment of plicae consists of antiinflammatory agents and rest. If this fails, removal of the plicae is warranted. At arthroscopy, medial plicae are seen best from the superomedial portal (your regularly unobstructed view down the medial gutter or medial half of the trochlea may be blocked by the plica), or the inferolateral portal. The superolateral portal has also been reported to be beneficial at giving a good view of the medial plica (37). The symptomatic plica will often look inflamed, thickened, and sometimes fibrotic. If you are looking from the superomedial view, your cautery, arthroscopic knife, or basket forceps may be placed through the inferolateral or inferomedial portal for removal (Figs. 5.25 and 5.26). After the plica is cut, the edges often retract due to the tension that the plica had been under. If you are viewing through an inferolateral portal, you can work through a superolateral or inferomedial portal. A shaver may be introduced to remove the remaining edges. Resection rather than division of the plica is preferred.

Results of plica excision vary in the literature. Broom and Fulkerson (3) reported 77% good/excellent results, with average follow-up of 17 months. Nottage et al (38) reported only a 9% failure rate; Jackson et al (39), 24%; and Dorchak et al (6), 25%. Many authors agree that the success rate for resection of a plica decreases with concomitant pathology (3). Broom and Fulkerson noted an association between pathologic plicae and abnormal patellofemoral mechanics. The main complication from plica resection is postoperative hemarthrosis.

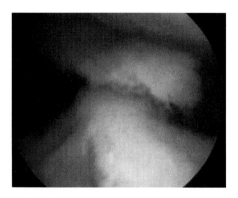

Figure 5.26. Inferomedial plica from superomedial portal view.

SUMMARY

Patellofemoral arthroscopy is an important aspect of general knee arthroscopy and permits definitive treatment in many cases. Along with evaluation and treatment of the patellofemoral joint, a look about the rest of the knee is mandatory. Evaluating articular lesions of the patella and trochlea, looking at patellar tracking, removing loose bodies, debriding articular surfaces, microfracture arthroplasty, arthroscopic lateral release, arthroscopic imbrication and plica removal are some of the options available to the arthroscopic surgeon. A good history and physical examination are the foundation of successful patellofemoral arthroscopic surgery. Taking the time to establish an accurate working diagnosis in the office before the time of surgery when the patient is under anesthesia will enhance your surgical results and patient satisfaction.

REFERENCES

1. Fu FH, Maday MG. Arthroscopic lateral release and the lateral patellar compression syndrome. Orthop Clin North Am 1992;23:601–612.
2. Fabbriciani C, Panni AS, Delcogliano A. Role of arthroscopic lateral release in the treatment of patellofemoral disorders. Arthroscopy 1992;8:531–536.
3. Broom MJ, Fulkerson JP. The plica syndrome: A new perspective. Orthop Clin North Am 1986;17:279–281.
4. Malek MM, Fanelli GC. Patellofemoral pain. An arthroscopic perspective. Clin Sports Med 1991;10:549–567.
5. Jackson RW, Kunkel SS, Taylor GJ. Lateral retinacular release for patellofemoral pain in the older patient. Arthroscopy 1991;7:283–286.
6. Dorchak JD, Barrack RL, Kneisl JS, Alexander AH. Arthroscopic treatment of symptomatic synovial plica of the knee. Long-term follow-up. Am J Sports Med 1991;19:503–507.
7. Small NC. An analysis of complications in lateral retinacular release procedures. Arthroscopy 1989;5:282–286.
8. Schreiber SN. Proximal superomedial portal in arthroscopy of the knee. Arthroscopy 1991;7:246–251.
9. Outerbridge RE. The etiology of chondromalacia patellae. J Bone Joint Surg 1961;43B:752–7571.
10. Fulkerson JP. Operative management of patellofemoral pain. Ann Chir Gynecol 1991;80:224–229.
11. Merchant AC, Mercer RL, Jacobsen RH, Cool CR. Roentgenographic analysis of patellofemoral congruence. J Bone Joint Surg 1974;56A:1391–1396.
12. Gillquist J, Hagberg G. A new modification of the technique of arthroscopy of the knee joint. Acta Chir Scand 1976;142:123–130.
13. Insall JN. Current concepts review. Patellar pain. J Bone Joint Surg 1982;64A:147–152.
14. Beguin J, Locker B. Chondropathie rotulienne. 2eme Journale Arthroscopie du Genou. Lyons, France; 1983;1: 89–90.
15. Noyes FR, Stabler CL. A system for grading articular cartilage lesions at arthroscopy. Am J Sports Med 1989;17: 505–513.
16. Dougados M, et al. The SFA system for assessing articular cartilage lesions at arthroscopy of the knee. Arthroscopy 1994;10:69–77.
17. Pidoriano AJ, Fulkerson JP, Buuck DA. Correlation of patella articular lesion with results from anteromedial tibial tubercle transfer. Presented at Arthroscopy Association of North America, 15th Annual Meeting; Washington, DC, April 1996.
18. Fulkerson JP. Patellofemoral pain disorders: Evaluation and management. J Am Acad Orthop Surg 1994; 2:124–132.
19. Federico DJ, Reider B. Results of isolated patellar debridement for patellofemoral pain in patients with normal patellar alignment. Am J Sports Med 1997;25(5):663–669.
20. Stuart MJ. Arthroscopic management for degenerative arthritis of the knee. Instr Course Lect 1999;48:135–141.
21. Jackson RW: Arthroscopic surgery and a new classification system. Am J Knee Surg 1998;11:51–54.
22. Goldman RT, Scuderi GR, Kelly MA. Arthroscopic treatment of the degenerative knee in older athletes. Clin Sports Med 1997;16:51–68.
23. Moseley JB, O'Malley K, Petersen NJ, et al. A controlled trial of arthroscopic surgery for osteoarthritis of the knee. N Engl J Med 2002;347:81–88.
24. Jackson R, Dieterich SC. Results of arthroscopic lavage and debridement of osteoarthritic knees based on the severity of degeneration. Arthroscopy 2003;19(1):13–20.
25. Romeo AA, Larson RV. Arthroscopic treatment of infrapatellar tendonitis. Arthroscopy 1999;15(3):341–345.
26. Merchant AC, Mercer RL. Lateral release of the patella. Clin Orthop 1974;103:40–45.
27. Shea KP, Fulkerson JP. Preoperative computed tomography scanning and arthroscopy in predicting outcome after lateral retinacular release. Arthroscopy 1992;8:327–334.
28. Henry JH, Goletz TH, Williamson B. Lateral retinacular release in patellofemoral subluxation: Indications, results, and comparison to open patellofemoral reconstruction. Am J Sports Med 1986;14:121–129.

29. Nonweiler DE, DeLee JC. The diagnosis and treatment of medial subluxation of the patella after lateral retinacular release. Arthroscopy 1994;5:680–686.
30. Lord M, Maltry JA, Shall LM. Thermal injury resulting from arthroscopic lateral retinacular release by electrocautery: Report of three cases and a review of the literature. Arthroscopy 1991;7:33–37.
31. Lankenner PA, Micheli LJ, Clancy R, Gerbino PG. Percutaneous lateral patellar retinacular release. Am Sports Med 1986;14:267–269.
32. Aderinto J, Cobb A. Lateral release for patellofemoral arthritis. Arthroscopy 2002;18:399–403.
33. Jouanin T, Dupont JY, Halimi P, Lassau JP. The synovial folds of the knee joint: Anatomical study. Anat Clin 1992;4:47–53.
34. Dandy DJ. Anatomy of the medial suprapatellar plica and medial synovial shelf. Arthroscopy 1990;6:79–85.
35. Dupont JY. Synovial plicae of the knee. In: Aichroth P, Cannon D, eds. The Knee. Vol 1. 1994; pp 5–19.
36. Patel D. Plica as a cause of anterior knee pain. Orthop Clin North Am 1986;17:273–277.
37. Brief LP, Laico JP. The superolateral approach: A better view of the medial patellar plica. Arthroscopy 1987;3:170–172.
38. Nottage WM, Sprague NF, Auerbach BJ, Shahriaree H. The medial patellar plica syndrome. Am J Sports Med 1983;11:211–214.
39. Jackson RW, Marshall DJ, Fujisawa Y. The pathological medial shelf. Orthop Clin North Am 1982;13:307–312.

6

Dysplasias

"The most valuable knowledge we can have is how to deal with disappointments."
—*Albert Schweitzer*

"Intoxicated with unbroken success we have become too self-sufficient to feel the necessity of redeeming and preserving grace, too proud to pray to the God that made us."
—*Abraham Lincoln, 1863*

Dysplasias include abnormalities of patellar and trochlear form and some malposition problems. In themselves, they do not necessarily cause symptoms. Many dysplasias are compatible with normal or near-normal function, just as normal morphology is not assurance of freedom from disease.

PATELLAR DYSPLASIAS

Aplasia

Complete absence of one or both patellae (Fig. 6.1) was reported as early as 1897 by Little (1) and Mayer (2). In 1899, Wuth (3) reported bilateral patella absence in all the male members of a family for three generations. Since then, many others have reported small series or isolated cases (4–6). The abnormality may exist as an isolated entity or in association with other congenital anomalies. Most commonly, it is part of the nail-patella syndrome, in which patellar malformation is associated with ungual dysplasia and iliac horns (7). Most patients function without difficulty, although Stuart (8) reported one female patient who lacked full knee extension by 50 degrees bilaterally.

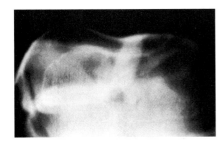

Figure 6.1. Despite the complete absence of a patella, the trochlear side of the patellofemoral joint looks completely normal. The sulcus shows good depth, and the lateral trochlear facet is more prominent than the medial, which is the normal characteristic.

129

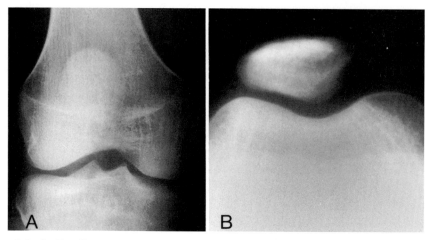

Figure 6.2. A, Patella parva. The patient is asymptomatic, but the patella is indeed unusually small. **B,** Axial view shows the patella well within the trochlear borders. The trochlea is nevertheless well developed.

Hypoplasia

In patella parva (Fig. 6.2), the entire patella is small. Such is the case in congenital dislocation, but cases occur without any apparent abnormal function. This form of dysplasia is often associated with quadriceps hypoplasia. It has been seen with apophysitis of the inferior pole of the patella (Sinding-Larsen-Johansson disease) (9, 10) in which the decrease in overall patellar size may put additional strains on the ligamentous and tendinous attachments.

Partial Hypoplasia

For the most part, this condition involves the medial facets. There appears to be much variation in patellar form consistent with normal function. Wiberg (11), in his classic and widely accepted 1841 article, proposed a three-part classification to encompass the majority of patellae encountered. It is based on the radiologic form on the axial view (Fig. 6.3, A to C).

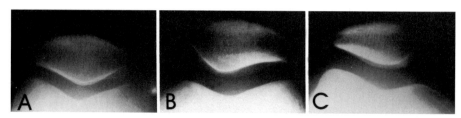

Figure 6.3. A, Wiberg Type I; **B,** Wiberg Type II; **C,** Wiberg Type III.

Type I

Both facets are gently concave, symmetric, and roughly the same size, although slight lateral predominance is common. Theoretically, this would appear to be the ideal patellar form. It is, however, the least common, occurring in only 10% of the population, according to Hennsge (12).

Type II

There is a subtle flow from I to II in which the medial facet is distinctly smaller than the lateral. The lateral facet remains concave, whereas the medial is either flat or slightly convex. The relative lateral facet predominance seems in accord with the general lateral predominance of the patellofemoral joint as a whole. This is the most common form, comprising 65% of Hennsge's series.

Type III

The medial facet is considerably smaller, with marked lateral predominance. Wiberg did not, in his original classification, specifically detail that the subchondral outline should be convex. However, the examples that he showed were convex, and subsequent authors have included medial facet convexity in the criteria for Type III. Even though this group comprises 25% of Hennsge's series, Wiberg regarded it as a frankly dysplastic form. Nevertheless, he was unable to show that it was associated with chondromalacia patellae with higher frequency than other forms. Also, other authors have noted no association between Type III and either chondromalacia (13, 14) or patellofemoral arthrosis (15).

Baumgartl (16) further described a rare type that appears to be a variation of Type III. It is characterized by a convex projection of the medial facet (Fig. 6.4). The importance of this type, according to Baumgartl, would appear to be a frequent association with osteochondritis dissecans of the medial femoral condyle. A look at contact prints of the knee in full flexion shows that the odd facet normally articulates here.

Ficat (17) proposed another classification based on the angle that the two major facets make with one another. With this method of measurement, there are four categories of abnormality:

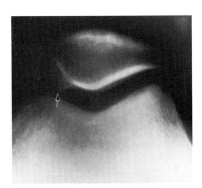

Figure 6.4. Baumgartl type with a medial excrescence (*arrow*).

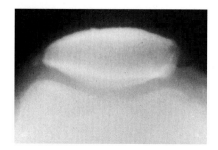

Figure 6.5. "So-called" pebble deformity.

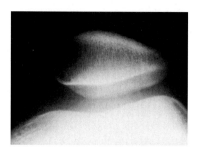

Figure 6.6. Alpine hunter's cap deformity. Here the patella is approaching a single articular facet. There is also considerable decrease in the depth of the trochlear sulcus.

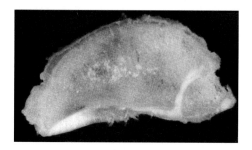

Figure 6.7. Example of a half-moon-shaped patella with a bipartite fragment that was removed because patient had severe pain.

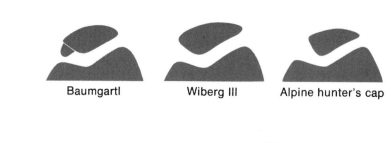

Baumgartl   Wiberg III   Alpine hunter's cap

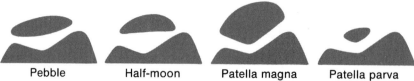

Pebble   Half-moon   Patella magna   Patella parva

Figure 6.8. Variations in patella form considered dysplastic.

1. An angle greater than 140 degrees gives a flattened, potentially unstable patella, a so-called "pebble-shaped" patella (Fig. 6.5).
2. With an angle from 90 to 100 degrees, one sees the category into which most Wiberg Type III patients will fall.
3. By 90 degrees, we have a hemipatella with one articular facet. This has been referred to as the Alpine hunter's cap deformity (Fig. 6.6) and is frequently observed in association with lateral instability. Not uncommonly, hypoplasia of the vastus medialis and even the medial facet of the trochlea can be seen with this patella form.
4. An acute angle with a single articular facet, with the patella in the form of a half moon as seen on the axial view, is often associated with marked permanent subluxation or dislocation of the patella (Fig. 6.7). The more important morphologic dysplasias of the patella are summarized in Figure 6.8.

Computed tomography and magnetic resonance imaging offer the alternative of defining articular cartilage contours as well as the subchondral bone. Staubli et al (18), in particular, pointed out the incongruity between osseous and chondral morphology. This is important in the interpretation of radiographic alignment, as the apparent congruity or incongruity of osseous structure relationships, such as the patella and the trochlea, may not adequately reflect the true articular relationship. Nonetheless, there are well-defined radiographic criteria of proper alignment based on osseous images (the Merchant congruence angle is a good example, based on good control data), and the validity of these relationships remains important in clinical practice.

Patella Fragmentation

Many diverse forms of patella fragmentation have been described by numerous authors. The basic configurations are summarized in Figure 6.9. The fragments would appear to result from an aberrant ossification center that failed to fuse with the main mass of the patella. However, the pathogenesis is obscure because it is known that the patella ossifies from a single ossific nucleus. It would be easier to understand if one accepted the pluricentric ossification theory of Schaer (19), but that does not, normally at least, appear to be the case.

Whatever the real ossification, one can pose the question of whether the real etiology might not be an increase in the constraint of muscle traction on a particular section of the patellar ossific nucleus at a critical time in its formation. This would perhaps better explain the overwhelming predominance for localization to the superolateral region of the patella. The lateral predominance of the patellofemoral joint, which plays such a significant role in the physiology and pathology of this articulation, is fully consistent with this concept.

Bipartite Patella

Although many forms of patellar fragmentation exist, all except bipartite patella (Fig. 6.10) are extremely infrequent. Since it was originally described in 1882 by Grüber (20), many cases have been published worldwide by so many authors that interest in this abnormality as a curiosity has waned, only now to be reawakened with the expansion of insurance claims that pose the medicolegal problem of separating a traumatic form from a congenital malformation.

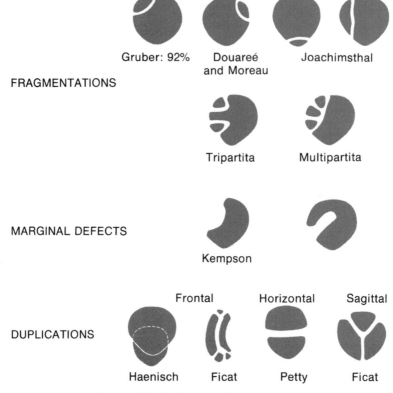

FRAGMENTATIONS

Gruber: 92%   Douareé   Joachimsthal
                 and Moreau

Tripartita   Multipartita

MARGINAL DEFECTS

Kempson

DUPLICATIONS

Frontal   Horizontal   Sagittal

Haenisch   Ficat   Petty   Ficat

Figure 6.9. Further patellar dysplasias.

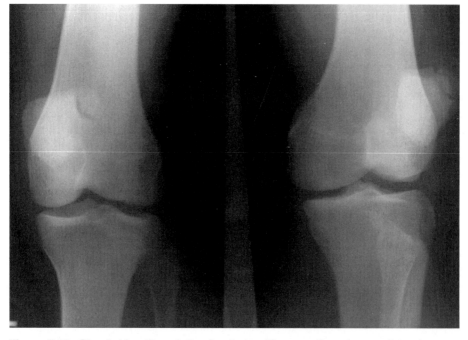

Figure 6.10. Classic bipartite patellar dysplasia with separation of superolateral corner.

The frequency rate of bipartite patella has been reported to be as low as 0.05% (21) in 20,000 soldiers to as high as 1.66% (22) in 1,378 patients. Anatomically, bipartite patella appears indistinguishable from a pseudarthrosis, with a cartilaginous bridge uniting the two fragments. In many respects, it is similar to a synchondrosis.

The clinical manifestation of bipartite patella presents several possibilities and some problems. Many, if not most, cases remain clinically silent, only to be fortuitously discovered at the time radiography is performed for other reasons. Also, there are some cases that will show up only on axial view. Bipartite patella may become spontaneously symptomatic just as other synchondroses become symptomatic, for example, the costochondral junction. The bipartite fragment may also be the site of early degenerative changes, which lead to symptoms.

A history of trauma frequently antedates symptoms and poses several possibilities. One may be dealing with a fracture of the superolateral corner. Factors favoring fracture would be (a) a history of significant direct trauma to this localized corner, (b) hematoma and swelling, (c) localized point tenderness and occasionally crepitus, and (d) a radiograph showing an irregular, sharply outlined line of separation. Of course, if films before the accident are available, the problem can be resolved.

Even when one can resolve the question of fracture versus bipartite patella, the determination of the role of injury is not made. The bipartite fragment may undergo symptomatic changes of posttraumatic chondromalacia, as elsewhere in the patella. The synchondrosis itself may be disrupted or strained, as manifested by localized direct tenderness and swelling, minimal effusion, painful restriction of motion, and possibly muscle atrophy. Those factors that support a previously existing bipartite fragment include (a) clearly defined radiolucency with rounded margins separating the fragments, (b) sclerosis of the margins, and (c) bilateral lesions. The latter is very helpful, but unilateral bipartite patella is by no means rare. Certainly, the most difficult situation is when the patient is seen for the first time for examination of the reported trauma after considerable delay because a true pseudarthrosis will have the same radiographic appearance as a bipartite patella.

Treatment

All patients with bipartite patella who have become symptomatic for whatever reason should undergo an attempt at conservative management. Depending on the severity of the symptoms, this might include immobilization in a cylinder cast or knee immobilizer, antiinflammatory therapy, and occasionally injection into an area of local tenderness, particularly if tenderness can be localized in the adjacent retinaculum. Surgical treatment is considered only after conservative management has failed. The smaller fragment is simply excised through a short lateral parapatellar skin incision. The lateral patellar retinaculum is not released. If the fragment is not mobile and articular cartilage is intact, a lateral retinacular release, in which the surgeon detaches the vastus lateralis insertion into the fragment (23), may be preferable in selected cases (Fig. 6.11). Although excellent results and healing of the fragment are reported with this approach, I prefer to *reattach* the released vastus lateralis tendon into the adjacent central quadriceps tendon. At surgery, the cartilage covering the fragment is frequently found to show significant degenerative changes and may require limited debridement when this procedure is necessary.

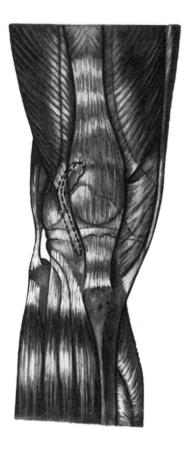

Figure 6.11. Mori has suggested release of the attachments to a bipartite patella fragment. Reprinted with permission from Mori Y, Okumo H, Iketani H, Kuroki Y. Efficacy of lateral retinacular release for painful bipartite patella. Am J Sports Med 1995;23(1): 13–18.

Marginal Patellar Defects

These defects are mentioned only for completeness of the chapter. They are extremely rare and of unknown clinical significance.

Patellar Reduplication

Double patellae are rare and may become evident in one of two forms. Petty (24) described a case of bilateral horizontal duplication with a 2-cm interval between the supe-

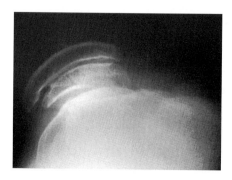

Figure 6.12. An example of patellar reduplication.

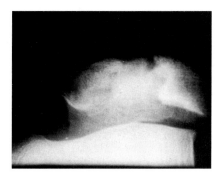

Figure 6.13. An example of reduplication in the sagittal plane, with patellar subluxation and trochlear dysplasia.

rior and inferior patellae, the patellae lying in the center of the extensor apparatus. The interest here lies in the apparent similarity with lemurs and tarsiers, small tree-living primates that are primarily climbers and jumpers (25, 26).

The second form, in which there is a reduplication in the frontal plane with the anterior patella more or less overlying the posterior one, has been reported by both Haenisch (27) and Ficat (17). The patient in Ficat's case presented with moderate symptoms of degenerative arthritis. Figure 6.12 shows patellar reduplication in the coronal plane. Reduplication is also possible in the sagittal plane (Fig. 6.13).

Hyperplasia or Patella Magna

Several factors can contribute to acquired patella magna. Infection and trauma with or without fracture are the most common causes. Calcification of the patellofemoral ligament may give the false impression of patellar enlargement. Also, medial and lateral osteophytes would have the same effect. Such osteophytes are covered on their contact surface with the femur by fibrocartilage, which enlarges the width of the patella, as seen on the axial view.

A rare congenital form exists, however, in which the patella surpasses a maximal measurement of 57 mm in width, but, more important, the patella surpasses the medial and lateral borders of the trochlear sulcus, thereby appearing too broad for its bed. The thickness is often increased as well but may be within normal limits. Patella magna seems to be associated with a high incidence of degenerative arthritis, although the congenital form is seen too infrequently for this association to be a certainty. Bennett (28) proposed an operation for reducing the volume by excising a vertical paramedian band in such a way as to recreate approximately a normal-sized facet.

SUPERIOR AND INFERIOR PATELLA MALPOSITION

Patella Alta

Radiographic criteria for the diagnosis of patella alta were considered in Chapter 4. Patella alta has been associated with recurrent subluxation and dislocation (29), chondromalacia, Sinding-Larsen-Johanssen apophysitis, recurrent effusion (16), and cerebral palsy (30, 31), in which walking is habitually in the knee-flexed position. It appears that increased tension on the patellar ligament results in its greater length, although Micheli et al (32) have correlated femoral growth rate with proximal patella migration, which suggests that overgrowth during the adolescent "growth spurt" may cause patella alta.

I believe that patella alta as an isolated entity will not require surgical treatment unless there is symptomatic delayed entry of the patella into the femoral sulcus with knee flexion. It is most important to separate problems of patellar tilt or subluxation from specific symptoms related to delayed patellar engagement of the trochlea. The Bernageau index, as referenced in the chapter on imaging, is probably the most accurate indicator of true patella alta. When adjustment of the patella level is necessary, the surgeon should proceed extremely cautiously because overdoing this adjustment can lead to problems with painful initial knee flexion. Most distalizations of the tibial tubercle require no more than 5 to 10 mm of tibial tubercle distalization. This is always preferable to patella tendon shortening.

Patella Baja or Infera

Although this condition may rarely occur spontaneously in otherwise normal children, it is a common finding in achondroplastic dwarfs, in whom it does not appear to cause any functional problem (Fig. 6.14). In fact, achondroplastic dwarfs can comfortably squat for long periods of time. Patellofemoral complaints are infrequent in a large group of patients with achondroplasia who were followed for other orthopedic problems. Poliomyelitis in childhood may also be responsible for patella baja.

The most frequent reason for this malposition, however, is as a complication of previous knee surgery or injury. Tibial tubercle transposition performed in a skeletally immature patient in whom the repositioned tubercle continues to grow distally with the tibia may cause patella baja. Noyes et al (33) and Paulos et al (34) have recognized the occurrence of patella infera as a postoperative complication of knee surgery. In such cases, open release of the captured infrapatellar fat pad and other infraarticular scar, followed

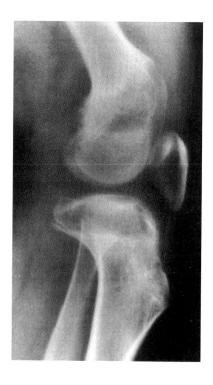

Figure 6.14. A lateral radiograph of the knee of a patient with achondroplasia.

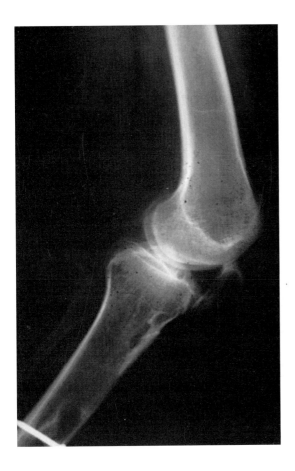

Figure 6.15. Severe patella infera as a complication of tibial tubercle surgery in a child.

by mobilization, may be indicated. Fortunately, excision of the infrapatellar fat pad does not seem to compromise patellar vascularity. Poorly performed tibial tubercle transfer surgery can be disastrous, resulting in extreme patella infera, as shown in Figure 6.15.

TROCHLEAR DYSPLASIAS

Hypoplasia of the Medial Condyle

This is frequently associated with hypoplasia of the medial patellar facet. However, dysplasias of both sides of the medial compartment are not always linked. With this particular dysplasia, computed tomography or magnetic resonance imaging may be particularly helpful.

This deformity will often appear only in the first 30 degrees of knee flexion because it is primarily a deformity of the proximal portion of the trochlea. The trochlea progressively deepens as it approaches the intercondylar notch. Therefore, the use of views taken in more than 30 degrees of flexion may result in a true hypoplasia being missed. Hypoplasia primarily affects the width of the medial condyle, but it may affect simply the height. The latter abnormality is more difficult to separate from a rotational malposition. Both types of medial hypoplasia are important in the various forms of patellar instability and chondromalacia.

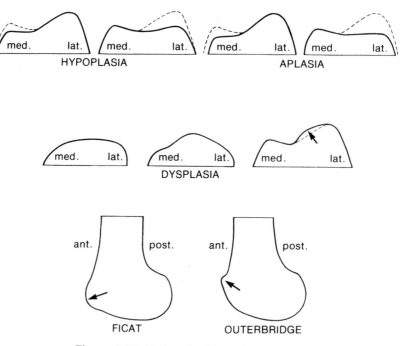

Figure 6.16. Various trochlear abnormalities.

Aplasia of the Medial Trochlea

This is a rare abnormality in which the proximal trochlea appears on the axial view or tomographic slice as an oblique slope running posteriorly from lateral to medial (Fig. 6.16). The patella usually consists of a single facet.

Global Dystrophy of the Trochlea

This exists whenever the opening angle of the sulcus is greater than 142 degrees. This, in fact, is not infrequent. It is not rare to encounter a trochlea that has no sulcus and presents a flat or even convex surface on the axial view. In these situations, if the patella is like-

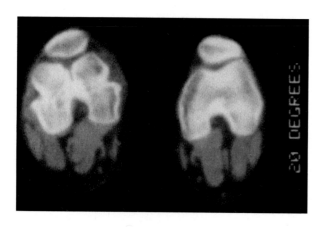

Figure 6.17. Posttraumatic trochlear dysplasia may occur after fracture. (Courtesy of David Burstein, Avon, CT.)

wise flat or concave, one can hope at least that a certain amount of congruence exists. However, stability is completely dependent on retinacular and muscle balance, and it is not surprising that this form of dysplasia is frequently associated with dislocation of the patella. One must consider that chronic patellar instability early in life may give rise to trochlear dysplasia. Also, intercondylar fracture may lead to trochlear dysplasia (Fig. 6.17).

SOFT-TISSUE DYSPLASIA

Soft-tissue dysplasia is undoubtedly a factor in many patients with patellar instability. Most commonly, the peripatellar retinaculum becomes adaptively dysplastic in association with chronic malalignment. A patella that is aligned such that the lateral facet is chronically tilted downward will eventually manifest adaptively shortened lateral retinaculum. This form of dysplasia, secondary to malalignment, probably occurs early in life when congenital structural malalignment exists. Similarly, one might think of the medial retinaculum as dysplastic if it is chronically stretched because of recurrent subluxation.

Hallisey et al (35) noted considerable variation in the angles of insertion of the vastus lateralis obliquus in cadaver dissections. This variability suggests that there may be angles of vastus lateralis obliquus insertion that are congenitally abnormal and thus predispose the patella to excessive lateralization. Also, there is variability in the angle of insertion of the vastus medialis obliquus. One might expect, therefore, that alteration of this muscle balance, either congenital or induced, might result in patellofemoral imbalance secondary to soft-tissue dysplasia. Similarly, in establishing surgical congruence of the patellofemoral joint, soft-tissue balance is important.

REFERENCES

1. Little EM. Congenital absence or delayed development of the patella. Lancet 1897;2:781–784.
2. Mayer HN. Congenital absence or delayed development of the patella. Lancet 1897;2:1384–1385.
3. Wuth EA. Uber angeborenen Mangel Sowie Herfunkt and Zweck der Kniescheibe. Langenbecks Arch Klin Chir 1899;58:900.
4. Bell J. Congenital absence of both patellae. J Bone Joint Surg 1955;37B:352.
5. Bernhang AM, Levine SA. Familial absence of the patella. J Bone Joint Surg 1973;55A:1088–1090.
6. Rubin G. Congenital absence of patellae and other patellar anomalies in three members of the same family. JAMA 1915;64:2062.
7. Most A. Fin fall von congenitalen bildungsanomalilen onychotrophia congenitala. Allg Med Cents Zig 1903;72:153.
8. Stuart. In: DePalma, ed. Diseases of the Knee. Philadelphia: JB Lippincott; 1954.
9. Johansson S. Fine bisher nicht beschriebene erkrankung der patella. Hygica 1922;84:161.
10. Sinding-Larsen C. A hitherto unknown affection of the patella in children. Acta Radiol 1927;1:1711.
11. Wiberg G. Roentgenographic and anatomic studies on the femoro-patellar joint. Acta Orthop Scand 1941;12:319–410.
12. Hennsge J. Die arthrosis deformans des patella gleitweges. Zentrabl Chir 1962;32:1381–1387.
13. Goodfellow JW, Hungerford DS, Zindel M. Patello-femoral mechanics and pathology. I. Functional anatomy of the patello-femoral joint. J Bone Joint Surg 1976;58B:287.
14. Outerbridge RE. Further studies on the etiology of chondromalacia patellae. J Bone Joint Surg 1964;46B:179–190.
15. Hungerford DS, Cockin J. Fate of the retained lower limb joints in WWII amputees. J Bone Joint Surg 1975;57B:111.
16. Baumgartl F. Das Kniegelenk. Berlin: Springer-Verlag; 1964.
17. Ficat P. Pathologie femoro-patellaire. Paris: Masson et Cie; 1970.
18. Staubli HU, Durrenmatt U, Porcellini B, Rauschning W. Articular cartilage surfaces and osseous anatomy of the patellofemoral joint in the axial plane. Sports Med Arthrosc Rev 2001;9:282–287.
19. Schaer J. Die patella biparitita. Ergeb Chir Orthop 1934;27:1.
20. Grüber W. Bildungsanomalie mit bildungshemmung begrundete bipartition beider patellae eines jungen subjektes. Virchows Arch Pathol Anag 1883;94:358.

21. Stucke K. Die patella partita in ihren beziehungen zum unfall and zer wehrdienst-beschadignung. Monatsschr. Unfallheilk 1950;53:238.
22. Blumensaat C. Patella partitia traumatische spaltpatella. Patellarfraktur. Arch Orthop Unfallchir 1932;32:263.
23. Mori Y, Okumo H, Iketani H, Kuroki Y. Efficacy of lateral retinacular release for painful bipartite patella. Am J Sports Med 1995;23(1):13–18.
24. Petty A. In: DePalma, ed. Diseases of the Knee. Philadelphia: JB Lippincott; 1954.
25. Vallois H. Etude anatomique de l'articulation du genou chez les primates. Thesis; Montpellier; France; 1914.
26. Vallois H. La valeur morphologique de la rotule chez les mammiferes. Bull Mem Soc Anthrop Paris, 1917;January 18.
27. Haenisch F. Verdoppelung der patella in sagitaller richtung. Fortschr Roentgenstr 1925;33:678 .
28. Bennett GE. Operation for hypertrophied patella. J Bone Joint Surg 1922;4:593–599.
29. Insall J, Goldberg V, Salvati E. Recurrent dislocation and the high-riding patella. Clin Orthop 1972;88:67–69.
30. Peltesohn S. Das verhalten der kniescheibe bei der little'schen krankheit. Dissertation. Leipzig, Germany; 1901.
31. Lotman DB. Knee flexion deformity and patella alta in spastic cerebral palsy. Dev Med Child Neurol 1976; 3:315–319.
32. Micheli LJ, Slater JA, Woods E, Gergino PG. Patella alta and the adolescent growth spurt. Clin Orthop 1986; 213:159–162.
33. Noyes F, Wojtys E, Marshall M. The early diagnosis and treatment of developmental patella infera syndrome. Clin Orthop 1991;265:241–252.
34. Paulos L, Wnorowski D, Greenwald A. Infrapatellar contracture syndrome. Am J Sports Med 1994;22(4): 440–449.
35. Hallisey M, Doherty N, Bennett W, Fulkerson J. Anatomy of the junction of the vastus lateralis tendon and the patella. J Bone Joint Surg 1987;69A:545.

7

Nonarthritic Anterior Knee Pain

*"If I were a policymaker, interested in saving money for health
care over the long haul, I would regard it as an act of high
prudence to give high priority to a lot more basic research in
biologic science."*

—*Lewis Thomas, The Lives of a Cell*

*"Man's productivity moves from potentiality to actuality in such
a way that everything actualized has potentialities for further
actualization."*

—*Paul Tillich*

Patellofemoral arthralgia is a descriptive term that simply means pain originating from
the patellofemoral joint. Because patellofemoral pain may occur also as a result of problems in the support structures around the patellofemoral joint, however, the term *anterior
knee pain* is more appropriate to consider all possibilities in and around the anterior knee.
This would seem to be a very simple matter but, in fact, the use of terms that imply understanding of etiology has led to a great deal of confusion in the real understanding of conditions that cause anterior knee pain. In the English literature, *chondromalacia patellae*
has been used inappropriately as a synonym for patellofemoral arthralgia, but it has
become clear that anterior knee pain may be a soft-tissue, retinacular problem in many
patients (1–3). Nerve injury in the lateral peripatellar retinaculum was first described in
1985 (2) and is undoubtedly a factor in the evolution of anterior knee pain, perhaps as
important as the "chondromalacia" to which anterior knee pain has been attributed commonly in years past. The term chondromalacia should be restricted to describe morphologic softening of patellar articular cartilage. Using the word chondromalacia has even
diverted attention from other sources of patellofemoral pain, providing a seemingly useful, but often inaccurate, "wastebasket" term to describe anterior knee pain. In fact, some
authors have gone so far as to describe patients with patellofemoral pain and normal
articular cartilage under the rubric of chondromalacia patellae (4). Use of the term anterior knee pain will underline the need to search further for a specific cause of pain in each
patient (5), remembering that there is not always a correlation between articular cartilage
lesions and pain (6). The term malalignment similarly describes only the condition of
patellofemoral incongruity, which can lead to overload of surfaces or strain in support
structure. Malalignment can exist without pain, and pain can exist without malalignment.
Nonetheless, abnormal alignment of the extensor mechanism can lead to chronic strain
and resultant pain in some patients, and this pain may have nothing to do with chondromalacia, subchondral bone, or synovial lining of the joint.

CLINICAL FEATURES

Symptoms

Pain

Anterior knee pain is often described as dull and aching or throbbing, but occasionally there may be episodes of acute, sharp pain. Pain is characteristically provoked by prolonged sitting with the knee flexed to 90 degrees, particularly in a theater or automobile where change of position is constrained by the physical setting. Going up and down stairs often precipitates pain. Squatting may be impossible. The surgeon should learn to characterize the pain and determine whether the specific pain described by a patient suggests neuroma (sharp, dysesthetic), articular damage (position related, aching, related to crepitation), synovitis (pinching, aching, swelling), referred (hard to localize), or another less common origin. Thomee et al (7) pointed out that patients with patellofemoral pain score higher on the "catastrophizing" scale. It is important, therefore, to note any hysterical tendency and be very specific in defining a pain source.

Crepitus

Some patients report uncomfortable grating while flexing or extending the knee. This complaint may be constantly present with knee movement. Occasionally, crepitus will be audible as well as sensed internally by the patient, although audible crepitus is a more common feature of patellofemoral arthrosis. Crepitus is not always present in patients with clinically significant anterior knee pain. Also, when it is present, it does not necessarily cause anterior knee pain. Nonetheless, crepitus may indicate a significant articular lesion or synovitis and should be interpreted in light of other clinical findings. Pain associated with crepitus, particularly with adding load to the articular lesion, may indicate an important source of pain.

Giving Way

This is another common symptom that may point to the patellofemoral joint; it consists of a sudden reflex relaxation of the quadriceps while performing some movement with the knee flexing or extending under load. Giving way is also a frequent complaint in association with ligamentous instability or meniscal lesions, but under those circumstances, the giving way is generally associated with a turning movement. Giving way of patellofemoral origin is most frequent while ascending stairs or walking down an incline. This may even occasionally lead to a fall. Quadriceps weakness alone is another common cause of giving way. One must also consider that sudden referred pain from the hip or back may cause giving way.

Locking

Patients may report locking of the knee related to a lesion on the patella or trochlea, but on closer questioning, they seldom mean anything more than a catching sensation on attempting to straighten the knee under load. These episodes of "locking" are usually transient, and one must not incorrectly diagnose a meniscal lesion. Asking the patient to define his/her meaning of locking will almost always bring out the difference, which is then confirmed on physical examination. True locking can occur when an articular cartilage fragment on the patella or trochlea everts and blocks normal motion. This can also occur in relation to a prominent synovial or fat pad lesion.

Swelling

Patients sometimes complain of knee swelling, although this is not a frequent physical finding. The complaints are often intermittent, and it is possible that a mild effusion may also be transiently present when there is significant patellar malalignment. In general, the presence of effusion will indicate synovial irritation from significant chondral disruption with free proteoglycan and cartilage fragments in the joint, a primary synovial disease, or trauma with bleeding. In most cases of synovitis, a corticosteroid injection will give relief, and arthroscopic intervention will not be necessary unless there are mechanical symptoms such as locking and catching.

Physical Findings

Careful history and precise examination are extremely important in determining a nonarthritic source of anterior knee pain (8). With the patient supine and the knee supported on the examining table in full extension with the quadriceps relaxed, the patella may be grasped with the examining thumb and finger and forced distally into the superior entrance of the trochlear sulcus. The examiner must be careful not to catch some of the suprapatellar synovial membrane, thus causing discomfort from pinching of the synovium between the articular surfaces. This can be avoided by drawing the patella into the sulcus before applying any pressure. Moving the patella distally and proximally in the sulcus (passively) with some pressure applied may bring out symptoms. This must be done carefully, with the knee slightly flexed to ensure articular contact. Any pain elicited must be differentiated from soft-tissue or retinacular pain. With the quadriceps relaxed, the patella can be tilted medially and then laterally in an attempt to differentiate the side or area of the patella that is causing the discomfort. The patella can also be tilted medially and laterally to palpate peripatellar retinaculum with the examining finger. Palpating specific facets is impossible without stressing the intervening retinaculum.

The retinaculum itself must be examined completely (1). First, the examiner should palpate the entire lateral retinaculum to see whether there is any specifically tender area (Fig. 7.1). Displacement of the patella in a lateral direction may be very helpful to place the lateral retinaculum on slight tension as the patella rides up the lateral trochlear facet (Fig. 7.2). This also permits the examiner to evaluate better the tension in the lateral retinaculum (tight lateral retinaculum is commonly associated with excessive patellar tilt). Tenderness has been noted particularly at the junction of the vastus lateralis and the lateral retinaculum in some patients with patellar malalignment.

Similarly, the examiner should proceed with gentle palpation of the medial retinaculum, distal quadriceps, and patellar tendon. Sometimes pain may be localized to the infrapatellar tendon region, completely separate from the patella itself.

Soft-tissue retinacular pain is common in many patients with anterior knee pain problems, and the source of this pain can be localized accurately if some time is devoted to careful clinical evaluation of the peripatellar soft tissues, including the quadriceps tendon, patellar tendon, and all retinacular structures (Fig. 7.3). Even patients who have had lateral retinacular release may have pain in a residual band of lateral retinaculum.

The patella should be compressed against the trochlea with the examining hand to test for articular pain. This should be done in varying degrees of flexion.

It is important to observe the course of the patella throughout the entire range of movement of the knee. With the patient supine and the quadriceps relaxed, the patella is drawn to the opening of the trochlear sulcus by the peripatellar retinaculum. Tightening the quadriceps produces a proximal and generally slightly lateral movement of the patella. It

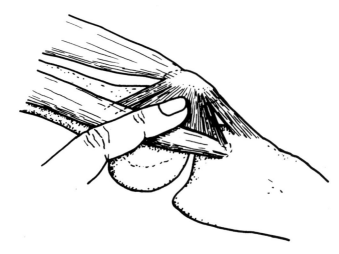

Figure 7.1. Careful palpation of the peripatellar retinaculum will often reveal localized tenderness in patients with patellar malalignment and anterior knee pain. Reprinted with permission from Fulkerson JP. Awareness of the retinaculum in evaluating patellofemoral pain. Am J Sports Med 1982;10:147.

should be noted if this proximal and lateral movement is excessive. Next, with the patient sitting on the edge of the examining table with the thigh well supported, beginning with the knee at 90 degrees of flexion, the course of the patella is carefully observed during active extension and then flexion. Of particular importance is the exit from, and reentry into, the trochlear sulcus. This should be smooth, with no abrupt or sudden movement. Lateral movement is normal in the last few degrees of extension, emphasizing the importance of obtaining tomographic studies of the patellofemoral joint with the knee slightly flexed to understand aberrations in contact pressure.

The Q angle may be measured, although the Q angle itself is not a reliable indicator of patellar malalignment. It should be regarded as one bit of information that may be correlated with other clinical findings to understand a malalignment problem as fully as possible. It is an error to treat a Q angle or to assume that a patient with a high Q angle will require tibial tubercle transfer in every case that resists conservative treatment. The Q angle is measured with the quadriceps relaxed and also with the patella localized in the trochlea. It is of interest to note the orientation of the patellar tendon with the knee flexed to 90 degrees. Under normal circumstances, the tibia has derotated, markedly reducing the Q angle in flexion (9, 10) (Fig. 7.4). The presence or absence of effusion should be noted. Effusion is more common when cartilage changes are more advanced and when there is synovial disease.

Next, the patient should roll into the prone position, and the examiner should evaluate knee flexion passively to see if the quadriceps is excessively tight (Fig. 7.5). This is also

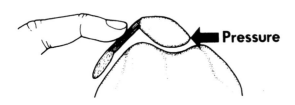

Figure 7.2. Gentle displacement of the patella will permit specific palpation of the peripatellar retinaculum away from the joint itself. Reprinted with permission from Fulkerson JP. Awareness of the retinaculum in evaluating patellofemoral pain. Am J Sports Med 1982;10:147.

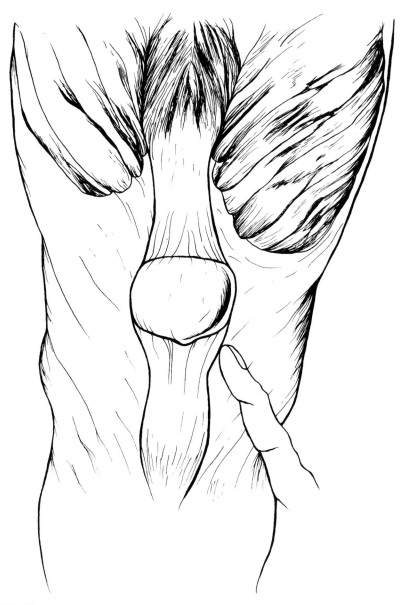

Figure 7.3. The surgeon must consider all components of peripatellar support structure when evaluating the patient with anterior knee pain. (Illustration by Phoebe Fulkerson.)

an ideal time to palpate the patellar tendon, particularly at its origin and insertion, as well as assessing hip rotation with the patient prone.

In any evaluation of a knee complaint, complete examination is necessary, including testing of the medial and lateral collateral ligaments, the anterior and posterior drawer signs, tests for rotatory stability, and evaluation for evidence of meniscus derangement or osteoarthritis. Insall (11) emphasized the importance of differentiating pain of patellar origin from other disorders of the knee.

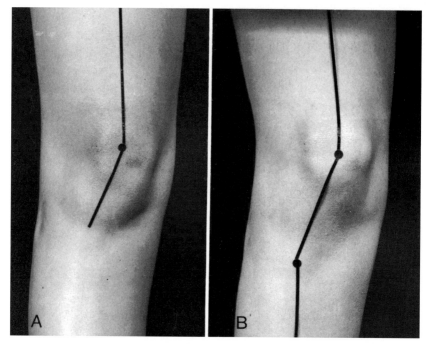

Figure 7.4. Q angle with the knee in full extension **(A)** is only slightly increased over normal. However, with the knee flexed at 30 degrees **(B)**, there is failure of both the tibia to derotate normally and the patellar tendon to line up with the anterior crest of the tibia. This is not an infrequent finding in patients with patellofemoral arthralgia.

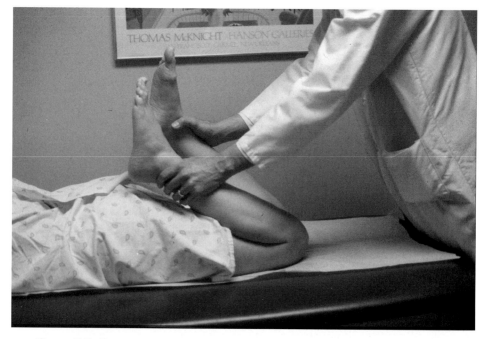

Figure 7.5. Prone quadriceps evaluation helps mobilize tight retinacular tissues.

RETINACULAR PAIN

Patients with patellofemoral malalignment frequently complain of nondescript aching or pain in the anterior knee. The association of this pain with softened articular cartilage has led historically to the assumption that this pain is caused by soft cartilage or chondromalacia. Several authors (6, 12–15) have documented the poor association between morphologically softened articular cartilage and pain in the anterior knee. Stougard (16), Casscells (17), and Emery and Meachim (18) demonstrated the frequency of softened articular cartilage at the time of autopsy. Pevsner et al (19) pointed out that there is normal age-related degeneration of patellar cartilage, further substantiating that intense anterior knee pain cannot be associated routinely with chondromalacia. Furthermore, articular cartilage is devoid of nerve fibers. Tenderness in the lateral retinaculum and vastus lateralis insertion is common in patients with patellofemoral pain (1). Johnson (15) later substantiated these findings. Recognizing that malalignment is frequently associated with such pain, it is apparent that recurrent stretching or abnormal retinacular stress might be associated with imbalance of the patellofemoral articulation (Fig. 2.13). Similarly, medial retinaculum might be recurrently stretched or abnormally stressed in patients with patellar imbalance.

We showed in 1985 that some patients with chronic anterior knee pain associated with malalignment show evidence of *small nerve injury* (2) in the lateral retinaculum (Fig. 7.6). In 1991, Mori et al (20) and Sanchis-Alfonso and Rosello-Sastri (21) later confirmed the presence of degenerative changes in retinacular nerves of patients with patellofemoral dysfunction. This is not really surprising when one recognizes that a chronic lateral tilt of the patella will eventually lead to adaptive shortening of the lateral retinaculum. On flexion of the knee, however, a shortened lateral retinaculum will come under excessive stress as the patella is drawn in the trochlea and the iliotibial band pulls posteriorly on the shortened lateral retinaculum, causing small nerve injury. *Such nerve injury may evolve from relative ischemia* from connective tissue induration.

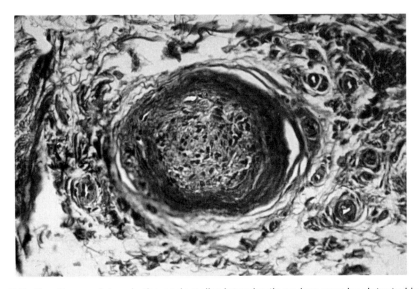

Figure 7.6. Small nerve injury in the peripatellar lateral retinaculum may be detected in some patients using Gomori trichrome stain of the retinaculum excised at the time of lateral release. A finding of nerve injury is most common in clinically tender portions of the lateral retinaculum.

Butler-Manuel et al (22) noted in 1992 that some patients with anterior knee pain, but without the usual features of reflex sympathetic dystrophy, will respond favorably to sympathetic blockade. One must carefully consider, therefore, the possibility that small nerve injury in these patients could potentially cause concomitant sympathetic stimulation.

Recognizing the pathomechanics of anterior knee pain will help the clinician identify accurately a source of pain in most patients, and careful evaluation of the patient with patellar malalignment should include a thorough examination of the peripatellar soft tissues. Commonly, pain has been noted in the inferomedial peripatellar area and the superolateral aspect of the patella where the lateral retinaculum interdigitates with the vastus lateralis tendon. If a retinacular pain source can be identified, injection of the painful retinacular band may confirm a diagnosis and, on occasion, give lasting relief of pain.

The clinician should pay particular attention to residual bands of lateral retinaculum in patients with continued pain after retinacular release. If a lateral retinacular release is done transecting all the lateral retinaculum except a specific painful band of the lateral retinaculum, pain may be intensified as stresses are transferred from transected, nonpainful portions of the retinaculum to a residual, painful component of the lateral retinaculum. Recognition of this condition may permit a fairly simple solution to persistent pain after lateral retinacular release in some patients.

PLICA OR SYNOVITIS

Anterior knee pain, particularly in the medial infrapatellar region, may be caused by a plical fold (23–25). Pain, particularly associated with a palpable tender band in the medial peripatellar area, may indicate a symptomatic plica causing anterior knee pain (Fig. 7.7). Although stretching and local treatment may give relief, arthroscopic resection of a thickened, inflamed plica may be necessary at times (24, 25). We (23) have pointed out that a symptomatic plica may, in some cases, be only an indicator of a more complex problem involving abnormal patellofemoral mechanics. Certainly, however, pain may

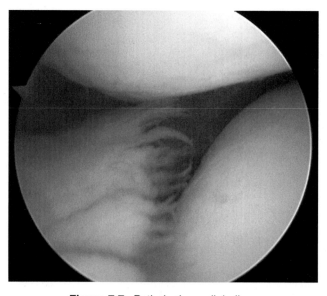

Figure 7.7. Pathologic medial plica.

occur as a result of direct injury to one of the plical folds, with secondary inflammation or fibrosis. Strover et al (26) have recommended arthroscopic resection of the pathologic plica using local anesthetic.

It is important to recognize the synovium as one of many sources of pain. There is little question that synovial irritation from any cause can be a primary or sole cause of pain in some patients. Simple corticosteroid injection into the knee can usually control such conditions.

PATELLAR TENDINITIS (JUMPER'S KNEE)

Some patients with anterior knee pain have distinct tenderness in the patellar tendon, particularly where it originates on the patella. This is particularly true in jumping athletes (basketball and tennis players seem to develop this problem more frequently than other athletes). Bear in mind also, however, that pain referred from the patella itself may be felt in the patellar tendon region.

Patellar tendinitis may be very difficult to treat, and the usual nonoperative treatment program may fail to bring improvement, even after several months. Hydrocortisone iontophoresis may be helpful, and alteration of the exercise program may eventually bring relief. A complete program of prone quadriceps stretching and eccentric quadriceps strengthening will help most patients, and a very localized injection of a small amount of corticosteroid will help some patients. The rare patient may require surgical exploration of the tendon, and a small amount of the painful tissue may be excised (Fig. 7.8).

It is important to recognize patellar tendinitis because the usual treatment programs for patellofemoral pain are not always helpful, and arthroscopy will add nothing to the treatment of this condition.

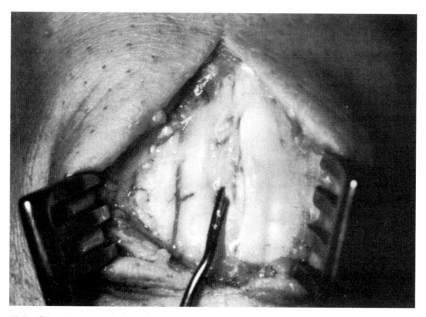

Figure 7.8. Chronic granulation tissue may perpetuate pain in the patellar tendon. Surgical excision of a limited area of granulation may be curative in patients for whom this procedure is deemed appropriate.

Prepatellar Bursitis

The symptoms may be very similar, but the patient generally has a history of prolonged kneeling, and there is not infrequently thickening of the skin over the patellar surface. In acute cases, the prepatellar bursa is swollen, boggy, and tender, and diagnosis represents no problem. However, in subacute cases, there may be less evidence in the physical findings, and a high index of suspicion can differentiate this from more serious patellofemoral problems (Fig. 7.9).

Retropatellar Tendon Bursitis

There is a small bursa outside the knee, just proximal to the tibial tubercle and behind the patellar tendon, that is occasionally the source of symptoms. These symptoms are remarkably similar to those of patellofemoral arthralgia. Physical examination, however, will generally reveal the bursa to be the source of symptoms. Palpation with the knee fully extended and the quadriceps relaxed will provoke acute, and sometimes exquisite, tenderness. When the quadriceps is contracted and the patellar tendon is tightened, the bursa is protected from the examining finger, and palpation will not provoke symptoms.

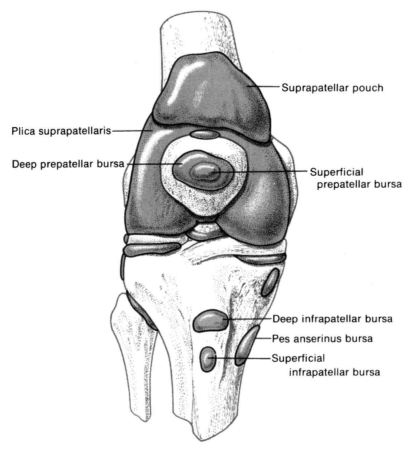

Figure 7.9. Bursae in the front of the knee can mimic many knee disorders. These bursae should be examined in the evaluation of patients with anterior knee pain.

Tenderness in this area may also result from fat pad syndrome or retinacular pain in the peripatellar tendon area. Corticosteroid injection into the tender area may be curative.

Pes Anserinus Bursitis

This bursa lies underneath the combined insertion of the sartorius, gracilis, and semi-tendinosus tendons into the proximal medial tibial metaphysis. It serves to reduce the friction between these tendons and the tibial metaphysis at the level of the medial collateral ligament insertion into the tibia. Because of its medial location, the symptoms are more likely to be confused with a medial compartment problem, including degenerative joint disease and meniscal lesions. Simple palpation will evoke tenderness and lead to the proper diagnosis. Beware of more serious problems, such as giant cell tumor or sarcoma of the proximal tibia. Do not neglect to take a radiograph.

Fat Pad Syndrome

The infrapatellar fat pads may be traumatized either by direct blow or by being caught between the femoral condyles and the tibial plateaus on extension (28). The latter mechanism is more common in genu recurvatum, in which the space for the fat pad is reduced. It is important to palpate the fat pad for tenderness and to compare it with the opposite side for texture. Symptoms arising from the infrapatellar fat pad are generally accompanied by tenderness to direct palpation and sometimes induration. It is important, however, not to confuse the synovitis that sometimes accompanies more advanced forms of patellofemoral arthralgia with the disease described by Hoffa (27). The fat pads are covered with synovial membrane and, therefore, if involved with a distinct synovitis, may also participate in general sensitivity. Therefore, it is important to rule out a generalized synovitis if attributing a knee complaint to the fat pad syndrome. Stretching the anterior knee with the patient prone may be very helpful in some patients, and at times, injection with corticosteroid or arthroscopic excision of impinging fat pad will be curative if symptoms cannot be otherwise eliminated.

Generalized Synovitis

The effusion accompanying many forms of patellofemoral disease is often minimal and not accompanied by significant synovitis. However, symptoms from a generalized knee synovitis may be similar to those noted by patients with patellofemoral disease. The effect of a prolonged synovial effusion is to create changes in articular cartilage, which makes the cartilage less capable of withstanding the mechanical forces of normal activity, and thus leading to secondary patellofemoral arthrosis in some patients.

MENISCAL LESIONS

Meniscal tears can cause chronic effusion and eventually patellar articular cartilage softening. Many patients point to the anterior knee when asked to localize knee pain, much as patients with abdominal pain will frequently point to the umbilicus. The astute clinician, however, will rely on a careful and thorough clinical examination to differentiate between meniscal pathology and patellofemoral pain. By carefully examining the peripatellar retinaculum, distal quadriceps muscle, patellar tendon, infrapatellar recesses, and patellar articular surfaces, one can generally localize a specific pain source in the patellar or peripatellar region as opposed to distinct tenderness along the medial or lateral joint line, which would be suggestive of a meniscal tear or arthritis. One must recognize, however, that snapping, popping, and even locking may occur with patellar problems. Again, clinical examination can often differentiate the source of a pop. Pain on full flexion of the knee with rotation and tenderness at the medial or lateral joint line is more suggestive of a meniscal tear. When differentiation is difficult, magnetic resonance imaging will be helpful.

CRUCIATE LIGAMENT DEFICIENCY AND RECONSTRUCTION

Like a meniscal tear, chronic effusion associated with cruciate ligament deficiency can lead eventually to patellar articular cartilage softening. Quadriceps atrophy in association with ligament insufficiency may also lead to patellar problems, particularly if there is patellar malalignment. Patellar crepitation and pain are common after cruciate ligament reconstruction (29) but may have originated before reconstruction when patellar articular cartilage had experienced insult from the original injury or instability with effusion. Shino et al (29), however, have shown that immobilization after anterior cruciate ligament (ACL) reconstruction leads to a high incidence of patellofemoral articular degeneration. Early mobilization of the knee after ACL reconstruction, as recommended by Shelbourne and Nitz (30), is important in minimizing patellofemoral degeneration after ACL reconstruction. Paulos et al (31) pointed out the importance of delaying ACL reconstruction until there is near-normal knee motion to help avoid infrapatellar contracture. Newer concepts of ACL reconstruction using allograft or quadriceps tendon without bone will also minimize risk of anterior knee pain postoperatively.

The clinician should consider rotatory instability in any patient with giving way of the knee. Sometimes one must differentiate between cruciate ligament injury and an unstable patella in the acutely injured patient who describes the knee "going out of place." There is no replacement for careful physical examination in making this differentiation, but magnetic resonance imaging is helpful when the knee is difficult to examine adequately.

HEMANGIOMA

Although very uncommon, hemangiomata can occur in skeletal muscle and have been reported in many locations in the body. We have found hemangiomata in the distal quadriceps muscle (Fig. 4.31) in two patients with anterior knee pain. If careful examination of the patient with anterior knee pain demonstrates muscle tenderness, one should consider the possibility of a hemangioma. Simple excision will be curative.

RUNNERS' KNEE

Cox (32) pointed out the occurrence of stress-related patellofemoral pain in runners. Gymnasts (33) have also described overuse problems in the anterior knee area. Irritation of the iliotibial band as it moves across the lateral femoral condyle is a common cause of such pain in active young athletes. If there is mild patellar malalignment, retinacular problems as previously described may occur and result in overuse pain. Devereaux et al (34) have pointed out that the vastus medialis insertion may also be a cause of overuse pain in athletes. Most of the anterior knee overuse problems in athletes can be localized by careful clinical evaluation (35).

ILIOTIBIAL FRICTION BAND SYNDROME

Some patients, particularly those who are very active in running sports, may develop pain along the lateral side of the knee that can mimic patellofemoral pain. Careful examination of the iliotibial band, where it slides over the lateral femoral epicondyle, will demonstrate tenderness in some of these patients. Rest stretching the iliotibial band, local hot packs, antiinflammatory medication, and orthotics may be helpful. It is most important to differentiate between a primary iliotibial band problem and a retinacular problem of synovitis associated with patellofemoral malalignment.

REFERRED PAIN

Back and hip problems can refer pain to the anterior knee. One should consider discogenic pain, sciatic pain, slipped femoral epiphysis in younger patients, Legg-Calvé-Perthes disease in 6 to 10 year olds, hip arthritis or dysplasia, and other disorders of the back and hip in the patient who complains of anterior knee pain.

With all the possible diagnoses in a patient presenting with anterior knee pain, it is important not to fall into the trap of saying that the patient has "internal derangement of the knee." Use of this term was condemned by Budinger (36) in 1908, and its use today is equally to be deplored. An awareness of the various specific diagnoses that can be the source of symptoms will be helpful in eliminating such wastebasket terminology. The abbreviation for internal derangement of the knee is IDK. This is also the abbreviation for I don't know!

REHABILITATION OF SOFT-TISSUE PROBLEMS

Before an appropriate rehabilitation program can be formulated, one must identify the specific source of pain. In those patients with predominantly soft-tissue pain related to malalignment, conservative rehabilitation is usually effective (37–39). Quadriceps strengthening has been a central component of rehabilitation in the patient with patellar malalignment. Some of the pain relief after quadriceps strengthening may be related to altered soft-tissue balance around the patella.

The program of extensor mechanism rehabilitation should avoid high-impact loading activities in case there is associated articular disease (40). Grood et al (41) noted that very large quadriceps forces are needed to raise a 7-lb weight through a range of motion and that the last 15 degrees of knee extension causes particularly high quadriceps force. Consequently, Grood et al (41) recommended exercise in the 15- to 50-degree range to avoid quadriceps stress. Because patellar contact stress is ordinarily greatest at 65 degrees of knee flexion, exercise at lesser degrees of knee flexion is desirable, and terminal extension exercises will maximize quadriceps demand (and thereby strengthening). The vector of quadriceps pull at 0 to 15 degrees of knee motion is such that there is little increased patellar articular load, despite maximal quadriceps stress.

Steinkamp et al (42) demonstrated that leg press exercise creates lower patellofemoral stress in the 30- to 0-degree range of motion when compared with knee extension exercise, the reverse being true in 60- to 90-degree range of motion. The type of exercise selected, therefore, should be specific to the pain-free range of motion.

Miller et al (43) noted that a program of isometric quadriceps exercises over a period of 3 months resulted in increased vastus lateralis and vastus medialis obliquus (VMO) activity without any notable alteration of muscle balance. On this basis, Miller et al recommended selective training of the VMO. Nonimpact loading during exercise may be accomplished through stationary cycling, swimming, isometric exercises, and activities such as cross-country skiing and running. Ericson and Nissell (44) noted that patellofemoral compressive force was approximately 1.3 times body weight when cycling at midlevel saddle height and 60 rpm. In general, for stationary bicycling, the seat should be set somewhat higher so that the knee is extended to −15 degrees during exercise. Biofeedback and electrical stimulation may be used selectively to help to build VMO strength. Isokinetic exercise is not usually necessary or even desirable in the rehabilitation of most patients with patellofemoral pain, but objective quadriceps strength gain should be documented by isokinetic testing to confirm that the patient has made an adequate effort. Isokinetic testing, however, can cause dangerous increases in patellar articular load and must be used cautiously. Certainly, patients who do not exhibit reasonable motivation in their rehabilitation are not patients who should be considered for surgery in most cases.

Braces may be helpful in the management of patients with patellofemoral pain of either soft-tissue or articular origin (Fig. 7.10). The author's Trupull wrap brace (DJ Ortho, Vista, CA) is extremely versatile and may be wrapped by each therapist or patient to address a specific painful area. For instance, patients can rotate the pad beneath the patella for patellar tendonitis and wrap it either tighter or looser as needed. The Trupull Advanced System employs the same concepts in a sleeve design.

Lysholm et al (45) noted that 88% of patients improved their performance on a Cybex isokinetic dynamometer when a patellar brace was used to treat patellofemoral arthral-

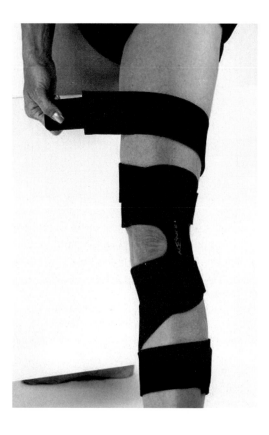

Figure 7.10. Simple brace support can be very helpful in the patient with patellofemoral pain or instability (Trupull Wrap, DJ Ortho, Vista, CA).

gia. Moller and Krebs (46) found similar symptomatic improvement of patellofemoral pain patients using patellar braces. Simple elastic sleeves with a patellar cutout, Levine straps, or a Trupull brace (DJ Ortho) can be very helpful in symptomatic management and may cause slight alterations in soft-tissue tensions, thereby giving relief. Osternig and Robertson (47) pointed out that prophylactic knee bracing can actually alter neuromuscular control around the joint. This suggests that true modification of patellar tracking may occur with brace use.

McConnell (48) reported good success in patients with patellofemoral pain using specific muscle strengthening and taping techniques to modify patellar tracking. This innovative approach warrants further investigation because it appears to be helpful in the management of retinacular and articular pain problems related to patellar malalignment (Fig. 7.11). The findings of Osternig and Robertson may apply here also. Although it does not appear that patellar tape actually changes patellar tracking mechanically to any significant degree, neuromuscular/proprioceptive responses to tape only create true functional improvement of patellofemoral function. There is little doubt that these techniques benefit patients.

Nonsteroidal antiinflammatory medication has been somewhat helpful in roughly half of all patients with patellofemoral pain (49). Although nonsteroidal antiinflammatory medications are not always helpful, they are worth considering if there is specific evidence of inflammation, persistent effusion, or need for pain management.

Some patients with anterior knee pain demonstrate a significant abnormality of gait either while walking or running. Tiberio (50) has shown that subtalar pronation is a factor in causing anterior knee pain. James et al (35), McKenzie et al (51), and others have noted that appropriate footwear and selective use of orthotics may be helpful in the patient with anterior knee pain. Inexpensive off-the-shelf orthotics are frequently helpful, particularly if there is significant pronation. Custom orthotics are sometimes necessary

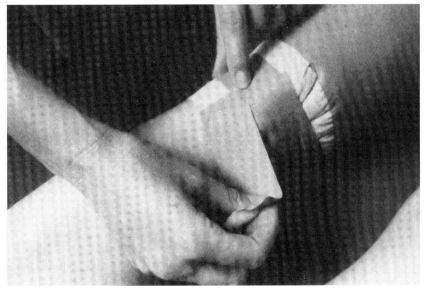

Figure 7.11. The McConnell taping techniques are helpful in managing many pain problems around the anterior knee.

when more complex lower extremity alignment problems exist and when the amount of wear, because of extensive athletic participation, requires a more durable orthosis.

In addition to the benefits of specific strengthening, physical activity can enhance self-esteem and help in the return of patients with anterior knee pain to improved levels of function. Some patients with resistant pain, arthritis, and limited access to physical therapy may also benefit from a resistance-controlled knee exercise and bracing system (Protonics, EMPI). Any rehabilitation program must be based on a thorough examination and understanding of each patient, with awareness of the peripatellar structures and the patella itself (52). A well-structured exercise program using a Trupull wrap selectively and emphasizing activities that do not create excessive contact stress on the patella should be the cornerstone of a good patellofemoral rehabilitation program.

REFERENCES

1. Fulkerson JP. Awareness of the retinaculum in evaluating patellofemoral pain. Am J Sports Med 1982;10:147.
2. Fulkerson JP, Tennant R, Jaivin JS, Grunnet M. Histologic evidence of retinacular nerve injury associated with patellofemoral malalignment. Clin Orthop 1985;197:196–205.
3. Dugdale TW, Barnett PR. Historical background: Patellofemoral pain in young people. Orthop Clin North Am 1986;17:211–219.
4. Darracott J, Vernon-Roberts B. The bone changes in chondromalacia patellae. Rheumatol Phys Med 1971;11:175.
5. Radin EL. A rational approach to the treatment of patellofemoral pain. Clin Orthop 1979;144:107–109.
6. Grana WA, Kriegshauser LA. Scientific basis of extensor mechanism disorders. Clin Sports Med 1985;4: 247–257.
7. Thomee P, Thomee R, Karlsson J. Patellofemoral pain syndrome: pain coping strategies and degree well-being. Scand J Med Sci Sports 2002 Oct;12(5):276–81.
8. Fulkerson JP. Patellofemoral pain disorders: Evaluation and management. J Am Acad Orthop Surg 1994;2(2):124–132.
9. Brantigan OC, Voshell AF. The mechanics of the ligaments and menisci of the knee joint. J Bone Joint Surg 1941;23:44.
10. Goodsir J. Anatomy and mechanism of the knee joint. In: Turner, ed. The Anatomical Memoirs of John Goodsir. Edinburgh: Adams and Charles Black; 1868.
11. Insall JN. Patellar pain syndromes and chondromalacia patellae. Instr Course Lect 1981;30:342–356.
12. Metcalf RW. An arthroscopic method for lateral release of the subluxating or dislocating patella. Clin Orthop 1982;167:9.
13. McGinty JB, McCarthy JC. Endoscopic lateral retinacular release: A preliminary report. Clin Orthop 1981; 158:120.
14. Bentley G, Dowd G. Current concepts of etiology and treatment of chondromalacia patellae. Clin Orthop 1984; 189:209.
15. Johnson R. Lateral facet syndrome of the patella. Clin Orthop 1989;238:148–158.
16. Stougard J. Chondromalacia of patella. Physical signs in relation to operative findings. Acta Orthop Scand 1975;46:685–694.
17. Casscells W. Arthroscopic and cadaver knee investigations. AAOS Symposium on Arthroscopy and Arthrography of the Knee. St. Louis: CV Mosby; 1978.
18. Emery IH, Meachim G. Surface morphology and topography of patello-femoral cartilage fibrillation in Liverpool necropsies. J Anat 1973;116:103–120.
19. Pevsner DN, Johnson JR, Blazina ME. The patellofemoral joint and its implications in the rehabilitation of the knee. Phys Ther 1979;59:869–874.
20. Mori Y, Fujimoto A, Okumo H, Kuroki Y. Lateral retinaculum release in adolescent patellofemoral disorders: Its relationship to peripheral nerve injury in the lateral retinaculum. Bull Hosp Joint Dis Orthop Inst 1991;51(2):218–229.
21. Sanchis-Alfonso V, Rosallo-Sastri E, Monteagudo-Castro C. Quantitative analysis of nerve changes in the lateral retinaculum. Am J Sports Med 1998;26:703–709.
22. Butler-Manuel P, Justins D, Heatley F. Sympathetically mediated anterior knee pain. Acta Orthop Scand 1992; 63(1):90–93.
23. Broom JM, Fulkerson JP. The plica syndrome: A new perspective. Orthop Clin North Am 1986;17:279–281.
24. Jackson R, Marshall D, Fujisawa Y. The pathological medial shelf. Orthop Clin North Am 1982;13:307–312.
25. Patel D. Arthroscopy of the plical-synovial folds and their significance. Am J Sports Med 1978;6:217–225.
26. Strover AE, Rouholamin E, Guirguis N, Behdad H. An arthroscopic technique of demonstrating the pathomechanics of the suprapatellar plica. Arthroscopy 1991;7(3):308–310.

27. Hoffa A. The influence of the adipose tissue with regard to the pathology of the knee joint. JAMA 1904;43:795.
28. Marder RA, Raskind JR, Carroll M. Prospective evaluation of arthroscopically assisted anterior cruciate ligament reconstruction. Patellar tendon versus semitendinosus and gracilis tendons. Am J Sports Med 1991;19(5): 478–484.
29. Shino K, Nakagawa S, Inoue M, Horibe S, Yoneda M. Deterioration of patellofemoral articular surfaces after ACL reconstruction. Am J Sports Med 1993;21(2):206–211.
30. Shelbourne D, Nitz P. Accelerated rehabilitation after ACL reconstruction. Am J Sports Med 1990;18:292–299.
31. Paulos L, Wnorawski D, Greenwald A. Infrapatellar contracture syndrome. Am J Sports Med 1994;22(4): 440–449.
32. Cox JS. Patellofemoral problems in runners. Clin Sports Med 1985;4:111–121.
33. Andrish JT. Knee injuries in gymnastics. Clin Sports Med 1985;4:111–121.
34. Devereaux MD, Parr GR, Lachmann SM, Thomas DP, Hazelman BL. Thermographic diagnosis in athletes with patellofemoral arthralgia. J Bone Joint Surg 1986;68B:42–44.
35. James S, Bates G, Osternig L. Injuries to runners. Am J Sports Med 1978;6:40.
36. Budinger K. Ueber traumatische knorpelrisse im kniegelenk. Dtsch Z Chir 1908;92:510.
37. Dehaven K, Dolan W, Mayer P. Chondromalacia patellae in athletes. Clinical presentation and conservative management. Am J Sports Med 1979;7:5–11.
38. Fisher RL. Conservative treatment of pain. Orthop Clin North Am 1986;17:269–272.
39. Paulos L, Rusche K, Johnson C, Noyes FR. Patellar malalignment: A treatment rationale. Phys Ther 1980;60: 1624–1632.
40. Hungerford DS, Lennox DW. Rehabilitation of the knee in disorders of the patellofemoral joint: Relevant biomechanics. Orthop Clin North Am 1983;14:397–402.
41. Grood ES, Suntay WJ, Noyes FR, Butler DL. Biomechanics of the knee-extension exercise. Effect of cutting the anterior cruciate ligament. J Bone Joint Surg 1984;66A:725–734.
42. Steinkamp L, Dillingham M, Markel M, Hill J, Kaufman K. Biomechanical considerations in patellofemoral joint rehabilitation. Am J Sports Med 1993;21(3):438–444.
43. Miller BN, Jurik AG, Tidemand E, Dal C, Krebs B, Aaris K. The quadriceps function in patellofemoral disorders. A radiographic and electromyographic study. Arch Orthop Trauma Surg 1987;106:195–198.
44. Ericson MO, Nissell R. Patellofemoral joint forces during ergometric cycling. Phys Ther 1987;67:1365–1369.
45. Lysholm J, Nordin M, Ekstrand J, Gillquist J. The effect of a patella brace on performance in a knee extension strength test in patients with patellar pain. Am J Sports Med 1984;12:110–112.
46. Moller RN, Krebs B. Dynamic knee brace in the treatment of patellofemoral disorders. Arch Orthop Trauma Surg 1986;104:377–379.
47. Osternig L, Robertson R. Effects of prophylactic knee bracing on lower extremity joint position and muscle activation during running. Am J Sports Med 1993;21(5):733–737.
48. McConnell J. The management of chondromalacia patellae: A long-term solution. Aust J Physiother 1986;32: 215–223.
49. Fulkerson J, Folcik M. Comparison of diflunisal and naproxen for relief of anterior knee pain. Clin Ther 1986; 9(suppl):59–61.
50. Timbero D. The effect of excessive subtalar joint pronation on patellofemoral mechanics. J Orthop Sports Phys Ther 1987;9:160–165.
51. McKenzie DC, Clement DB, Taunton JE. Running shoes, orthotics, and injuries. Sports Med 1985;2:334–347.
52. Fulkerson J. Evaluation of the peripatellar soft tissues and retinaculum in patients with patellofemoral pain. Clin Sports Med 1989;8:197–202.

8

Patellar Tilt Compression and the Excessive Lateral Pressure Syndrome

"Disease is from old and nothing about it has changed. It is we who change as we learn to recognize what was formerly imperceptible."

—Jean Marie Charcot (1825–1893)

Patellar tilt compression is characterized clinically by pain and radiographically by patellar tilt, as evidenced on the Maldague lateral radiograph, axial patellofemoral radiograph, computed tomography (CT), or magnetic resonance imaging (MRI). In the original edition of this book, Ficat and Hungerford (1) described the excessive lateral pressure syndrome (ELPS). It is important now to recognize that patellar tilt occurs *with or without* associated subluxation and may eventually cause ELPS. The concept of ELPS, however, is important because chronic lateral patellar tilt can have devastating effects on articular cartilage. Chronic alteration of pressure on the medial facet and overload on the lateral facet (Fig. 8.1) will lead to arthrosis in many patients, but associated tightness of the lateral retinaculum may result in persistent retinacular pain even before there is evidence of articular cartilage disruption (Fig. 8.2). Surprisingly, however, some people live for many years, or even a lifetime, with patellar tilt and never experience symptoms. The clinician therefore must be sure in every patient to understand the origin of pain, and *not treat tilt or any malalignment unless it is clearly the cause of the patient's pain.*

Tilt compression is a clinical radiographic condition of the patellofemoral joint that can lead to retinacular strain (peripatellar effect) and ELPS (articular effect) in some patients. A cause-and-effect relationship, therefore, can be defined between tilt compression (cause) and retinacular strain (effect) or ELPS (effect). Understanding this cause-and-effect relationship will help the clinician to understand the pathogenesis of articular disruption in patients with chronic patellar tilt (with or without associated subluxation). Pure subluxation (without associated tilt) is less common and more typically creates a clinicopathologic picture of instability. Subluxation is discussed in Chapter 9. Nonetheless, subluxation is often associated with tilt, so there may be factors of both excessive compression (tilt) and patellar instability (subluxation) in some patients.

CLINICAL FEATURES

Signs and Symptoms

One group of physical findings needs to be underscored and enlarged. With the normal knee fully extended and the quadriceps relaxed, there is passive medial and lateral

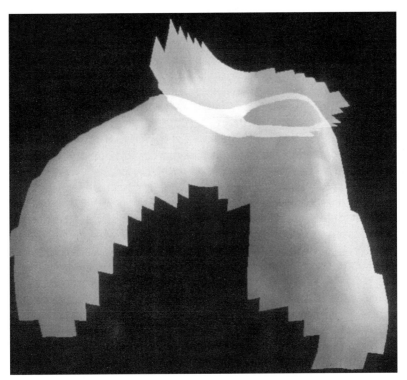

Figure 8.1. Stereophotogrammetry of the patellofemoral joint shows rotational malalignment (tilt) of the patella and lateral facet stress concentration. (Courtesy of Dr. Van Mow, Columbia Presbyterian Medical Center, New York, NY.)

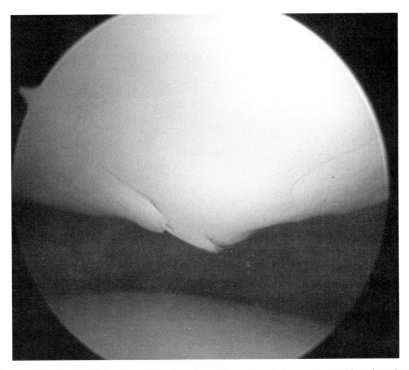

Figure 8.2. Central lateral patellar facet cartilage breakdown caused by chronic tilt.

"play" of the patella (Fig. 8.3). This passive movement shows a particular amount of individual variability, but it is usually approximately a centimeter in each direction and may be more. Examining knees for this play will provide an appreciation for the normal limits. Examination of the sound knee provides useful comparison. One should remember, however, that both knees may show radiographic abnormality even though only one is symptomatic. Similarly, patellofemoral pain often occurs as a result of overuse despite perfectly normal alignment. Medial and lateral movement is limited by the retinacula, particularly the meniscopatellar and patellofemoral ligaments, reinforced laterally by the fascia lata. It is common to subluxate the patella passively in a lateral direction during physical examination, searching for evidence of instability or signs of apprehension. One should also displace the patella in a medial direction, searching for excessive lateral tethering. The quality of the retinacula can be appreciated by palpation. This is done best by subluxating the patella toward the side to be palpated, much as would be done to palpate the facet, but this time paying attention to the quality of the respective retinacular ligaments.

As far as the tilt compression syndrome is concerned, there are two major patterns: (a) Transverse play is markedly reduced due to global capsular thickening and retraction. This finding is more common in reflex sympathetic dystrophy. (b) Transverse play is restricted in comparison with the sound side. This may be in either or both directions, but it is most commonly a restriction of medial displacement. In this group, lateral retinacular pain is fairly common. Such restriction may or may not be associated with patellar subluxation.

The patient with patellar tilt compression may complain of generalized anterior knee pain. On careful clinical examination, however, tenderness in the lateral retinaculum (2), particularly where the vastus lateralis tendon interdigitates with the proximal lateral retinaculum, may be noted. This is common in the younger patellofemoral pain patient who

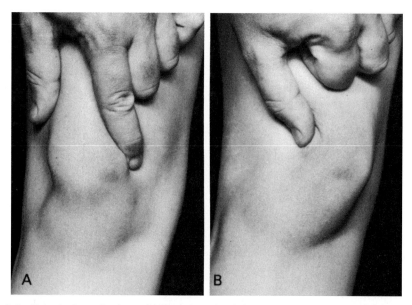

Figure 8.3. Extent of passive lateral **(A)** and medial **(B)** displacement of the patella that is possible with the knee in full extension and the quadriceps relaxed. This represents the play of the patella.

has not yet developed significant articular cartilage erosion or histologic evidence of nerve injury in the lateral retinaculum (3). Tightness of the lateral retinaculum perpetuates the problem and can be evaluated objectively, with experience, by raising the lateral edge of the patella past the horizontal plane, with the knee supine (4, 5). Meanwhile, some medial peripatellar tenderness may be present, most likely related to medial stretching and imbalance or medial facet breakdown caused by the lateral tilt condition. This may be particularly prominent in those patients with subluxation in addition to tilt.

Although rehabilitation may improve patellar balance through vastus medialis obliquus strengthening and stretching of the quadriceps and lateral retinaculum, some patients with tilt compression will manifest articular changes with ELPS (6), including distal *medial* patellar degeneration, presumably related to deficient contact pressure on this medial articular cartilage as the tilted patella enters the trochlea from full extension, such that there is only lateral contact. By the time the medial patella is pulled into the trochlea, the contact zone has shifted onto more proximal articular cartilage. Chronic patellar tilting, with associated retinacular shortening, can lead to considerable lateral facet overload and deficient medial contact pressure. Eventually, then, many patients with tilt compression syndrome will manifest crepitation in the patellofemoral joint, which is truly articular. Some patients will develop effusion related to release of free proteoglycan in the joint, and loose bodies or painful crepitus may occur. When the patient with tilt compression manifests signs of intraarticular disease, it is likely that ELPS has developed. Climbing stairs may become particularly difficult; crepitation is frequently noted, and physical activity is limited. Retinacular pain may accompany the articular problems and may even be the predominant source of pain. By this time, if the patient has had chronic retinacular pain, a pattern of small nerve injury in the painful retinaculum may be found if the segment of painful retinaculum is sent for Gomori trichrome stain and evaluation by a pathologist (3). Such retinacular nerve injury, first described in 1985, may form a basis for the later development of chronic pain and even reflex sympathetic dystrophy.

NATURAL HISTORY OF THE TILT COMPRESSION SYNDROME

Patellar tilt compression problems may present initially in the early teen years, with anterior knee pain aggravated by physical activities. Such patients have had congenital tilting of the patella that was not clinically apparent earlier in life. With time and longitudinal bone growth, however, the magnitude of stress on a chronically tilted patella may become substantial if the retinaculum does not adapt and stretch with growth and therapy. The patella that has been chronically tilted, even to a mild degree, may eventually manifest findings consistent with an *adaptively shortened lateral retinaculum.* If a patella tilts down chronically to the lateral side (Fig. 8.4), the retinaculum becomes short, relative to what is normal. As the size of the patient increases, the vector of posterior pull on this already shortened lateral retinaculum becomes greater with knee flexion, and overload on the lateral retinaculum (which is now tight) may become enough to cause retinacular overload, stretching, and compression of small sensory nerves within the lateral retinaculum, resulting in pain and accentuation of lateral facet compression. Many of the early pain problems experienced by patients with patellar tilt will be most apparent in the lateral retinaculum and peripatellar connective tissue supports. Histologic study of lateral retinacular biopsy specimens from patients with patellar tilt and pain, first reported in 1985 (3), showed fibroneuromatous degeneration of small nerves in the lateral retinaculum. This finding was common in patients with chronic patellar malalignment.

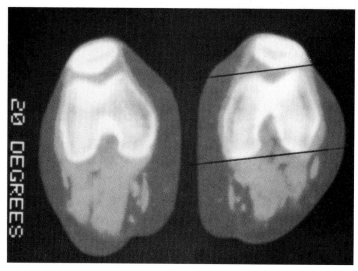

Figure 8.4. If a patella tilts chronically to the lateral side, there will be adaptive retinacular shortening. With knee flexion then, it is likely that abnormal strain will occur in this retinaculum.

As this process proceeds, lateral facet overload and deficient medial facet contact may lead to articular cartilage degeneration on both the medial and lateral facets. Often, the first sign of articular trouble is at the *critical zone* (Fig. 8.5). ELPS is primarily the result of chronic lateral patellar tilt, adaptive lateral retinacular shortening, and resultant chronic imbalance of facet loads. Although full ELPS may develop rapidly in young patients, it is more commonly found in older patients, particularly female patients, with

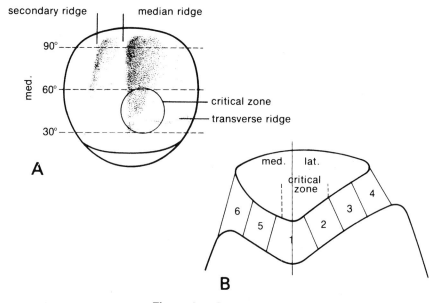

Figure 8.5. Patellar map.

a long history of anterior knee pain. The chronic lateral facet overload can lead to a devastating loss of lateral facet articular cartilage.

In summary, then, tilt compression syndrome will usually proceed through a period of soft-tissue pain related to chronic strain and small nerve injury (3) and eventually lead to patellar cartilage degeneration.

RADIOGRAPHIC FEATURES

Loss of patellar cartilage under load will be noted radiographically as "joint line narrowing." To make comparisons of radiographs and surgical findings as well as to facilitate meaningful comparisons for future studies, Ficat's patellar map may be helpful (Fig. 8.5). One has to be careful in overinterpreting plain films because of the normal variation in patellar cartilage thickness and image overlap inherent in any axial radiograph. Lateral joint line diminution may be clearly visible on an axial view (Fig. 8.6). The lateral radiograph (posterior condyles superimposed) may also reveal tilt (Fig. 8.7). However, traditional radiographic views are sometimes normal. Therefore, radiographs alone cannot rule out a tilt compression syndrome in the patient with patellofemoral pain. Nonetheless, because this condition relates to mechanical dysfunction, the clinician should seek objective proof of a significant mechanical imbalance.

Axial View Arthrography (Fig. 8.8)

In the original edition of this book, Ficat and Hungerford (1) wondered, as did Wiberg (7) in 1941, "why with all the interest in arthrography there has been so little interest in using it to evaluate the patellofemoral joint." To perform an invasive study such as arthrography without axial views in patients with knee pain of less than obvious origin is as erroneous as ordering only an anteroposterior view or not viewing the lateral compartment by radiography when medial compartment pathology is anticipated. One should

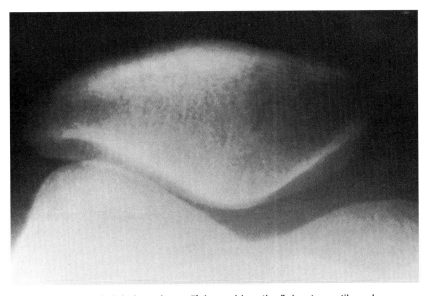

Figure 8.6. Axial view shows "false subluxation" due to cartilage loss.

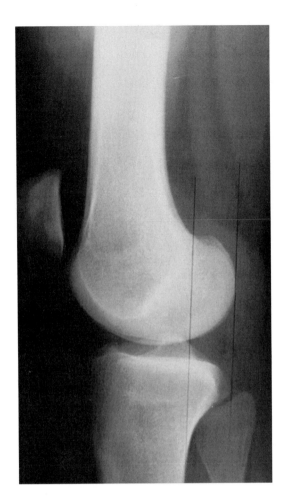

Figure 8.7. The lateral radiographic (posterior condyles superimposed) will reveal tilt if the central ridge and lateral facet overlie each other such that normal alignment (central ridge posterior to the lateral facet) is lost (see Chapter 4).

always obtain good quality axial views when performing knee arthrograms. Today, however, knee arthrograms are almost always done in conjunction with CT or MRI.

CT and MRI

Tomographic imaging, as described in Chapter 4, is particularly important in the evaluation of patients with patellar tilt compression syndrome. The posterior condyle refer-

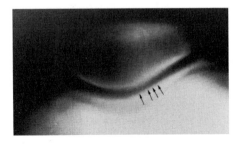

Figure 8.8. Axial view arthrography shows lateral patellofemoral cartilage damage and narrowing (*arrows*). With the advent of magnetic resonance imaging, however, patellofemoral arthrography is rarely indicated.

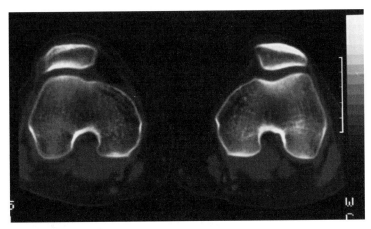

Figure 8.9. These computed tomography images show how the trochlear image can vary substantially, depending on how the tomographic slice is taken. The posterior condyles provide a more consistent reference plane for determining tilt.

ence line is symmetric and reproducible for determining the patellar tilt angle. This reference line can only be obtained with a properly oriented tomographic image of the patellofemoral joint. The anterior trochlear anatomy varies so much that a determination of tilt using a line across the trochlea carries some risk of inaccuracy (Fig. 8.9).

CT offers the option of serial images with the knee in increasing flexion. This can be very helpful in determining whether a patient has progressive tilt (increasing tilt with increased knee flexion) or transient tilt (tilt of the patella in early knee flexion that corrects with further flexion). In the asymptomatic control studies available (5), the patellar tilt angle using CT was never less than 7 degrees, even at full extension. With the knee flexed 10 to 20 degrees, the patellar tilt angle was not less than 12 to 14 degrees in asymptomatic normal volunteers (20 knees). CT is also very helpful postoperatively, when necessary, to see whether appropriate correction has been accomplished (Fig. 8.10).

MRI provides articular cartilage images but generally does not usually allow images in different degrees of knee flexion, unless kinematic MRI is available. This is not usually the case and cost is generally prohibitive.

Indirect Signs of Excessive Pressure

With excessive lateral pressure related to chronic lateral patellar tilt, there will ultimately be changes in the osseous portions of the patellofemoral joint, including medial osteopenia (diminished contact) and subchondral sclerosis (related to overload) as well as lateral joint space narrowing.

Subchondral Bone

Increased density in the subchondral bone layer may be evident early in the syndrome, mainly under the lateral facet (Fig. 8.11). Also, there may be some decrease in medial facet subchondral density as it becomes relatively unloaded. The cancellous portions of bone are equally involved and serve as an indirect sign of excessive lateral compartment load. These are not inevitable changes, and cartilage softening has been encountered

**PATELLAR TILT ANGLE IMPROVEMENT FOLLOWING
LATERAL RELEASE OR ANTEROMEDIALIZATION**

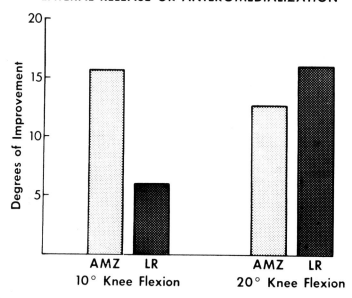

Figure 8.10. Computed tomography before and after lateral release or anteromedial tibial tubercle transfer demonstrates substantial reduction of abnormal patellar tilt postoperatively. Of course, this will occur only if abnormal tilt was present preoperatively. *AMZ*, anteromedialization; *LR*, lateral release. Reprinted with permission from Fulkerson J, Schutzer S, Ramsby G, Bernstein R. Computerized tomography of the patellofemoral joint before and after lateral release or realignment. Arthroscopy 1987;3(1):19–24.

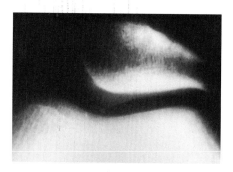

Figure 8.11. Subchondral plate of the lateral side is markedly thickened. Relative medial compartment porosis is also evident.

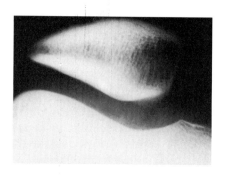

Figure 8.12. Trabeculae of the patellae are seen to be oriented perpendicular to the lateral facet rather than perpendicular to the equator of the patella.

without them. Subchondral cysts are evidence of advanced cartilage changes, even though they may be present without significant joint narrowing. Surprisingly, there are even some patients with subchondral bone sclerosis who live with very little pain. Usually, however, pain increases as the joint deteriorates. Subchondral bone is richly innervated (8, 9). Schneider et al (10) regard subchondral hypertension as one cause of patellar pain; relief of such pain is sometimes reduced by drilling.

Lateralization of Cancellous Trabeculae (Fig. 8.12)

It will be recalled that the trabeculae of the patella normally run perpendicular to the equator of the patella. With tilt compression, there may be a change in this orientation as the trabeculae become more perpendicular to the lateral facet. As the lateral vector increases due either to lateral tethering or to increased Q angle, the resultant force (the summation of the resultant of flexion and the lateral tilt vector) is more perpendicular to the lateral facet. Both the sclerosis and lateralization would appear to be a simple expression of Wolff's law (11).

Patellar Dysplasias

It is likely that excessive lateral pressure during embryonic growth and development will modify the shape of the patella, which ossifies rather late, as well as the trochlea. This would follow the law of Delpech (12) enunciated in 1829, concerning the influence of compression and tensile forces on an epiphysis. Hueter (13) and Volkmann (14) recognized these factors in 1862. Compression retards epiphyseal growth, whereas decreased pressure of traction stimulates epiphyseal growth. This has been referred to as the Hueter-Volkmann law and has been confirmed experimentally by several authors (15, 16). Relative elongation and flattening of the lateral facet as seen in the Wiberg Type III patella and the Alpine hunter's cap deformity are examples.

Hypoplasia of the Lateral Trochlea

This is likely a result of excessive modulating force during growth, similar to what occurs on the patellar side. Retardation of lateral trochlear development (or flattening of the lateral trochlea) because of excessive lateral facet compression is most likely caused by chronic lateral tilt and/or lateral translation (subluxation) of the patella.

Lateral Margin Fracture (Fig. 8.13)

These are different from bipartite patella in that the margins are irregular and the separation is greater. However, if the fracture fragments are brought together on the radiographic view, one has the impression of a patella too wide for the sulcus. These may also represent a fatigue fracture from excessive lateral pull on the patella (17), secondary to a shortened retinaculum. With repeated knee flexion, the "fixed" patella is unable to subluxate, and eventually a lateral margin fracture may occur.

Lateral Margin Osteophytes

Macnab (18) signaled the importance of traction in osteophyte production. The osteophyte may extend the lateral border of the patella, giving the impression of wrapping

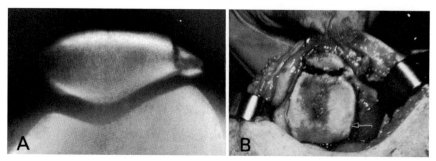

Figure 8.13. A, Lateral marginal fracture indicates excessive lateral tension, in this case associated with a very minor injury. **B,** Operative view of the same patient. The fracture margin is outlined by methylene blue. The distal portion of the lateral facet shows marked fibrillation (*darkened area*). The *arrow* marks the proximal portion of the patella at the median ridge.

around the lateral condyle. As in the lateral margin fracture, such osteophytes are most likely a result of chronic excessive lateral traction from a secondarily shortened retinaculum that exerts pathologic pull on the patella on flexing the knee. They are almost always associated with articular degeneration related to hyperpressure as well (19–21).

Soft-Tissue Changes

The lateral retinaculum may become visible on a slightly underpenetrated view, testifying to the thickening of this fibrous tissue. CT gives a better view of the peripatellar retinaculum (Fig. 8.14). Ultimately, however, MRI gives the best view of retinacular and soft-tissue structures. The indirect radiographic features are summarized in Figure 8.15. Around the knee, the quadriceps tendon and both medial and lateral retinacula are more densely innervated by Type IVA nerve endings than is synovium (8). Witonski and Wagrowski-Danielewicz (22) showed that pain substance (substance P) is present in the knee retinaculum of patients with knee pain. Neural growth factor produced in response to ischemia (23) (tension in the lateral retinaculum) is a likely cause of the retinacular nerve changes in patients with patellofemoral pain. These changes were first described in 1985 (3). Sanchis-Alfonso and Rosello-Sastre (24) later substantiated these findings and noted associated immunohistochemical changes.

ETIOLOGY

Excessive Lateral Ligamentous Tension

There are many reasons to believe that the lateral retinaculum causes and perpetuates many patellofemoral problems. Certainly bone, synovium, and fat pad are important also, but the retinaculum is far more important than commonly recognized. There are several ways in which this may come about. First, we develop the arguments for implicating the lateral soft-tissue structures.

Clinical Evidence

Many cases of ELPS demonstrate a clear difference in transverse passive movement. In these cases, the lateral retinaculum can be palpated and found to be thickened,

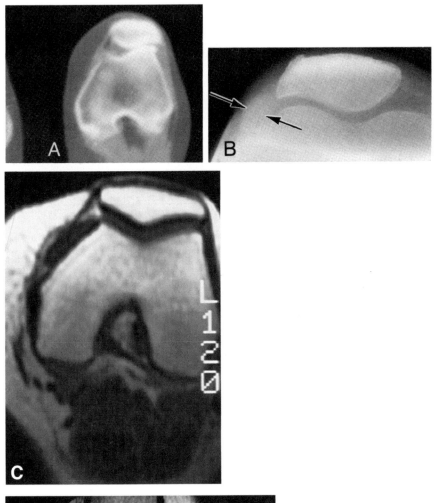

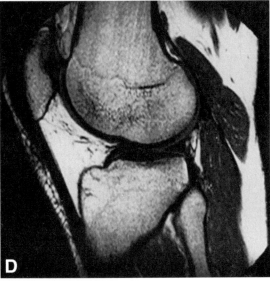

Figure 8.14. A, Peripatellar retinaculum can be demonstrated
using computed tomography. Magnetic resonance imaging (MRI) will
also provide a view of the peripatellar retinaculum. **B,** Retinacular
thickening may be visible occasionally on an axial view also. **C,** MRI of
retinaculum. **D,** MRI shows patellar
tendon.

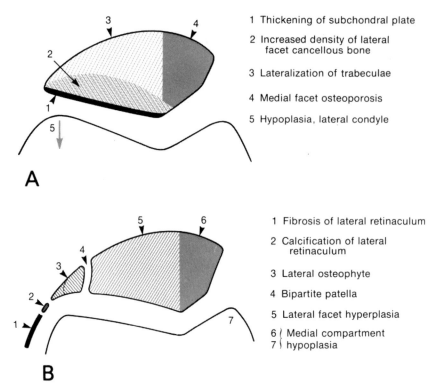

1 Thickening of subchondral plate

2 Increased density of lateral facet cancellous bone

3 Lateralization of trabeculae

4 Medial facet osteoporosis

5 Hypoplasia, lateral condyle

A

1 Fibrosis of lateral retinaculum

2 Calcification of lateral retinaculum

3 Lateral osteophyte

4 Bipartite patella

5 Lateral facet hyperplasia

6 } Medial compartment
7 } hypoplasia

B

Figure 8.15. A, Indirect radiographic signs of excessive lateral pressure. **B,** Indirect radiographic signs of excessive lateral ligamentous tension.

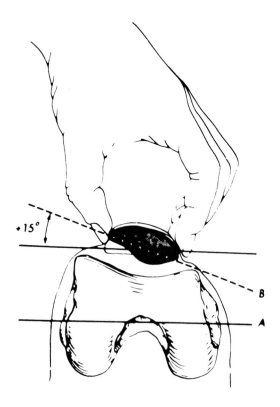

Figure 8.16. The clinician should be able to elevate the lateral facet 15 degrees or more from the horizontal plane in a normal knee. Reprinted with permission from Kolowich P, Paulos L, Rosenberg T, Farnsworth S. Lateral release of the patella: Indications and contraindications. Am J Sports Med 1990;18(4):359–365.

indurated, and retracted. In these forms, the diagnosis, when searched for systematically, is not difficult. However, more frequently, the lateralizing forces of the lateral retinaculum are brought into play only during flexion and extension. In these cases, the transverse "play" in full extension may be normal. Flexion, however, results in excessive tightening of lateral soft-tissue structures as the patella is brought into and over the trochlea. This may escape clinical detection but is evident in other aspects of the complete evaluation. Careful evaluation of lateral "tether" by elevating the lateral facet manually, as described by Kolowich (4), may be the most reliable clinical test for tilt (Fig. 8.16).

Anatomic-Pathologic Evidence

The dysplasias nearly always show evidence of excessive lateral modulating forces during skeletal development; lateral predominance (e.g., Wiberg Type III, Baumgartl type) single lateral facet, half-moon patella, and congenital dislocation with secondary valgus deformity of the knee are examples. Autopsy studies (19–21) show ulceration of patellar cartilage to be centered on the median ridge and the lateral facet, indicating that this is the localization for the effect of excessive forces. (The findings of surface changes elsewhere in the joint are not an argument against predominantly lateral excessive pressure.)

The direct evidence comes from specimens removed at surgery. If the lateral retinaculum is found to be tender preoperatively, the histology may show evidence of small nerve fibrosis.

Radiographic Evidence

There is surprisingly little correlation of axial radiographic tilt with pain in the literature (25). Much of this has to do with uncontrolled technique, axial views in too much flexion, and lack of control data on asymptomatic knees. Schutzer et al (26), however, did provide control data, using CT, confirming distinct alignment differences in patients with patellofemoral pain compared with 20 asymptomatic control knees. Bipartite patella may be a type of stress fracture, with failure to reunite, or it may be the pathologic development of a secondary center, also under the influence of excessive stress. Of bipartite patella, 90% of cases are localized to the superolateral corner of the patella, at the tendinous insertion of the vastus lateralis. Tripartite patella is rare, but those that we have seen have shown the second fragment to be localized to the inferolateral border of the patella in the region of the insertion from the fascia lata. Rohlederer (27) reported a case of fusion of the bipartite fragment to the rest of the patella after simple release of the lateral retinaculum. It would be difficult to conceive a more elegant experimental situation to lend support to these concepts. Moreover, the development of a bipartite fragment may represent a method of reduction of the excess lateral pressure during growth. It is certain that many, if not most, bipartite patellae remain asymptomatic, only to be revealed at the time of injury or fortuitously by radiographs for other reasons.

Operative Findings

Confronted with a patient who has patellofemoral clinical, physical, and radiologic findings suggesting pain and tilt compression syndrome, the clinician may seek confirmation of the concept at the operating room table. Figure 8.17 shows the spontaneous separation of the lateral retinaculum with the knee in full extension. It has not been

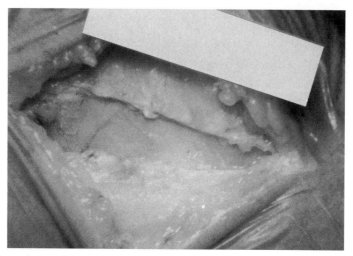

Figure 8.17. This patient with excessive lateral pressure syndrome has the knee in full extension after retinaculum section; there is a spontaneous separation of 1.5 cm.

uncommon to observe a separation of 1.5 cm with the knee flexed to 90 degrees. The dynamic test for lateral tension is to reattach the lateral retinaculum after it has been released with a single 2-0 suture. On flexing the knee to 90 degrees, the suture will normally hold unless there is excessive tension in the lateral retinaculum. Under this excessive tension, the suture will either break or pull out of the soft tissue. These observations confirm the considerable tension that can develop in these lateral structures. In the majority of cases, excessive retinacular tension is a major factor contributing to ELPS. Such tension might reasonably explain the ischemic damage to retinacular nerves, which has been histologically proven (3, 8, 24).

Therapeutic Results

"The proof of the pudding is in the eating," said Don Quixote. The final argument is the most convincing. By relieving excessive lateral tension through surgical section of the lateral retinaculum, without any other surgical maneuver, it is possible to relieve many patients of their symptoms. Also, CT of patellofemoral joints before and after lateral release for patellar tilt in patients with pain shows that abnormal tilt is usually reversed to normal alignment (28), which again supports the belief that a tight lateral retinaculum causes and perpetuates patellar tilt. After considering all the evidence, the clinician is led to the conviction that excessive tension in the lateral retinaculum is, indeed, a major contributing factor in most cases of ELPS.

Causes of Excessive Lateral Ligamentous Tension

Development

Abnormal tension in the lateral retinaculum probably develops in the course of growth, only to be clinically revealed after an injury or with the passage of time. This concept is not so strange if one thinks about the more apparent anomalies that may remain clinically silent for many years, that is, genu varum, femoral anteversion, dysplasia of the hip, and so on. It also explains three clinical situations that are not rare: (a) A radiograph taken immediately or soon after an injury shows clearly evident lateral joint line narrowing. ELPS, therefore, pre-existed the injury. (b) Conservative measures may render a patient with ELPS symptom free; however, the radiographic evidence remains unchanged. (c) There may be radiographic evidence of excessive lateral tilt on the clinically "normal" side. Thus, it appears that excessive lateral tilt may preexist clinical symptoms, only to be revealed when additional factors add to the disequilibrium, such as ischemic (23) or traumatic small nerve injury and elaboration of substance (22). This imbalance may affect the synovium (8), retinaculum (3, 13, 24), bone (8), or possibly even the fat pad (29).

It is most likely, however, that lateral retinacular shortening occurs secondary to chronic lateralization and/or tilt of the patella. If there is a persistent lateral malalignment, there will be adaptive shortening of the lateral retinaculum. This adaptively shortened retinaculum will not only perpetuate, but may actually aggravate, an existing patellar lateralization or tilt of the patella. The adaptively shortened retinaculum ultimately *causes* articular problems (ELPS), particularly as the child grows into adolescence and adulthood.

Acquired Form

K-wire or screw fixation for fracture treatment, local trauma, or capsulitis (dystrophy) may lead to the formation of abnormal lateral tethering forces that may be at the origin of excessive lateral tension. The same thing may happen also on the medial side. However, this is much less common. One must remember the potential impact in retinacular tissues whenever patellar alignment or repair surgery is necessary.

Congenital Form

We have seen that abnormal fascial bands may be responsible for congenital or recurrent dislocation of the patella. They may also, in a lesser form, be responsible for the excessive lateral tension that leads to ELPS. The latter two causes account for approximately 10% of cases.

Disruption of Medial Stabilizers

Anything that diminishes the factors that naturally stabilize valgus forces normally operating on the patellofemoral joint will cause a disequilibrium in favor of the lateral forces. Rupture of the medial retinaculum is the most common of these factors. Diminution of the retentive power of the medial retinacular structures may follow medial arthrotomy, patellar subluxation, or dislocation. Chronic effusion may bulge out the medial capsular structures, rendering them less effective. Atrophy of the vastus medialis reduces this medial stabilization. Tearing of the medial patellofemoral ligament after dislocation can lead to instability because this is part of the medial retinaculum.

Residual Retinacular Band

After lateral retinacular release, a small number of patients continue to have pain despite release for appropriate indications and minimal arthrosis. On clinical examination of such patients, the author has noted bands of tender retinaculum, usually either proximal or distal to the release, in some patients. A very localized injection of 1% lidocaine into the tender portion of the band may give complete relief of the patient's pain.

If a band of tender retinaculum is left after lateral release, pain may not only persist, it may *intensify* because other retinacular supports have been removed, and therefore, the residual tender band may experience increased loads. Transection of the painful residual band usually brings prompt relief.

Treatment of Patients with Tilt Compression (Nonoperative)

Nonoperative treatment of patients with patellar tilt should focus on mobilization of tight quadriceps and lateral retinaculum, medial quadriceps and hip external rotator strengthening, gait and foot pronation correction, hamstring and quadriceps stretching, bracing or taping, and antiinflammatory treatment of any intraarticular synovitis secondary to articular breakdown. It is particularly important in these patients to recognize that there is likely to be focal lateral facet overload, so isokinetic strengthening or resistance weight training through a range of motion must be approached cautiously. The rehabilitation program should incorporate selective medial quadriceps strengthening and taping, as discussed in Chapter 12. Trupull bracing (DJ Ortho, Vista, CA) (Fig. 8.18) is most helpful in controlling lateral instability or maintaining a stretch on tight lateral retinaculum to enhance the rehabilitation program.

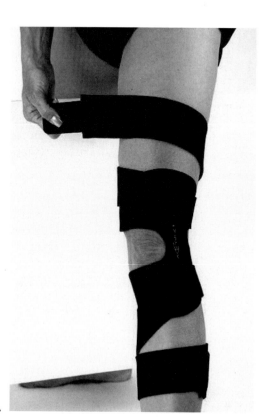

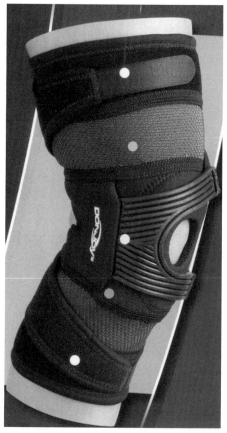

A   B

Figure 8.18. The Trupull patellofemoral braces (DJ Ortho, Vista, CA) provide secure, easily adjustable support for the patella (braces patented by author). **A,** Trupull wrap. **B,** Trupull advanced system.

When chronic tilt has progressed to medial and lateral facet arthrosis, nonoperative treatment may be less successful but still worth pursuing. Lateral facet collapse will not resolve with nonoperative rehabilitation, but retinacular strain may respond to stretching. Synovitis should improve with antiinflammatory medication. Correction of pronation may alter articular load distribution slightly. Hvid et al (30) noted that the stage of chondromalacia did not affect the outcome of nonoperative rehabilitation at an average of 5.7 years from onset, further substantiating the importance of retinaculum.

In short, nonoperative treatment of patients with tilt compression syndrome should be designed for each specific patient, focusing on each component of the disorder and avoiding any treatment that might aggravate the problem.

LATERAL RELEASE FOR THE PATIENT WITH TILT COMPRESSION SYNDROME

Years ago, lateral retinacular release was shown to be effective for the relief of many patients who have patellofemoral pain (31–38). Although initial studies did not differentiate the tracking patterns of such patients, it has become more apparent that lateral retinacular release may reduce lateral tension on the patella, thereby reducing load on the patellar articular surfaces.

Most patients with patellar tilt *but little arthrosis* (39) should benefit from lateral retinacular release (Fig. 8.19). Lateral retinacular release will reduce abnormal tilting of the patella (increasing the lateral patellofemoral angle as described in Chapter 4) provided the lateral facet has not collapsed (28). Huberti and Hayes (40), however, noted that there was little or no change of patellar contact pressure in a cadaver laboratory model when there was no specific prerelease tilt of the patella. Vuorinen et al (41) noted specifically that operations that modify patellar mechanics are most successful in treating patients with patellar articular cartilage lesions. *It is important, therefore, that lateral release be done only when it will have a mechanically beneficial effect (such as relieving documented tilt).*

When the lateral facet has collapsed as a result of ELPS, lateral release will be less effective in reducing tilt (29). If pain in the patient who has lateral facet arthrosis is pre-

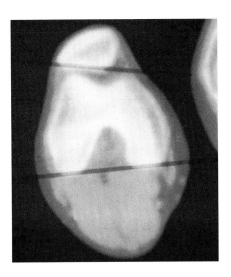

Figure 8.19. The patellar tilt angle in this patient is 4 degrees with the knee flexed 20 degrees. If there are minimal articular cartilage damage and patellofemoral pain that will not respond to a full nonoperative course of treatment, lateral release should be very helpful.

dominantly noted in the retinaculum [presumably caused by retinacular neurofibrosis (3)], lateral retinacular release may still be very helpful. If pain is more related to arthrosis (Outerbridge Grades 3 to 4), the surgeon may consider anteromedial tibial tubercle transfer (42, 43) to unload the lateral patella at the same time that lateral retinacular release is accomplished. This decision is best made on clinical grounds. Certainly, when lateral retinacular release has failed to benefit a patient with lateral patellar tilt and lateral facet arthrosis, anteromedial tibial tubercle transfer becomes a desirable alternative (see Chapter 13 for technical details).

TECHNIQUE OF LATERAL RETINACULAR RELEASE

Diagnostic arthroscopy is extremely helpful in defining and quantitating articular damage in the patient who has patellofemoral disease. The initial arthroscopy, preceding lateral release, should rule out other intraarticular pathology, debride synovitis, correlate patellar tracking with radiographic findings, quantitate and characterize articular lesions, and rule out loose bodies elsewhere in the knee.

The surgeon may choose then to perform an arthroscopic lateral retinacular release, provided the tourniquet is released and hemostasis achieved. A short 3- to 4-cm long incision immediately adjacent to the lateral patella also provides easy access for lateral release. A nerve stimulator may be placed on the femoral nerve proximally to stimulate a quadriceps contraction under anesthesia and thereby simulate dynamic patellar tracking. The lateral retinaculum and *synovium* are incised with a scalpel under direct vision, and particular care is taken to release the lateral retinaculum enough to allow reverse tilting of the patella (lifting away from the lateral trochlea). Excessive release is inappropriate and may occasionally lead to a problem of medial dynamic subluxation of the patella. Rarely, an overly aggressive lateral release can even result in quadriceps rupture. Partial release of any tight retropatellar tendon fat pad while raising the lateral edge of the patella is helpful. This helps to divert the lateral release at this level *away* from the lateral meniscus and ensures that any minor component of infrapatellar contracture is released. Particular care is taken to *avoid the lateral meniscus.* The vastus lateralis obliquus (see Chapter 1) may be released along the fatty plane that separates it from the main vastus lateralis tendon. *Care is taken to avoid the main tendon of the vastus lateralis.* The procedure, when performed this way, permits release of both static and dynamic lateral patellar supports and enables the surgeon to evert the patella such that open debridement or arthroplasty may be undertaken selectively, taking care to preserve intact articular cartilage wherever possible. One should ensure that an adequate release has been achieved (44). If the surgeon has defined a consistently painful segment of the lateral retinaculum, this portion should be excised and sent for histologic examination with Gomori trichrome stain (3) with the intent of looking for small nerve injury in the lateral retinaculum. Through a short incision, the surgeon can achieve excellent hemostasis, and postoperative hemarthrosis becomes unlikely. It is our impression that this short lateral incision introduces no significant morbidity when compared with arthroscopic lateral release, and technical accuracy, including release of the vastus lateralis obliquus and hemostasis, can be maximized. Nonetheless, we do arthroscopic lateral release, without a tourniquet. If bleeding is excessive, we will extend the lateral incision and maximize hemostasis with open visualization.

After release, patellar tracking may be observed passively and actively, using femoral nerve stimulation by the anesthesiologist, if desired. The subcutaneous tissue and skin are closed, and a compressive wrap is applied, after which *motion and weight bearing are started immediately.*

Complications of Lateral Retinacular Release

Busch and DeHaven (45) reviewed some "pitfalls" of lateral retinacular release. Although this procedure will work well for the majority of patients with persistent pain associated with tilt and less severe articular degeneration, Ogilvie-Harris and Jackson (46) noted that results are not as good when there is more advanced patellar arthrosis.

Hemarthrosis is the most common complication of lateral release. This usually resolves after aspiration of the knee, but occasionally one may need to open the lateral peripatellar region to coagulate an arterial bleeder. The best approach is to avoid this complication by tourniquet release and complete hemostasis at the time of lateral release, open if necessary.

Hughston and Deese (47) pointed out that medial subluxation may complicate lateral release. It is important to recognize this potential complication, but we have found that this rarely occurs if a proper lateral release is done without releasing the main vastus lateralis tendon and the patient has documented prerelease lateral rotation (tilt).

Other complications (48, 49) of lateral release include residual patellar subluxation (Fig. 8.20) infection, deep venous thrombosis, prolonged weakness, reflex sympathetic dystrophy, dehiscence, and compensation abuse. If a patient has residual feelings of instability, it is most important to establish whether there is medial subluxation, in which case,

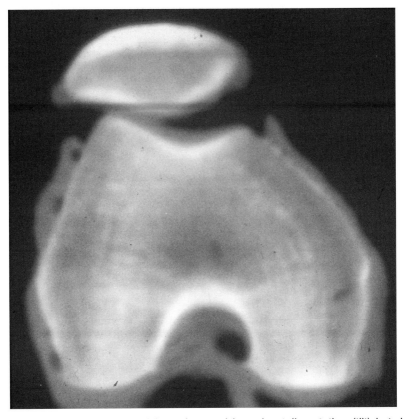

Figure 8.20. Lateral release diminishes abnormal lateral patella rotation (tilt) but does *not* consistently or predictably correct patella subluxation. This computed tomography image shows a cadaver knee demonstration of lateral release for tilt and subluxation (with deficient medial retinaculum). In this situation, tilt is corrected, but subluxation is not. (Courtesy of Dr. William Post, Morgantown, WV.)

the patient will experience the patella *moving laterally from too far medially back into the trochlea in early knee flexion* (50).

CASE HISTORIES

Patient 1 (32-Year-Old Female Hairdresser)

This patient had spontaneous onset of pain in both knees, in the left more than the right, 3 years before first being seen. One and one-half years after the onset, she noted swelling in both knees at the end of the day standing at work, which was associated with a sense of heaviness in the knees. Going up and down stairs particularly increased the pain. *On examination:* Flexion/extension was full, there was no ligamentous laxity, and there were no meniscal signs. There was pain on compression of the lateral facet and on extension of the knee against resistance. The patella tracked normally on clinical examination. Crepitus could be felt on moving the patella both longitudinally and transversely in the trochlea. Transverse movement (i.e., the patellar play) was decreased. The patient was unable to squat. Physical signs were identical on both sides. *Radiograph:* Antero-posterior, lateral, and axial views were all within normal limits. *Operative findings* (Fig.

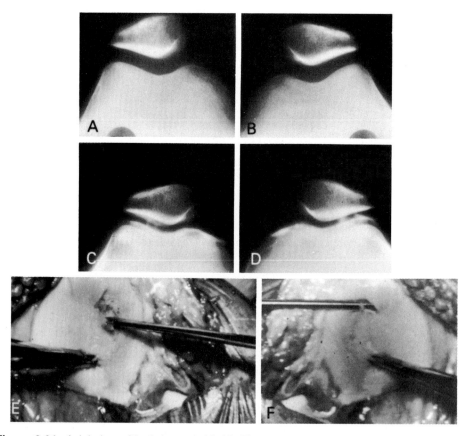

Figure 8.21. Axial view of both knees with **(A, B)** and without **(C, D)** contrast material compared with operative findings **(E, F)** (patient 1).

8.21): In the right knee, there were Outerbridge Grade 3 findings on the lateral facet, with fissures and softened cartilage. The patellar surface was debrided of loose cartilage; on the left knee, there were Outerbridge Grade 3 to 4 changes, more extensive than in the right knee, affecting the entire medial and lateral facets, with one long horizontal fissure extending from the median ridge into the lateral third of the lateral facet. Secondary stellate fissures reached subchondral bone along nearly the entire lateral border; patellar debridement was coupled with microfracture arthroplasty, using Steadman picks. Limited synovectomy was also done. The patient started immediate range of motion and was kept on crutches for 6 weeks with toe-touch weight bearing only. The postoperative course was uncomplicated. The patient returned to work 2 months after the surgery. *Follow-up at 1 year:* The patient continued to work but also continued to have pain and swelling at the end of a day's work and some difficulty with stairs. Because of the advanced arthrosis, this patient eventually may be a candidate for patellar anteriorization. The right knee would be particularly amenable to steep anteromedial tibial tubercle transfer to shift contact stress from the arthritic lateral facet onto better medial cartilage and reduce overall load. In retrospect, a CT scan might have revealed tilt of the patella in early flexion, at which time a decision to do lateral release in addition to debridement would have been appropriate. In view of the advanced cartilage changes, initial tibial tubercle anteromedialization might have eliminated the need for reoperation. Because there was no documented lateral rotation (tilt) of the patella, it is doubtful that lateral release would have helped much, if at all. Taking the less invasive approach is certainly reasonable, but the patient should be warned that there is risk of recurrent difficulty. Some patients who are substantially disabled may opt for more definitive surgery.

Patient 2 (16-Year-Old Girl)

This patient had spontaneous onset of bilateral anterior knee pain 3 years before consultation. Pain had gradually increased in severity and was worse at the end of the day. She was completely unable to participate in sports. *Examination:* There was mild ligamentous laxity, no meniscal signs, and no significant quadriceps atrophy. The knee showed a full range of movement, but transverse patellar play was reduced, and there was a *tender and tight lateral retinaculum bilaterally.* Extension against resistance was painful. The patella was noted to have a more definite lateral excursion at the end of extension than normal. Anteroposterior and lateral radiographs were normal; the axial patellar view showed no subluxation, but the 15-degree knee flexion midtransverse CT cuts showed 4-degree patellar tilt angles bilaterally (radiographic proof of abnormal rotation or tilt). A 6-month rehabilitation program failed, and, therefore, a lateral retinacular release was performed on the right knee. There was softening of the entire lateral facet and the median ridge, with small fibrillations of the surface. The trochlea appeared to be more prominent than usual. The patient returned with pain in the other knee identical in all respects to the right side. The patient had the same procedure, at which time softening in the area of the median ridge in the critical zone was noted (Fig. 8.22). The patient was seen in follow-up and had relief of symptoms on both sides, with a return to normal rotation on a repeat CT study 1 year after surgery.

Patient 3 (30-Year-Old Man)

This patient had a lateral release because of persistent patellofemoral pain associated with tilt but was referred because of persistent, *increased* anterior knee pain. On exami-

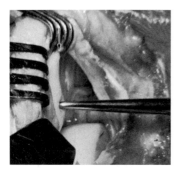

Figure 8.22. Softening localized to area noted by the instrument (*arrow* marks lateral patellar margin).

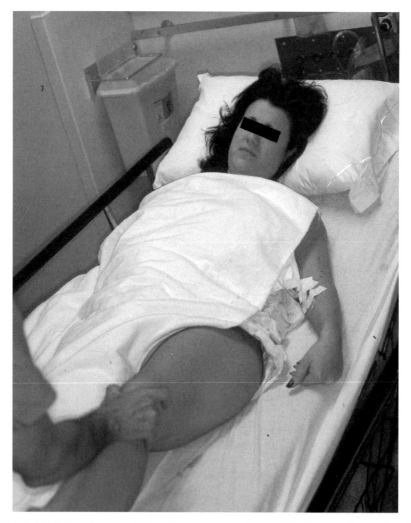

Figure 8.23. Medial subluxation test. This is a provocative test that is negative in the absence of medial subluxation. The patella is held medially with the knee in extension and then released on abrupt knee flexion. Reproduction of the patient's symptom strongly suggests a problem of medial patella subluxation.

nation, he had clinically normal patellar alignment, with no crepitation in the patellofemoral joint. Further examination revealed a single tender band of residual lateral retinaculum running from the distal patella to the tibia. Injection of the tender portion of this band gave complete relief of the patient's pain. The patient was referred back to the operating surgeon, with a recommendation that the residual band of painful retinaculum be released.

Patient 4 (27-Year-Old Woman)

This patient became much worse, with painful giving way of the knee, soon after a lateral release had been done. A referring orthopedist was contemplating medial patellofemoral ligament reconstruction despite normal radiographs because the patient was complaining of the patella moving laterally. On clinical examination, the patient had a positive medial subluxation test [the patella held medially with the knee extended and released on knee flexion (50)] (Fig. 8.23), confirming a diagnosis of medial patellar subluxation (the patella slipping from too far medially back into the trochlea) with daily activity. She was greatly relieved after a lateral tenodesis was done.

REFERENCES

1. Ficat P, Hungerford D. Disorders of the Patellofemoral Joint. Baltimore: Williams & Wilkins; 1977.
2. Fulkerson J. Evaluation of peripatellar soft tissues and retinaculum in patients with patellofemoral pain. Clin Sports Med 1989;8(2):197–202.
3. Fulkerson J, Tennant R, Jaivin J, Grunnet M. Histological evidence of retinacular nerve injury associated with patellofemoral malalignment. Clin Orthop 1985;197:196.
4. Kolowich P, Paulos L, Rosenberg T, Farnsworth S. Lateral release of the patella: Indications and contraindications. Am J Sports Med 1990;18(4):359–365.
5. Fulkerson J, Kalenak A, Rosenberg T, Cox J. Patellofemoral pain. AAOS Iinstr Course Lect 1992;XLI.
6. Ficat P, Ficat C, Bailleux A. Syndrome d'hyperpression externe de la rotule (SHPE). Rev Chir Orthop 1975;61: 39–59.
7. Wiberg G. Roentgenographic and anatomic studies on the femoro-patellar joint. Acta Orthop Scand 1941;12: 319–410.
8. Biedert R, Kernan V. Neurosensory characteristics of the patellofemoral joint: what is the genesis of patellofemoral pain? Sports Med Arthrosc Rev 2001;9:295–300.
9. Reimann I, Christensen B. A histologic demonstration of nerves in subchondral bone. Acta Orthop Scand 1977; 48:345–352.
10. Schneider U, Graf J, Thomsen M, Wenz W, Niethard F. Das hypertensionssyndrom der patella. Z Orthoop Ihre Grenzgeb 1997;135:70–75.
11. Wolff J. Uber die innere architectur der knochen und ihre bedeutung fur die frage von knochenwachstum. Virchows Arch Pathol Anat 1870;50:389.
12. Delpech JM. De L'orthomorphie, Par Rapport a L'espece Humaine. Paris: Gabon; 1829.
13. Hueter C. Anatomische studien an den extremitatengelenken neugeborener und erwachsener. Virchows Arch Pathol Anat 1862;25:575.
14. Volkmann R. Chirurgie erfanhrungen uber knochenverbiegungen und knochen wachstum. Arch Pathol Anat 1862;24:512.
15. Arkin AM, Katz JF. Effects of pressure on epiphyseal growth. The mechanism of plasticity of growing bone. J Bone Joint Surg 1956;38A:1056.
16. Wilkinson JA. Femoral anteversion in the rabbit. J Bone Joint Surg 1962;44B:386.
17. Devas MB. Stress fractures of the patella. J Bone Joint Surg 1960;42B:71–74.
18. Macnab I. The traction spur. J Bone Joint Surg 1971;53A:663.
19. Emery IH, Meachim G. Surface morphology and topography of patello-femoral cartilage fibrillation in Liverpool necropsies. J Anat 1973;116:103–120.
20. Casscells SW. Gross pathological changes in the knee joint of the aged individual. A study of 300 cases. J Bone Joint Surg 1975;57A:1033.
21. Ficat C. La degenerescence du cartilage de la rotule. De la chondromalacie a l'arthrose. Semin Hop Paris 1974; 50:3201–3209.
22. Witonski D, Wagrowski-Danielewicz M. Distribution of substance P nerve fibers in the knee joint of patients with anterior knee pain syndrome. Knee Surg Sports Traumatol Arthrosc 1999;1:177–183.

23. Lee T, Kato H, Kogurek, Itoyama Y. NGF immunoreactivity after transient focal cerebral ischemia in rats. Brain Research 1996;713:199–210.
24. Sanchis-Alfonso V, Rosello-Sastre. A neuroanatomic basis for anterior knee pain in the active young patient. Am J Sports Med 2000;28:725–731.
25. Post W. Clinical assessment of malalignment: does it correlate with patellofemoral pain? Sports Med Arthrosc Rev 2001:9:301–305.
26. Schutzer S, Ramsky G, Fulkerson J. CT classification of patellofemoral pain patients. Orthop Clin North Am 1986;17:235–248
27. Rohlederer K. L'arthrose de la surface articulaire de la rotule. Rev Chir Orthop 1964;50:361–368.
28. Fulkerson J, Schutzer S, Ramsby G, Bernstein R. Computerized tomography of the patellofemoral joint before and after lateral release or realignment. Arthroscopy 1987;3(1):19–24.
29. Krenn V, Hofmann S, Engel A. first description of mechanoreceptors in the corpus adiposum infrapatellare of man. Acta Anat 1990;137:187–188.
30. Hvid I, Andersen LL Schmidt H. Chondromalacia patellae. The relation to abnormal patellofemoral joint mechanics. Acta Orthop Scand 1981;52(6):661–666.
31. Dzioba RB, Strokon A, Mulbry L. Diagnostic arthroscopy and longitudinal open lateral release: A safe and effective treatment for "chondromalacia patellae." Arthroscopy 1985;1(2):131–135.
32. Grana W, Hinkley B, Hollingsworth S. Arthroscopic evaluation and treatment of patellar malalignment. Clin Orthop 1984;186:122–128.
33. Krompinger J, Fulkerson J. Lateral retinacular release for intractable lateral retinacular pain. Clin Orthop 1983; 179:191–193.
34. Larson RL, Cabaud HE, Slocum DB, James SL, Keenan T, Hutchinson T. The patellar compression syndrome: Surgical treatment by lateral retinacular release. Clin Orthop 1978;134:158–167.
35. Metcalf R. An arthroscopic method for lateral release of the subluxating or dislocating patella. Clin Orthop 1982;167:9–18.
36. Merchant A, Mercer R. Lateral release of the patella: A preliminary report. Clin Orthop 1974;103:40–45.
37. Schonholtz G. Lateral retinacular release of the patella. Arthroscopy 1987;3:269–272.
38. Scuderi G, ed. The Patella. New York: Springer-Verlag; 1995.
39. Outerbridge RE. The etiology of chondromalacia patellae. J Bone Joint Surg 1961;43B:752–757.
40. Huberti HH, Hayes WC. Contact pressures in chondromalacia patellae and the effects of capsular reconstructive procedures. J Orthop Res 1988;6(4):499–508.
41. Vuorinen OP, Paakkala T, Tunturi T, Harkonen M, Salo K, Tervo T. Chondromalacia patellae. Results of operative treatment. Arch Orthop Trauma Surg 1985;104(3):175–181.
42. Fulkerson J. Anteromedialization of the tibial tuberosity for patellofemoral malalignment. Clin Orthop 1983; 177:176–181.
43. Fulkerson JP, Schutzer SF. After failure of conservative treatment for painful patellofemoral malalignment: Lateral release or realignment? Orthop Clin North Am 1986;17(2):283–288.
44. Fu FH, Maday MG. Arthroscopic lateral release and the lateral patellar compression syndrome (review). Orthop Clin North Am 1992;23(4):601–612.
45. Busch M, DeHaven K. Pitfalls of lateral retinacular release. Clin Sports Med 1989;8(2):279–290.
46. Ogilvie-Harris D, Jackson R. The arthroscopic treatment of chondromalacia patellae. J Bone Joint Surg 1984; 66B:660–665.
47. Hughston J, Deese M. Medial subluxation of the patella as a complication of lateral retinacular release. Am J Sports Med 1988;16:383–388.
48. DeLee J. Complications of arthroscopy and arthroscopic surgery. Arthroscopy 1985;1:214–220.
49. Small N. Complications in arthroscopy: The knee and other joints. Arthroscopy 1986;4:253–258.
50. Fulkerson J. A clinical test for medial patella tracking. Tech Orthop 1997;12:165–169.

9

Patellar Subluxation

"I find the great thing in this world is not so much where we
stand, as in what direction we are moving."
—*Oliver Wendell Holmes*

A patella may articulate abnormally such that it is transiently or permanently medial or lateral to its normal tracking course. In general, subluxation (or lateral translation) of the patella will involve transient lateral movement of the patella early in knee flexion such that the patient will experience a feeling of instability or pain; however, some patients may have chronic lateral tracking of the patella. It is most important to differentiate between this form of abnormal patellar alignment and *tilt* because there can be lateral translation with or without tilt (lateral rotation) and tilt with or without lateral translation. In order to be clear to those with different definitions of *subluxation,* in this book the terms *subluxation* and *translation* will be used interchangeably, whereas *tilt* will refer specifically to *rotation* of the patella out of the coronal plane.

Subluxation may be considered minor, major, or permanent and may be either congenital or secondary to injury or trauma. Awareness of the nature of a patient's subluxation will be helpful in formulating a treatment plan and prognosis.

TYPES OF SUBLUXATION (TRANSLATION)

Minor Recurrent Lateral Subluxation

In this case, the patella deviates little from the normal patellar course and is not associated with any gross or perhaps even clinically apparent relocation. These minor forms are often the result of a functional imbalance between the articular surfaces of the patella and the femoral trochlea. Larsen and Lund (1) have noted that patellofemoral incongruence is common after extensor mechanism rupture, and even less dramatic traumatic events may leave residual subluxation. One also must consider that there are many asymptomatic people in the normal population who have minor subluxation and no clinically significant symptoms.

Major Recurrent Lateral Subluxation

In this condition, the patella comes nearly astride the lateral trochlear facet and then suddenly returns to the patellofemoral groove with an audible snap. Episodes of near dislocation occur particularly at the beginning of flexion or semiflexion and recur with a variable rhythm. They may occur infrequently, perhaps associated with strenuous activity, and may be associated with patella alta (2). Episodes may occur with each flexion of

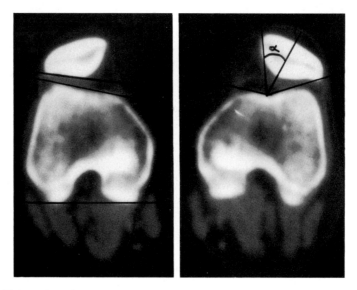

Figure 9.1. This patient demonstrates bilateral subluxation and tilt. Although there is no sign of arthrosis here, this combination usually leads to patellar articular cartilage degeneration.

the knee or intermittently. Most often, they occur at frequent intervals. It is possible that one of these episodes may proceed to a complete dislocation, a possible complication of recurrent subluxation. For our purposes, a patella will not be considered dislocated unless it is completely displaced out of the femoral trochlea. It is likely that many cases of major recurrent subluxation are included in series describing recurrent dislocation, which explains why some authors have reported them in combined series (3).

Persistent Lateral Patella Displacement

This form of lateral displacement is stable, in that the lateral subluxation (displacement) is persistent throughout knee flexion. There is little tendency toward recentering of the patella with progressive flexion, and there is always associated tilt (4) (Fig. 9.1). This form may progress rapidly to cartilage degeneration, and most examples already show significant degenerative change at the time of clinical presentation.

At the time of initial presentation, degenerative changes are common, but malalignment is usually greater if there has been significant cartilage loss. The mean age in Ficat's experience was 50 years, whereas Merle D'Aubigne and Ramadier (5) reported a mean age of 62 years.

There are two primary mechanisms for the development of a permanent stable form of lateral displacement: (a) congenital or dysplastic origin or (b) acquired, either through faulty mechanics or surgery. Persistent lateral patella displacement usually leads to arthrosis because of abnormal unit loading of articular cartilage.

ETIOLOGY

Recurrent subluxation is relatively common. Several authors have reported this condition predominantly in women (3, 6, 7), but Hughston (8) emphasized the notion that it also occurs in athletic men. That author found in his series of 60 patients that 25 (42%) were men, all of whom were athletes. Of the 35 women in his series, 10 were athletes. We believe that recurrent patellar subluxation or dislocation may occur after traumatic patellar displacement in athletes of either sex but that women have a greater inherent predisposition to spontaneous malalignment-related patellar instability. Bennett et al (9) have noted that differences in vastus medialis obliquus orientation in women may contribute to their increased tendency to have patellar subluxation. Like recurrent dislocation, it is a disorder of the second decade, although there are individuals who have minor recurrent subluxation for many years before any significant pain or dysfunction occurs.

Congenital Subluxation

Most patients with patellar subluxation are born with extensor mechanism imbalance. Subluxation may result from congenital deficiency of the femoral trochlea, malalignment of the lower extremity related to excessive valgus, excessive hip anteversion, external tibial torsion, pronation of the foot and ankle, or another extremity alignment problem. Soft-tissue imbalance, particularly deficiency of the vastus medialis obliquus or excessive vastus lateralis obliquus pull on the patella, may cause or accentuate extensor mechanism subluxation. Connective-tissue laxity will aggravate any pre-existing extensor mechanism malalignment. Many patients with mild patellar subluxation undoubtedly go unrecognized and, in fact, may have little risk of developing arthrosis or pain if subluxation is minimal and there is no significant tilting of the patella to pathologically increase lateral facet load. Most clinicians realize that minor degrees of subluxation occur in some asymptomatic individuals.

Secondary Subluxation

Patellar subluxation may occur after extensor mechanism injury, knee surgery (Fig. 9.2), or below-knee amputation (10). Dysplasia of the trochlea is less common in secondary subluxation, but treatment still is aimed at restoration of normal alignment.

Trauma is certainly not necessary to cause patellar subluxation, but when it can be extracted from the history, it is nearly always a rotational stress or direct blow (from the

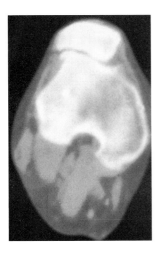

Figure 9.2. This patient had long-standing permanent patellar subluxation and tilt after medial arthrotomy. This led eventually to lateral facet arthrosis. Anteromedial tibial tubercle transfer gave excellent relief to the patient by transferring most articular contact load onto the intact medial facet.

side). The athlete may plant a foot and change direction, with internal rotation of the femur on the fixed tibia in slight flexion and a powerful contraction of the quadriceps. This movement accentuates the lateral vector that normally exists in the extensor apparatus and can cause lateral displacement or dislocation of the patella.

Natural History

Many patients with simple patellar subluxation without tilt (Type I malalignment) show little or no sign of articular cartilage degeneration. Often, these patients have lax ligaments. When there is tilt associated with subluxation (Type II malalignment), progression of articular cartilage deterioration is more prominent because of the increased lateral facet loading. Type I malalignment may show little or very slow progression of articular cartilage softening and degeneration.

Recurrent subluxation may proceed to a frank dislocation at any time that then would render the patella more susceptible to recurrent dislocation related to tearing of the medial patellofemoral ligament. Even a trivial injury can cause dislocation of the unstable subluxating patella. In a sense, then, the patient with patellar subluxation is in a precarious position, limited functionally by apprehension and insecurity on the one hand and risk of dislocation with minor mishaps on the other.

Patellar subluxation (lateral translation) can occur as subluxation alone; subluxation with patellofemoral arthrosis; or subluxation with both patellofemoral arthrosis and tibial-femoral arthrosis.

In asymptomatic individuals, a relative equilibrium has been established, and they are not prone to the giving way and general sense of insecurity characteristic of the recurrent subluxation and dislocation syndromes. Lateral subluxation may not be clinically apparent, and the knee often tracks smoothly in flexion and extension despite lateral tracking of the patella (Fig. 9.3). Many of these people have little or no associated tilt.

When subluxation is accompanied by lateral facet arthrosis, there may be aching pain (typically anterior), trouble with stairs, giving way, and swelling—in short, all the symptoms of patellofemoral arthrosis. Flexion frequently is limited, and a mild fixed flexion contracture is not uncommon. Quadriceps atrophy is often impressive, particularly the vastus medialis. Difficulty with stairs represents the most frequent chief complaint. Obesity often precipitates or aggravates the problem.

As contact studies have shown, flexion of more than 90 degrees brings the patella into direct contact with the tibiofemoral weightbearing area of the femur. Degeneration sometimes spreads to involve the lateral tibiofemoral compartment, and patellofemoral disease often precedes tibiofemoral changes (11). Any significant genu valgum is likely to exacerbate the degeneration of both lateral and patellofemoral compartments, which explains the predominance of knock-kneed elderly women in this end-stage group (Fig. 9.4).

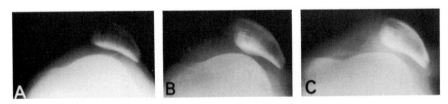

Figure 9.3. Despite substantial patellar subluxation throughout knee flexion and extension, some patients have remarkably little pain or evidence of arthrosis.

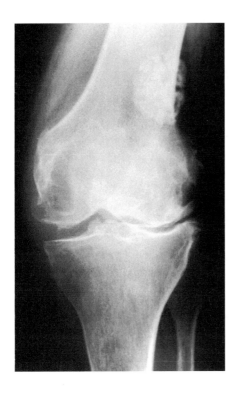

Figure 9.4. Anteroposterior view of the knee in a 58-year-old obese woman with genu valgum, severe lateral compartment arthrosis, and permanent lateral patella subluxation.

This disorder is very frequently bilateral, although the clinical and radiologic stages are frequently not symmetric (Fig. 9.5). However, *as is characteristic clinically of arthrosis in general, the correlation between symptoms and radiologic changes is not always high.* Minor injury may be responsible for pushing the disorder over the clinical threshold.

Although "staging" subluxation may be helpful, it is probably better to describe the specific alignment disorder in each patient, quantitating the relative amounts of subluxation and tilt, and grade the amount and location of arthrosis (4). Of paramount importance is the individual evaluation and classification of each patient. Radiographic changes do not always correlate with pain. Objective observations of abnormal alignment

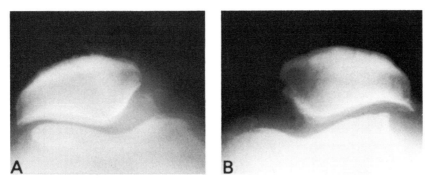

Figure 9.5. A and **B,** Patient with bilateral subluxation.

or cartilage wear are important only insofar as they correlate with the patient's pain or instability.

CLINICAL FEATURES OF SUBLUXATION

History

The most important clinical features are giving way and a feeling of instability or pain. These clinical symptoms are associated with many patellofemoral disorders and are perhaps most frequently mistaken for a torn medial meniscus. Subluxation often is accompanied by tilt, so many of these patients will complain of tightness or discomfort around the patella and may report a history consistent with patellar arthrosis in the later stages of subluxation. The patient may not be specific in describing episodes of subluxation but reports that "something" jumps in the knee or that something is out of place momentarily, causing a sensation of instability and, particularly, of insecurity in performing certain movements. A history of locking is unusual. When elicited, it inevitably means something different from the locking associated with a meniscal tear. The patient generally means a temporary stiffness in the knee that may appear after prolonged sitting and generally disappears after movement. Sometimes there may be a symptomatic flap of synovium or articular cartilage. Pain is generally localized anteriorly, behind the medial aspect of the patella or at the distal pole. Usually crepitus becomes an important complaint only after the clinical entity has persisted for some time, which suggests that subluxation alone, particularly if not accompanied by tilt or dislocation, may spare articular cartilage in some patients. The patient with patellar subluxation frequently complains of apprehension and limitation in sports because of the feeling of insecurity or instability. Episodes of giving way are common, and effusion frequently will accompany such episodes. Snapping and popping often are noted by these patients, although such findings may be less prominent early in the clinical course and in minor recurrent subluxation.

Physical Findings

When pain occurs, it is frequently difficult to localize. Retinacular pain (12, 13) may occur, either in the medial or lateral retinaculum. Some patients also demonstrate patellar tendon or distal patellar apophyseal tenderness, probably because of alteration of normal stresses in this area. Occasionally, the clinician will note tenderness in the distal quadriceps, particularly at the vastus lateralis obliquus or vastus medialis obliquus insertion. Care should be taken to palpate all soft-tissue components around the patella, including the medial infrapatellar ligament and all components of the lateral retinaculum (13). Apprehension is common on displacing the patella in a lateral direction. Hypermobility of the patella, which reflects excessive ligamentous laxity, may be pronounced. Patella alta is notable in some patients. Medial or lateral parapatellar tenderness often is present. Effusion exists only after an acute episode or when secondary cartilage damage has complicated the disorder. Muscle atrophy is very common but generally not as marked as with recurrent dislocation. Minor crepitus may be felt during flexion and extension of the knee under the weight of the leg.

Hughston (8) has described a lateral orientation of the patella with the knee flexed to 90 degrees. Gentle palpation during flexion and extension may reveal a slight lateral overhand of the patella. Occasionally, particularly when the patient is flexing and extending the knee under load (squatting), subluxation can be observed. The patella momentarily perches on the lateral trochlear facet and then suddenly relocates with an audible snap.

It is rare to detect this because it usually occurs under functional circumstances that the patient cannot consciously reproduce. However, the patient should be made aware of what to look for so that he/she may more accurately interpret the episodes when they occur and thus facilitate the correct diagnosis.

An abnormal patellar course is a characteristic sign of patellar instability. The importance of observing the course of the patella from the fully extended knee with the quadriceps set to full flexion and back again has been underlined for many patellar abnormalities. It is particularly important to observe the entrance and exit into the trochlea at between 10 and 20 degrees of flexion. The abnormalities here are many, but some that we have encountered are as follows: (a) an abrupt lateral movement at the termination of extension; (b) a trajectory described by Ficat (14) as "bayonet," which is characterized by an abrupt lateral translation just before full extension and then further extension in a straight line (the entire course is one of two vertical lines connected by an abrupt lateral translation); (3) an atypical semicircular route as if the patella were pivoting around the lateral trochlear facet; and (4) a trajectory in which there is a short medial displacement, just before the final slight external movement associated with full extension. A pattern of patella entry into the trochlea from a slightly *medial* position may suggest a medial subluxation disorder—this can be very subtle.

This list is in no way exhaustive and may even vary with a given case, dependent upon what muscles are brought into play and what movements are carried out with regard to rotation or varus/valgus stress during extension. Perhaps the diversity of observations explains some of the confusion that exists in attempting to classify subluxations and dislocations of the patella. There is a complex interplay of alignment factors, starting with hip and foot rotational alignment and ending with proximal and distal extensor mechanism alignment vectors. It must be remembered, of course, that, at the time of examination, the patellar course may be entirely normal, yet during functional activities, pathologic patellofemoral mechanics may persist. Once a clinical impression is formed, however, one should try to confirm the suspected malalignment pattern radiographically, functionally, and by reproduction of the symptom.

Many patients with simple patellar subluxation have little or no evidence of articular disease (Fig. 9.6). Is it not uncommon to find at arthroscopy that the patellar articular sur-

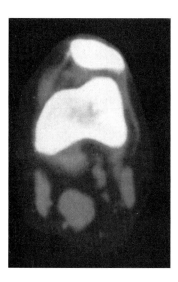

Figure 9.6. Patellar subluxation may occur without any evidence of articular cartilage damage in some patients.

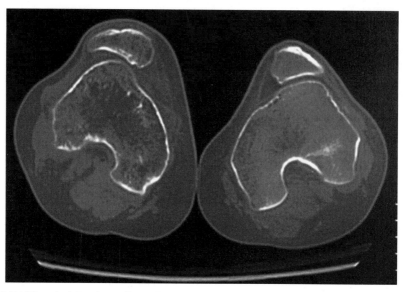

Figure 9.7. Chronic lateral patellar subluxation will lead to dysplastic changes, which usually include elongation and deterioration of the lateral facet, distal medial and central cartilage degeneration, lateral subchondral sclerosis, and flattening of the lateral trochlea.

face is perfectly normal despite considerable apprehension related to instability. However, some patients with patellar subluxation, particularly if there is associated tilt, eventually will develop dysplastic changes (Fig. 9.7), articular cartilage softening, and erosion. Recurrent subluxation accompanied by tilt will lead to lateral facet arthrosis more commonly because of the lateral overload. Once dislocation has occurred, articular damage is common at the medial patellar facet or the lateral trochlea; therefore, procedures that add load to the medial patella must be avoided as much as possible.

Diagnosis

A positive diagnosis of recurrent subluxation can be somewhat difficult, as is always the case at the boundary between normal and abnormal. The diagnosis incorporates the history; the careful physical examination of both knees, particularly the course of the patella in flexion and extension; and the evaluation of radiographs. Computerized tomography (CT), as described in Chapter 4, is particularly helpful in differentiating subluxation from tilt. When a young patient presents with complaints of discomfort, swelling, insecurity, and a poorly defined functional abnormality, vis-á-vis the knee, whether trauma is part of this history or not, the clinician should think systematically about whether the patient manifests predominantly a pattern of subluxation-instability, tilt-compression, or a combination of both.

The patient with hypermobility of the patella and a feeling of insecurity or instability may be more likely to have some degree of patellar subluxation, whereas the patient with a tight, laterally fixed patella and lateral retinacular tenderness is more likely to have a problem with tilting of the patella.

Radiologic Features

Standard tangential radiographs may readily demonstrate subluxation, and either the Laurin 20-degree axial view or the Merchant view, as described in Chapter 4, may show subluxation, particularly if it is more advanced. Some patients with normal tangential (axial) radiographs, however, have significant subluxation that may be detected using CT. Also, there are patients who *appear* to have subluxation on an axial view because of image overlap, but CT will not reveal *actual* subluxation! Flexion of the knee can draw the unstable patella deep into the femoral trochlea so that subtle subluxation problems may be missed. CT may show signs of a patella that is slow to centralize in the trochlea, with notable subluxation on the 10- and 20-degree knee flexion tomographic cuts. This may be important information in the patient who has failed conservative treatment because such patients may have considerable *functional* instability with athletic activities despite normal standard radiographs at 45 degrees of knee flexion. CT can be very helpful also in determining if there is tilt associated with subluxation. Schutzer et al (15) have defined the limits of normal versus abnormal using a group of 20 asymptomatic knees as controls. Lateral patella subluxation (lateral translation) radiographically is clearly related to clinical lateral patella malalignment and related pain.

Medial subluxation is a functional problem and not usually detected on standard axial views.

Patellar Dysplasia

Radiographically, there are patients with lateral facet predominance (Wiberg Type III, alpine hunter's cap deformity) and tilt in association with subluxation (Fig. 9.8). Developmentally, a patella that is laterally aligned will form in response to molding pressures such that the result may be lateral facet predominance. It is more likely that this form of dysplasia is secondary, rather than a *cause* of patellar degeneration. The lateral facet deformity noted in some patients with patellar malalignment is analogous to femoral head dysplasia in congenital dislocation of the hip. The onset of pain is similar also in the sense that there are people with substantial hip dysplasia and no pain. At some point the imbalance leads to enough strain or tissue disruption that pain ensues.

Trochlear Dysplasia

The lateral trochlear facet is frequently flat in patients with subluxation. However, such is not always the case. CT with tomographic cuts centered on the mid-transverse patella at progressively increasing knee flexion angles will provide a good indication of trochlear morphology in the functional range of motion. Many patients with patellar instability, however, will show no gross evidence of trochlear dysplasia, particularly patients with connective tissue laxity.

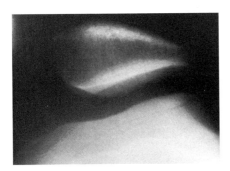

Figure 9.8. Alpine hunter's cap dysplasia associated with a very shallow trochlear sulcus in a patient with recurrent dislocation of the patella.

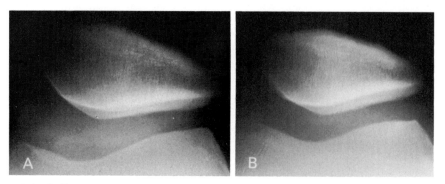

Figure 9.9. A, The 30-degree axial view shows mild subluxation. **B,** Further flexion leads to perfect centering.

Displacement

Deviation of the patella from its normal femoral groove may be seen on standard tangential (axial) radiographs. We only rarely have observed lateral subluxation on the 60-degree flexion film when the patella was centered on the 20- and 40-degree flexion views. Instability is usually manifest in the first 30 degrees of flexion, which indicates the value of the 20-degree flexion view and CT in early knee flexion. Those who fail to obtain these studies undoubtedly will miss some significant subluxations. It is unfortunate that an axial radiograph cannot be taken in less flexion, but this is the technical limit. CT is necessary to appreciate fully the details of patellar tracking and to avoid image overlap. Evidence of subluxation can be identified using CT between 0 and 30 degrees as the patella is centering in the trochlear groove. These images may show one of several possibilities: (a) a slight lateral subluxation on the 20- to 30-degree flexion view, with perfect recentering of the patella on further flexion (Figs. 9.9 and 9.10); (b) Type II lateral subluxation (with associated tilt) (Fig. 9.11); (c) a patella that sits astride the lateral trochlear facet (Fig. 9.12) but recenters on further flexion.

In addition, and perhaps most important, one can determine most accurately with CT whether there is tilt associated with subluxation. Using the posterior condyles to determine tilt relative to the lateral facet is possible only with tomography. Although CT is not necessary for all patients with subluxation, it may be very helpful in surgical planning. Magnetic resonance imaging (MRI) has not yet proved any more helpful than CT in this regard, although serial slices of the patella may help in understanding the condition of the articular cartilage. It is our opinion, however, that MRI is unnecessary in the majority of patients with patellofemoral pain, unless one needs information on cartilage or ligaments. CT, however, is frequently helpful in differentiating tilt and subluxation and offers align-

Figure 9.10. A, Axial views of a patient complaining only of right knee instability show marked subluxation on 30-degree view only of both patellae. Perfect recentering is evident on the 60- and 90-degree flexion views, which underscores the need for obtaining radiograms or computerized tomography with knee flexion of 20 to 30 degrees. **B,** Computerized tomographic view of subluxation without tilt.

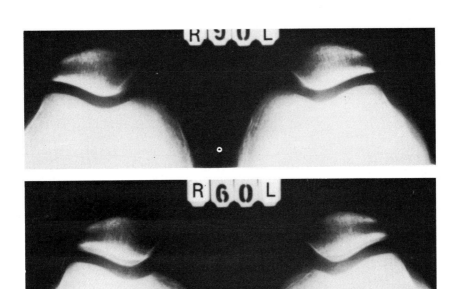

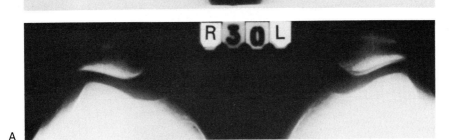

A

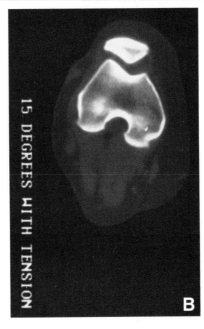

B

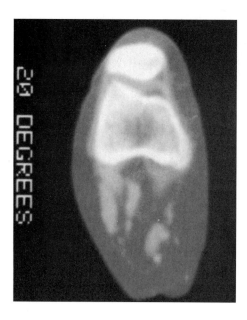

Figure 9.11. Mild tilt and subluxation at 20 degrees of knee flexion. Often, subluxation improves with further flexion, but tilt may either improve or worsen.

ment data comparable to that available with MRI but with ability to obtain images in greater degrees of knee flexion.

Soft-Tissue Calcifications

Calcification is noted sometimes on the axial views and may occur in association with recurrent subluxation (Fig. 9.13). Sometimes these calcifications are well defined,

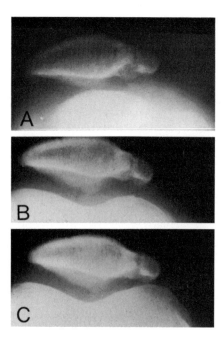

Figure 9.12. At 30 degrees of knee flexion **(A)**, the patella is lateral, but on further flexion **(B and C)**, the patella centralizes.

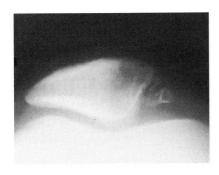

Figure 9.13. Medial retinacular calcification in a patient who, by history, has never had a dislocation. The history, however, was compatible with recurrent subluxation.

appearing as a discrete medial osteophyte, and need to be carefully distinguished from an artifact. Trillat et al (3) compared them quite correctly to Pellegrini-Stieda disease of the knee in that they are the soft-tissue reaction to repetitive ligamentous trauma. They represent a post-traumatic soft-tissue calcification and are seen frequently, perhaps even more frequently than with frank dislocations. These calcifications are differentiated from marginal fractures in that the medial border of the medial facet is intact. Moreover, they are covered with synovial membrane and are, therefore, extraarticular.

Medial Subluxation

Medial subluxation of the patella (16, 17) is caused most commonly by excessive medialization of the extensor mechanism in realignment surgery or lateral retinacular release in which there was little or no patellar lateralization preoperatively. Rarely, this may occur even after lateral retinacular release in a patient with preoperative patellar lateralization or excessive tilt. In such cases, reattachment of the vastus lateralis obliquus may reestablish normal patellar tracking. In patients with hypermobile joints, however, particularly if the trochlear groove is shallow, achieving "balance" of the patella in the trochlea may be extremely difficult.

Medial subluxation as an isolated entity, without previous surgery, is extremely rare or nonexistent, in the author's opinion. Radiographic studies (18) have shown that *tilting of the patella can simulate medial subluxation by causing rotation of the central ridge of the patella in a medial direction.* In an asymptomatic volunteer group, the lower limit for congruence angle was −26 degrees by computerized tomography. Consequently, one should exercise *extreme* caution in making a diagnosis of medial patellar subluxation on the basis of radiographs. Dupont (19) has described a variant in which the patella is lateral with the knee extended and medial with the knee in flexion. Medial subluxation is a clinical condition that will be best diagnosed on physical examination using a provocative test.

A clinical test for medial patellar subluxation involves holding the patella in a slightly medial direction with the knee in extension and then flexing the knee to see if the patient's symptom is reproduced with a sudden entry of the patella into the trochlea from medial to lateral (Fig. 9.14). In patients with symptomatic medial subluxation of the patella, this simple maneuver usually will cause considerable discomfort and reproduction of the painful instability sensation (17). Medial subluxation is prone to misdiagnosis because the patient experiences the patella moving *laterally, from too far medial back into the trochlea* upon knee flexion. This may be incorrectly interpreted as persistent lateral instability unless the examiner is thinking about the possibility of medial functional

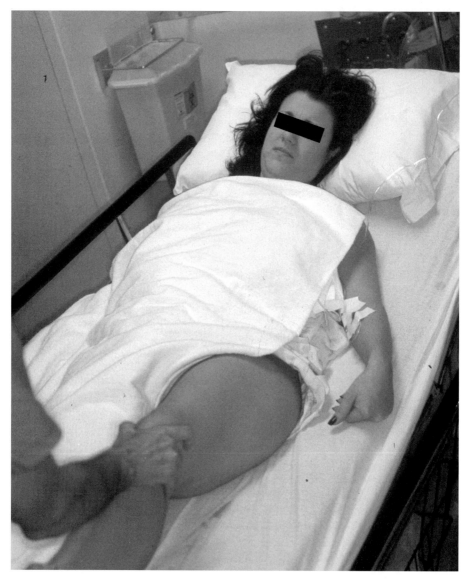

Figure 9.14. Medial subluxation test. Hold the patella slightly medial, knee extended. Then abruptly flex while letting go of the patella. In a patient with medial subluxation, this will yield a dramatic reproduction of the patient's symptom.

instability. The text outlined here reproduces the patient's symptom and is by far the most reliable test available.

TREATMENT

Nonoperative Treatment

Nonoperative treatment of patients with patellar subluxation centers on maintaining patellar stability to minimize symptoms and diminish risk of dislocation. Medial quadri-

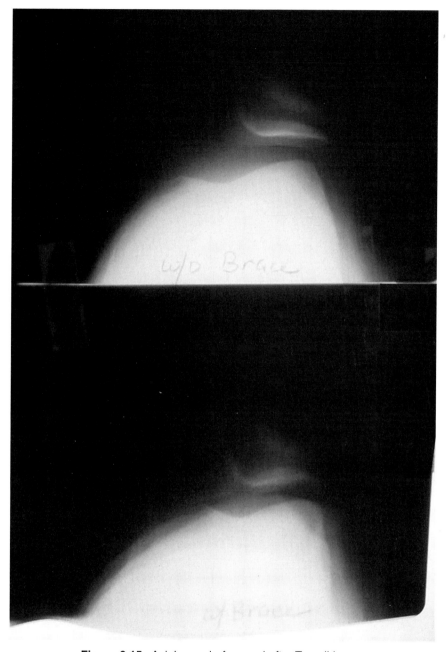

Figure 9.15. Axial x-ray before and after Trupull brace.

ceps strengthening and Trupull bracing (see Figures 8.18 and 9.15) to hold the patella will be helpful. Taping may add some feeling of security. Orthotics may improve lower-extremity alignment and diminish valgus thrust at the knee, thereby reducing the risk of patellar dislocation or symptoms of subluxation. Plyometric training and emphasis on hip external rotator strength, particularly in females, should help add a sense of lower

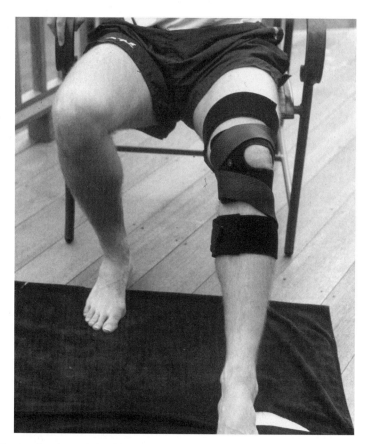

Figure 9.16. Application of the Trupull brace to provide lateral support, controlling medial patella subluxation.

extremity and extensor mechanism stability. The program must be individualized because of the "numerous etiologic factors associated with patellofemoral pain" (20). In the patient with *medial* patella subluxation, the Trupull brace is most effective for short-term management (Fig. 9.16).

Most patients with symptomatic minor subluxation will improve or become asymptomatic with nonoperative treatment. Some patients with more severe subluxation also respond to nonoperative treatment. When disabling symptoms and significant activity limitation persist after well-structured nonoperative treatment, however, surgery may be indicated to align the extensor mechanism.

Operative Treatment

The number of different techniques for patellar realignment and stabilization reported in the literature is astonishing. In 1959, Cotta (21) numbered 137 surgical methods directed at solving the problem of the unstable patella. Many of these methods have not enjoyed great success and rarely are used today.

In essence, however, control of patellar subluxation is not extremely complicated in most cases. Occasionally, the surgeon may encounter a very shallow trochlea or unusual dysplasia of the extensor mechanism such that stabilization of the subluxating patella is difficult, but most patients with less prominent subluxation causing functional limitation will respond to simple lateral release and medial imbrication (arthroscopic or open). Less commonly, a more extensive proximal and distal realignment may be necessary to compensate for more severe dysplasia or malalignment. It is such patients, in my experience, who sometimes need a reconstruction of the medial patellofemoral ligament (22).

Lateral Retinacular Release

Lateral retinacular release rarely is indicated as an isolated procedure in patients with subluxation. Because studies (23) have indicated that lateral release alone will not always correct subluxation, the surgeon must be careful to determine if something more than lateral release is necessary in the patient with patellar subluxation. Femoral nerve stimulation by percutaneous electrode may help the surgeon assess patellar tracking under anesthesia. Lateral retinacular release becomes particularly desirable in the patient with tilt and subluxation because the tilt component may respond particularly well to lateral release. Nonetheless, if there is residual patellar subluxation after lateral retinacular release, particularly if such subluxation is confirmed by femoral nerve stimulation under anesthesia, an Elmslie-Trillat procedure or medial patellofemoral ligament (MPFL) imbrication may be indicated selectively as long as this can be done without adding load to a medial patella lesion. Brief (24) emphasized the fact that lateral release alone fails to correct the patellar hypermobility that often accompanies subluxation. Occasionally, and particularly if there is significant patellar arthrosis (Outerbridge Grades 3 to 4), a surgeon may prefer to include anteromedial tibial tubercle transfer to unload the patella and improve patellar alignment (see Chapter 13). In a cadaver model, lateral retinacular release will correct patellar tilt but does not always correct subluxation (25). The best candidate is one with lateral compression syndrome, tilt laterally, and tight lateral retinaculum and without significant chondrosis. Subluxation alone is not a reliable indication for doing a lateral release alone.

Capsulorrhaphy

Representing a relatively simple surgical procedure and sufficient for many patients, capsulorrhaphy consists of weakening the lateral retinaculum (simple release) and strengthening the medial retinaculum (imbrication). Insall et al (26) reported experience with a technique of capsulorrhaphy that avoids a suture line in the medial retinaculum in a position where it might cause conflict with the medial femoral condyle on full flexion. It is important that the lateral release be sufficient, extending from the tibial tubercle, across the entire lateral retinaculum, and releasing the vastus lateralis obliquus only, without cutting into the main vastus lateralis tendon. This procedure may be done arthroscopically (see Chapter 5).

Fascioplasty

Several authors have described attempts to reinforce the weakened medial retinacular structures by grafting a variety of materials, including fascia lata, preserved skin (27), and nylon, to mention a few. These techniques mostly have been abandoned, having never gained wide popularity. Hauser (28) has reviewed these procedures extensively. More recently, there has been some interest in tendon graft reconstruction of the MPFL, but these techniques are not proven and risk adding excessive loads to the medial patella.

Osteotomy

Valgus osteotomy has been reported by Heywood (29) as being ineffective for control of recurrent dislocation of the patella. He noted five recurrences in seven patients who had osteotomies. Osteotomy may be necessary because of functional tibial or femoral overloading in one compartment, but it is not indicated as a primary treatment for recurrent subluxation of the patella. Tiege (30) has proposed femoral derotation to control patella instability, but this has not been necessary in my practice.

Myotendinous Procedures

Tendons may be transferred into the extensor mechanism either from above or below, and methods for some of these tendon transfers are summarized in Figure 9.17. Advancement of the vastus medialis has been widely recommended in conjunction with medial imbrication, particularly for the skeletally immature patient. Gracilis, semitendinosus, and sartorius tendons have all been used in a variety of ways. When the tendon is inserted from above, it is designed to act as a dynamic component; when the tendon is inserted from below, the intended effect is tenodesis. Baker et al (31) revived the original semitendinosus tenodesis described by Galliazzi in 1921 and reported good and excellent results in 81% of 53 cases. We have not found this procedure to be necessary and are concerned that it may be insufficient regarding isometry. Lateral release and careful medial imbrication, taking care to restore medial patellofemoral ligament continuity, may be appropriate for some difficult cases that require surgery before epiphyseal closure. In such cases, tibial tubercle procedure can result in anterior epiphyseal closure and genu recurvatum or distal migration of the tubercle with continued growth of the tibia. Such complications must be avoided.

Krogius (32) described a technique that has become popular in Europe. The skin incision is medial parapatellar. A strip of medial capsule with attachment of the vastus medialis is developed, creating a medial retinacular defect. A lateral retinacular release is then carried out, and the medial defect is closed. The myofascial strip that has been developed is then sutured into the lateral defect that has been created by the medial plication. The author reported good results with this technique. In our experience, however, lateral retinacular release and medial imbrication without excising any medial capsule has proved satisfactory in the majority of skeletally immature patients. This procedure, however, requires considerable attention to detail, and the surgeon must be careful *not to overtighten* the medial capsule because this will increase medial facet loading and lead to articular degeneration. I prefer to use sutures to *anchor* the vastus medialis obliquus to the central quadriceps tendon (CQT) above the patella and at the CQT-patella junction. Galliazzi's procedure (29) may be helpful in the skeletally immature patient (Fig. 9.18), but I have not found this procedure to be necessary. One must consider the possibility that this technique could create aberrant stresses on the patella, depending on the degree of knee flexion.

Patellectomy

If patellectomy is indicated for the arthritic sequelae of malalignment *and the patella has been surgically centered and stable,* then simple patellectomy can be appropriate.

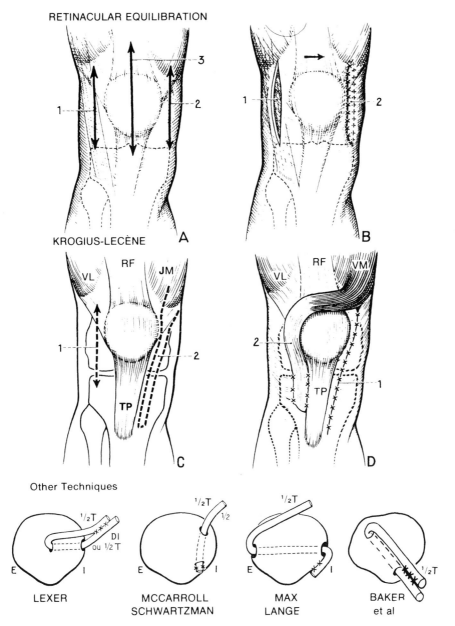

Figure 9.17. Several popular methods of extensor mechanism equilibration. Reprinted with permission from Ficat P. Pathologie Femoro-Patellaire. Paris: Masson et Cie, 1970.

However, it must be remembered that the extensor apparatus without a patella can subluxate and dislocate as well. Benoist and Ramadier (33) have underscored this observation with the report of their results of only nine good and excellent results in 19 patients with simple patellectomies for recurrent subluxation and dislocation, whereas there were 17 good and excellent results of 19 in patellectomy associated with transplantation of the tibial tubercle. In the case of patellofemoral arthrosis in which a patellectomy is contem-

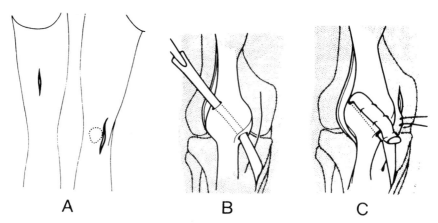

Figure 9.18. The Galliazzi semitendinosus tenodesis provides medial support for major or permanent patellar subluxation in the skeletally immature patient. Reprinted with permission from Baker RH, Carroll N, Dewar P, Hall JE. Semitendinosus tenodesis for recurrent dislocation of the patella. J Bone Joint Surg 1972;54B:103–109.

plated, anterior displacement to facilitate the extensor moment arm may be appropriate. West and Soto-Hall (34) have reported on 31 of 33 patients who had patellectomies with good or excellent results. Heywood (29) was more pessimistic, reporting 10 unsatisfactory results in 29 patients with patellectomies and only one excellent result. In general, however, the surgeon should avoid patellectomy in patients with patellar subluxation (35) unless arthrosis is severe and other alternatives, such as anteromedial tibial tubercle transfer, cannot give relief (Chapter 13). Centralization and proper alignment of the extensor mechanism are imperative before performing patellectomy. Isolated patellofemoral replacement surgery may replace patellectomy as the procedure of choice in end-stage patella arthritis.

Patellar Ligament Procedures (Historical)

Roux (36) in 1888 was the first to report tibial tubercle transplantation coupled with lateral release and medial plication in the treatment of recurrent patellar dislocation. His single case report was apparently dramatically effective. Hauser (28), in 1938, apparently unaware of Roux's single case report, reviewed the literature for the procedures popular at that time and reported four cases of medial tibial tubercle transplantation—all with successful outcomes in short-term follow-up. In each case, lateral retinacular release and medial plication were carried out. Since Hauser's original report, a variety of modifications have been reported. At long-term follow-up (average, 8 years), Barbari et al (37) found that less than 50% of patients were free of pain following a Hauser procedure. Hauser's operation was widely popular in the United States but has now become contraindicated in the majority of patients because it places the tibial tubercle posterior and actually increases contact pressure on the patella (38) (Fig. 9.19). MacNab (7), reporting an average 10-year follow-up on 10 patients, mostly after medial tibial tubercle transplantation, attributed the lack of good results to preoperative patellar cartilage damage, and it seems likely that load may have been transferred in many cases onto significant articular lesions given the known occurrence of medial lesions in patients with patellar

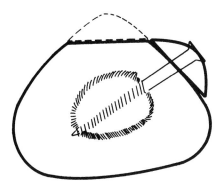

Figure 9.19. Procedures that transfer the tibial tubercle in a medial direction *down* the medial slope of the tibia are rarely, if ever, indicated. Reprinted with permission from Cox JS. Evaluation of the Roux-Elmslie-Trillat procedure for knee extensor realignment. Am J Sports Med 1982;10:303.

instability and pain. Loff and Friedebold (39) found a direct correlation between preoperative joint status and postoperative results. Crosby and Insall (40) reported not only a recurrent dislocation rate of 20% after tibial tubercle transfer in 69 patients but also a high incidence of late osteoarthritis. This late osteoarthritis was most likely the result of the medial patella overloading that occurs with the Hauser procedure. Although there was a 25% incidence of redislocation after 12 proximal soft-tissue procedures, there was no late osteoarthrosis seen. More recently, Juliusson and Markhede (41) noted that only 12% of 40 patients whose knees underwent a Hauser procedure showed objectively satisfactory results. This is clearly unacceptable.

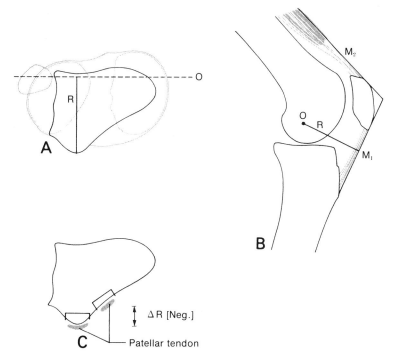

Figure 9.20. A, Transection through the tibia at the level of the tibial tubercle, with the tibial plateau superimposed for orientation. O = axis of knee flexion; R = extensor lever arm. **B,** Lateral view of extensor mechanism and the knee. M_1, M_2 = quadriceps vectors (see Chapter 2). **C,** Transected view of proximal tibia showing *detrimental* effect of tibial tubercle medialization using such methods.

The observation by Goutallier and Debeyre's (42) on the detrimental biomechanical effect of posteromedial transfer of the tibial tubercle by the Hauser technique (Fig. 9.20) may account for poor late results after the Hauser procedure. Posterior placement of the tibial tubercle has no place in the management of patella instability today.

Goldthwait (6) reported a technique whereby the patellar tendon is split and the lateral half is detached from the tibial tubercle, passed behind the medial half, and sutured to the medial capsule. The net result is to change the resultant vector of traction of the patellar tendon. This procedure has never gained widespread popularity and carries significant risk of adversely affecting patellar contact pressure distribution by pulling down the lateral facet; it is no longer useful given better alternatives.

Distal Realignment

When there is minimal arthrosis and proximal realignment alone is insufficient, distal realignment of the extensor mechanism, without anteriorization, is most appropriate (43–45).

Subluxation may be persistent despite lateral retinacular release (22), particularly because lateral release is an inappropriate procedure for patella instability. Nonetheless, patients with patellar subluxation have been shown to improve in some cases after lateral retinacular release alone (46), probably because of reduced tilt and lateral pressure associated with the subluxation. Although medial imbrication will provide all of the additional balance that is needed in many patients, distal realignment (medialization of the tibial tubercle) may be necessary in some patients (skeletally mature) to assure appropri-

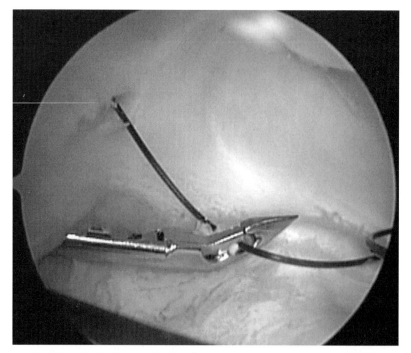

Figure 9.21. Arthroscopic medial imbrication requires a penetrating grasper to retrieve sutures (#2–5), which are tied externally with a knot tier (technique of Pienovi).

ate patellar tracking. The surgeon must recognize that excessive medial imbrication to support the patella medially can overload the medial facet and aggravate an already degenerating patella. Therefore, distal realignment becomes an important consideration in extensor mechanism realignment for subluxation. Nonetheless, the author (JPF) does not recommend tibial tubercle transfer when a careful medial imbrication can control subluxation without adding load to a medial lesion. In many cases, this will be done arthroscopically (Fig. 9.21).

The Roux-Elmslie-Trillat procedure, as reviewed by Cox (47) and Andrish (48), is the preferred distal realignment technique because it provides pure medialization without transferring the tibial tubercle posteriorly. This procedure also allows very secure fixation and early motion, which is so important in these patients. The technique of Goutallier and Debeyre (42) is similar in concept (Fig. 9.22). Also, if there is Outerbridge

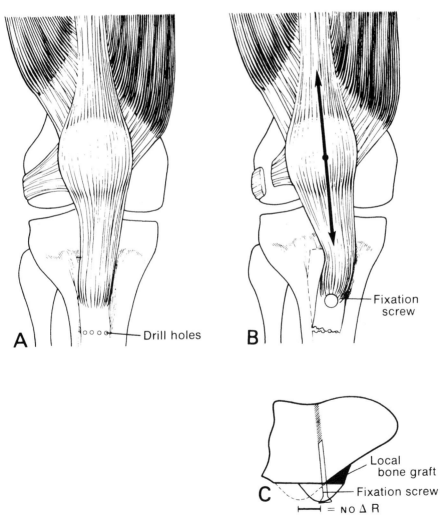

Figure 9.22. Method of medial tibial tubercle transfer fashioned after the method of Elmslie and modified by Goutallier and Debeyre (42). This minimizes diminution of the extensor lever arm.

Grades 3 to 4 lateral facet degeneration, the traditional Trillat procedure can be modified to provide anteromedial tibial tubercle transfer by making the osteotomy oblique, as originally described in 1983 (49) (see Chapter 13). Shelbourne et al (50) have pointed out that correction of congruence by the Elmslie-Trillat procedure will not deteriorate with time. Wootton et al (51) reported satisfactory results in the knees of 68 patients following an Elmslie-Trillat procedure for patellar dislocation or subluxation.

The Trillat procedure may be performed through an anterior or anterolateral incision approximately 10 to 15 cm long and extending from the midlateral patella to approximately 5 cm distal to the tibial tubercle. The lateral retinaculum is incised as described in the section on lateral retinacular release. The patella is inspected, and a decision is then possible as to whether the Trillat procedure or an anteromedial tibial tubercle transfer is more appropriate (Fig. 9.23). If there is distal or lateral facet breakdown, anteromedialization may be indicated.

If the decision is to do a Trillat procedure, the anterior compartment musculature is reflected posteriorly by subperiosteal elevation and a flat osteotomy is made deep to the tibial tubercle such that a bone pedicle (approximately 5 cm long and tapered anteriorly) is formed. The bone pedicle is hinged distally and rotated in a medial direction, maintaining good bone–bone contact until the desired amount of patellar tendon medialization is achieved. The bone pedicle is fixed then with two screws, preferably into the posterior tibial cortex as in the anteromedial tibial tubercle transfer. Cox (47) reported that only 7% of his patients experienced subluxation after this procedure.

Postoperatively, a Hemovac drain is used for 24 hours, and the patient remains on crutches for approximately 6 weeks, but knee motion is started immediately after surgery, assuming secure fixation of the bone pedicle.

In the final analysis, what is most important is to correct accurately the specific extensor mechanism malalignment noted preoperatively and to avoid any surgery that might aggravate the situation in any way. As a general rule, the surgeon should do the least surgery possible to achieve realistic correction of patellar tracking and restoration of satisfactory patellar articular cartilage contact stress distribution. In addition, any source of chronic retinacular or synovial pain caused by the imbalance must be identified preoperatively and released or resected (52).

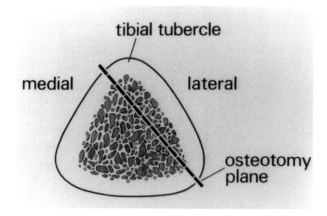

Figure 9.23. Creating an oblique osteotomy deep to the tibial tubercle will permit anterior as well as medial tibial tubercle displacement. One must beware of the anterior tibial artery and the deep peroneal nerve at the posterolateral corner of the osteotomy.

REFERENCES

1. Larsen E, Lund PM. Ruptures of the extensor mechanism of the knee joint. Clinical results and patellofemoral articulation. Clin Orthop 1986;213:150–153.
2. Kujala UM, Friberg O, Aalto T, Kvist M, Osterman K. Lower limb asymmetry and patellofemoral joint incongruence in the etiology of knee exertion injuries in athletes. Int J Sports Med 1987;8:214–220.
3. Trillat A, Dejour H, Coutette A. Diagnostic et traitement des subluxations recidivantes de la rotule. Rev Chir Orthop 1964;50:813–824.
4. Fulkerson J. Patellofemoral pain disorders. J Am Acad Orthop Surg 1994;2(2):124–132.
5. Merle D'Aubigne R, Ramadier JO. La subluxation de la rotule dans l'arthrose du genou. Rev Chir Orthop 1959; 45:437–153.
6. Goldthwait JE. Slipping or recurrent dislocation of the patella: With the report of eleven cases. Boston Med Surg J 1904;150:169–174.
7. MacNab I. Recurrent dislocation of the patella. J Bone Joint Surg 1952;34A:957.
8. Hughston JC. Subluxation of the patella. J Bone Joint Surg 1968;50A:1003–1026.
9. Bennett W, Doherty N, Hollisey M, Fulkerson J. Insertion orientation of terminal vastus lateralis obliquus and vastus medialis obliquus muscle fibers in human knees. Clin Anat 1993;6:129–134.
10. McIvor JB, Gillespie R. Patellar instability in juvenile amputees. J Pediatr Orthop 1987;7:553–556.
11. Casscells SW. Gross pathological changes in the knee joint of the aged individual. A study of 300 cases. J Bone Joint Surg 1975;57A:1003.
12. Fulkerson J, Tennant R, Jaivin J, Grunnet M. Histologic evidence of retinacular nerve injury associated with patellofemoral malalignment. Clin Orthop 1985;197:196–205.
13. Fulkerson J. Evaluation of the peripatellar soft tissues and retinaculum in patients with patellofemoral pain. Clin Sports Med 1989;8:197–202.
14. Ficat P. Pathologie Femoro-Patellaire. Paris: Masson et Cie, 1970.
15. Schutzer SF, Ramsby GR, Fulkerson JP. Computed tomographic classification of patellofemoral pain patients. Orthop Clin North Am 1986;17:235–248.
16. Hughston J, Deese M. Medial subluxation of the patella as a complication of lateral retinacular release. Am J Sports Med 1988;16:383–388.
17. Fulkerson JP. A clinical test for medial patella tracking. Tech Orthop 1997;12:165–169.
18. Fulkerson JP, Wright J, Legeyt M, Cautilli RA Jr. Precise criteria of normal and abnormal patellofemoral joint alignment using three dimensional computerized tomography. Orthopedic transactions. J Bone Joint Surg 1993-1994;17(4):1062.
19. DuPont JY. Presentation d'Une Forme Rare de Subluxation Rotulienne. J Traumatol Sport 1996;12:77–89.
20. Wilk K, Reinold M. Principles of patellofemoral rehabilitation. Sports Med Arthrosc Rev 2001;9:325–336.
21. Cotta H. Zur Therapie der Habitullen Pattellaren Luxation. Arch Orthop Unfallchir 1959;51:256–271.
22. Fithian D, Meier S. The case for advancement and repair of the medial patellofemoral ligament in patients with recurrent patellar instability. Oper Tech Sports Med 1999;7:81–89.
23. Fulkerson J, Schutzer S, Ramsby G, Bernstein R. Computerized tomography of the patellofemoral joint before and after lateral release or realignment. Arthroscopy 1987;3:19–24.
24. Brief LP. Lateral patellar instability: Treatment with a combined open-arthroscopic approach. Arthroscopy 1993;9(6):617–623.
25. Post WR, Fulkerson J, Shea K. A cadaver model of patellofemoral realignment. J Bone Joint Surg 1994;8(3):742.
26. Insall J, Falvo KA, Wise DW. Chondromalacia patellae. J Bone Joint Surg 1976;58A:1–8.
27. Bonvallet JM. Resultats de la reflection a la peau de l'aileron rotulien interne dans les luxations recidivantes de la rotule. Chirurgie 1973;99:124–128.
28. Hauser EW. Total tendon transplant for slipping patella. Surg Gynecol Obstet 1938;66:199.
29. Heywood AWB. Recurrent dislocation of the patella. J Bone Joint Surg 1961;43B:507–517.
30. Tiege R. Personal communication (2003).
31. Baker RH, Carroll N, Dewar P, Hall JE. Semitendinosus tenodesis for recurrent dislocation of the patella. J Bone Joint Surg 1972;54B:103–109.
32. Krogius A. Zur operativen behandlung der habituellen luxation der kniescheibe. Zentralbl Chir 1904;31:254.
33. Benoist JP, Ramadier JO. Luxations et subluxations de la rotule. Rev Chir Orthop 1969;55:89–109.
34. West FE, Soto-Hall R. Recurrent dislocation of the patella in the adult. J Bone Joint Surg 1958;40A:386–393.
35. Kelly M, Insall J. Patellectomy. Orthop Clin North Am 1986;17(2):289–295.
36. Roux D. Luxation Habituelle de la Rotule. Rev Chir Paris 1888;8:682–689.
37. Barbari S, Raugstad TS, Lichtenberg N, Refvem D. The Hauser operation for patellar dislocation. 3-32-year results in 63 knees. Acta Orthop Scand 1990;61:32–35.
38. Hehne HJ. Biomechanics of the patellofemoral joint. Clin Orthop 1990;258:73–85.
39. Loff P, Friedebold G. Die habituelle patellarluxation als präarthrotische deformität. Ergeb Chir 1969;52:60.
40. Crosby EB, Insall J. Recurrent dislocation of the patella. J Bone Joint Surg 1976;58A:9–13.
41. Juliusson R, Markhede G. A modified Hauser procedure for recurrent dislocation of the patella. A long-term follow-up study with special reference to osteoarthritis. Arch Orthop Trauma Surg 1984;103:42–46.

42. Goutallier D, Debeyre J. Le recentrage rotulien dans les arthroses femoro-patellaires lateralisees. Rev Chir Orthop 1974;60:377–386.
43. Fulkerson JP. Operative management of patellofemoral pain. Ann Chir Gynaecol 1991;80(2):224–229.
44. Post W, Fulkerson J. Distal realignment of the patellofemoral joint. Orthop Clin North Am 1992;23:631–643.
45. Cautilli R, Fulkerson J. Operative treatment of patellofemoral disorders. Distal realignment. Sports Med Arthr Rev 1994;2:250–262.
46. Henry JH, Goletz TH, Williamson B. Lateral retinacular release in patellofemoral subluxation. Indications, results, and comparison to open patellofemoral reconstruction. Am J Sports Med 1986;14:121–129.
47. Cox JS. Evaluation of the Roux-Elmslie-Trillat procedure for knee extensor realignment. Am J Sports Med 1982; 10:303–310.
48. Andrish, J. The Elmslie-Trillat procedure. Tech Orthop 1997;12:170–177.
49. Fulkerson J. Anteromedialization of the tibial tuberosity for patellofemoral malalignment. Clin Orthop 1983; 177:129–133.
50. Shelbourne D, Porter D, Rozzi W. Use of a modified Elmslie-Trillat procedure to improve abnormal patellar congruence angle. Am J Sports Med 1994;2:318–323.
51. Wootton JR, Cross MJ, Wood DG. Patellofemoral malalignment: A report of 68 cases treated by proximal and distal patellofemoral reconstruction. Injury 1990;21(3):169–173.
52. Kasim N, Fulkerson J. Resection of clinically localized segments of painful retinaculum in the treatment of selected patients with anterior knee pain. Am J Sports Med 2000;28:811–814.

=10=
Patellar Dislocation

*"I expect to pass through this world but once. Any good
therefore that I can do or any kindness that I can show for any
fellow creature, let me do it now. Let me not defer or neglect it,
for I shall not pass this way again."*

—*Ralph Waldo Emerson*

Patellar dislocation may occur as a direct traumatic event in the patient with normal patellar alignment, or it may occur in the patient with preexisting malalignment, particularly if there is significant baseline subluxation (Fig. 10.1). Subluxation with or without associated tilt will predispose a patient to patellar dislocation. Patellar dislocation also occurs after total knee replacement (1).

Whether patellar trauma is direct such that articular cartilage is damaged by extreme and sudden compression or indirect by twisting the knee with lateral vector stress on the patella causing dislocation, acute articular injury is common.

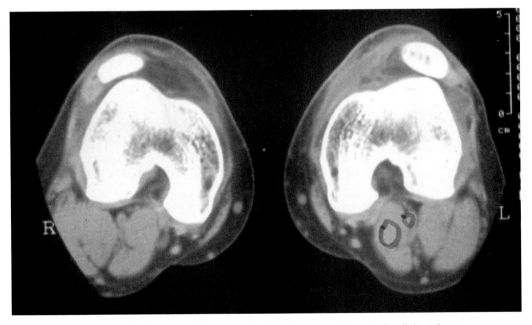

Figure 10.1. Computed tomography showing complete patella dislocations.

ETIOLOGY OF PATELLAR DISLOCATION

There is normally some tendency for the patella to displace laterally. On extension of the knee, this tendency is balanced *passively* by the medial patellofemoral ligament and by a buttress effect of the lateral femoral trochlea. The patella is balanced *functionally* by the orientation of the distal vastus medialis fibers. In the case of acute or recurrent dislocation, there is a breakdown of this equilibrium. In certain cases, an imbalance in the extensor mechanism can be primarily responsible for patellar dislocation, but there are usually some associated bony morphologic changes related to ongoing instability.

Bony Abnormalities

Trochlear Abnormalities

Brattstrom (2), using a complicated radiologic technique for assessing the trochlear surface of the distal femur, determined in 131 patients with recurrent dislocation of the patella that, on the average, the trochlear facet (sulcus) angle was 10 degrees greater in dislocators than in a normal population (200 similarly studied controls). Vainionpaa et al (3) confirmed the presence of abnormally high sulcus angles in patients with patellar dislocation. Brattstrom (2) thought that this was the most important factor in patients with recurrent dislocation, even though fully half of the patients studied had a normal sulcus angle. His technique allowed him to conclude that the change in the trochlear sulcus angle is due to a rising depth of the sulcus rather than to a decrease in the prominence of the facets. Measurement of the angle is not subject to distortion by rotation as is measurement of the relative prominence of the lateral facet, vis-á-vis the medial facet.

Today, one may obtain an accurate appraisal of trochlear anatomy using computed tomography (CT) or magnetic resonance imaging (MRI). By obtaining serial sections of the patellofemoral joint, centering the cut at the midtransverse patella, and obtaining tomographic slices at 10-degree increments of knee flexion, one can achieve an excellent radiographic picture of trochlear anatomy as it relates to patellar tracking and trochlear damage from patellar dislocation. Nietosvaara et al (4) noted that the trochlear fracture from patellar dislocation occurs mostly on the edge of the articular surface at the middle third of the condylar arc. With CT, one also can define the extent of trochlear dysplasia preoperatively (Fig. 10.2). Radiographic studies should look closely at this area for evidence of change.

Patellar Abnormalities

Not all series reporting recurrent dislocation have paid sufficient attention to patellar form. Baum and Bensahal (5), however, measured a patellar depth coefficient and found 35 of 59 patellae were abnormally shallow. As far as patellar form is concerned, these authors encountered 42 cases of Wiberg Type III patellae in their series of 59 patients. Similar percentages have been reported by Rohlederer (6) (76%) and Loff and Freidebold (7) (86%). Abnormal patellar morphology may be more *effect* than *cause,* however. If a patella is chronically malaligned, particularly during skeletal development, it is likely there will be secondary morphologic changes. Dislocation, therefore, is a result, in most cases, of chronic malalignment. Trauma dislocation, of course, can occur when anatomy and alignment are completely normal.

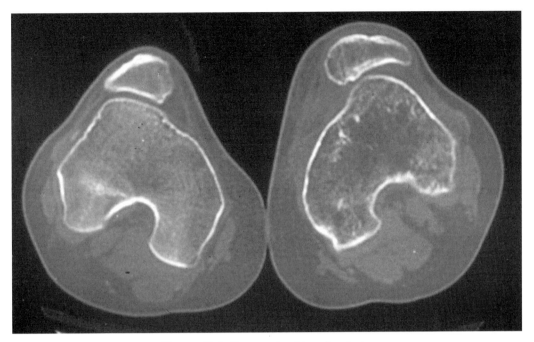

Figure 10.2. Extreme trochlea dysplasia.

Abnormal Bony Relationships

External Tibial Torsion

Brattstrom (2) was not able to document any statistically significant difference in rotation or torsion between his patient and control groups. Heywood (8) reported two cases in his series of 54 patients.

Femoral Anteversion

When femoral anteversion presents as a toe-in gait without compensatory external tibial torsion, patellar problems are not common. Some patients, however, who have excessive femoral anteversion and external tibial torsion will show signs of patellar instability and may be at increased risk of dislocation.

Lateral Location of the Anterior Tibial Tubercle

This has been thought to be an important factor by many authors, particularly Trillat et al (9), based more on clinical impressions than on precise measurements. Dupuis (10), in his monograph on tibial torsion, measured the distance between a vertical line from the center of the patella to a vertical line from the tibial tubercle. However, these measurements are of little value because the patella may likewise be laterally situated with a laterally placed tuberosity. Because of tibial translation and rotation with knee flexion, there is no one measurement that will consistently indicate a proper relationship of the patella to the tibial tubercle.

Genu Valgum

Heywood (8) reported genu valgum in 7 of his 106 cases, and Hughston (11) found it in 1 of 111 cases. Bizou (12) concluded that genu valgum is not a prominent cause of patellar dislocation. The large number of young children with significant genu valgum without patellar problems supports the validity of Bizou's conclusion.

Soft-Tissue Abnormalities

Patella Alta

This abnormal relationship of the patella to the trochlea is due, in the majority of cases, to a patellar tendon that is abnormally long (Fig. 10.3). The relationship of patella alta to dislocation is the subject of some difference of opinion. Brattstrom (2) does not record this finding in his series. Ficat and Bizou (13) considered patella alta to be a significant factor in more than half of their cases. Insall et al (14) also thought that patella alta is an important etiologic factor. As in other abnormalities, it is clear that patella alta is not universally associated with dislocation because many patellae that dislocate are normally situated. Although patella alta may be observed in association with patellar malalignment or dislocation, patella alta is less of a problem than other alignment and structural factors.

Medial Stabilizers

The medial patellofemoral ligament reinforced by the vastus medialis would appear to be important in preventing dislocation (15). These may be weakened or torn. Koskinen and Kujala (16) have noted that the vastus medialis inserts more proximally in patients with patellar dislocation when compared with normal subjects. A primary dislocation, whether traumatic or due to constitutional factors, may so weaken the medial stabilizers that subsequent dislocations become likely. Recurrent dislocation has also been reported by several authors in syndromes of generalized ligamentous laxity including chondroosteodystrophy, Ehlers-Danlos syndrome, and Marfan syndrome (10, 17). In these instances, the medial stabilizers are insufficient to resist the normal lateral tendency imposed by the Q angle.

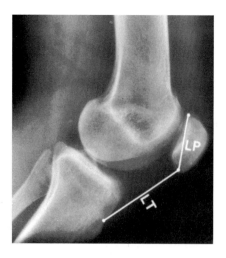

Figure 10.3. Radiograph of patella alta in a 20-year-old woman with multiple episodes of patellar dislocation. *LT/LP* = 1.67.

Recurrent dislocation may occur after isolated vastus medialis paralysis, secondary to poliomyelitis. Other patients may manifest atrophy or hypoplasia of the vastus medialis. In the latter case, the muscle fibers attach only to the superior aspect of the patella as opposed to the superior and medial borders (11).

Lateral Retinacular Factors

Abnormal fibrous insertion of the vastus lateralis, abnormal fascial bands from the vastus lateralis, and abnormally tight lateral retinaculum may play important roles in dislocation of the patella. Jeffries (18) reported three cases of abnormal attachment of fascia from the iliotibial tract to the superolateral border of the patella. However, in reviewing 76 cases, Heywood (8) did not see any cases in which this was the cause. All of this serves to underline the importance of many factors that contribute to the basic functional equilibrium of the extensor mechanism of the knee. Tight lateral retinaculum undoubtedly perpetuates lateral displacement of the patella while accentuating tilt (rotation) and will increase the risk of dislocation.

Hereditary Factors

Many authors have mentioned the tendency for recurrent dislocation to run in families. Bowker and Thompson (19) reported an incidence of 25% in their series of 48 patients, and Crosby and Insall (20) found 28% with positive family histories in their series. Down's syndrome also predisposes to patellar dislocation (21, 22), and there is a possible relationship between Turner's syndrome and recurrent patellar dislocation (23). Recurrent patellar dislocation also occurs in Kabuki make-up syndrome (24).

DIRECT PATELLAR TRAUMA WITHOUT DISLOCATION

Any direct blow to the patella may result in articular cartilage injury. Although the pattern of cartilage degeneration subsequent to direct trauma may simulate that noted in patients who have malalignment, the posttraumatic course and subsequent treatment will often be different. In general, the clinician will approach direct trauma to the patella without dislocation as any other direct articular injury. Certainly, if there is a fracture, immobilization with reduction and fixation of the fracture will be necessary. Open reduction with tension band wiring after alignment of distracted and displaced articular fragments is generally most satisfactory (25).

Subsequent to blunt trauma (26), with or without fracture, articular cartilage breakdown is common. Many patients notice some crepitation, but many have little associated pain. Unfortunately, some of these patients eventually develop erosion of articular cartilage to bone and true arthrosis of the patellofemoral joint. It is important for the clinician to recognize when a patient has articular degeneration related to trauma as opposed to malalignment. In the former group, treatment should be directed to the articular surface itself, and procedures such as lateral retinacular release generally are not helpful. Lateral release should not be the treatment of choice for patients with blunt articular injury to the patella and subsequent arthrosis. In fact, some patients will become worse after lateral retinacular release when there is no preexisting tilt (rotation) of the patella. The lateral retinaculum is an anteroposterior-oriented structure, and cutting it can even *accentuate* lateral patella displacement.

Treatment of the patient with articular cartilage damage but no malalignment must be directed specifically to the articular surface, assuming that reflex sympathetic dystrophy has not evolved as a result of the injury. Selective microfracture arthroplasty or articular debridement may be helpful using arthroscopic technique in some patients if there is a localized lesion with exposed bone and some good or satisfactory surrounding articular cartilage to which contact stresses may be transferred. When patellar articular injury is extensive and there is no evidence of reflex sympathetic dystrophy, some patients may benefit from tibial tubercle anteriorization or anteromedialization. This is most desirable if proximal articular cartilage on the patella is intact, because anteriorization of the tibial tubercle will result in a proximal shift of contact stresses as well as unload the joint (27). As a last resort, patellectomy may be the procedure of choice to remove a badly damaged and widely eburnated patella when the trochlea is intact, but patellectomy as a treatment for patella instability is contraindicated. One will replace a dislocating patella with a dislocating extensor mechanism.

ACUTE PATELLAR DISLOCATION

Patellar malalignment, particularly subluxation, will increase the chance that a complete patellar dislocation will occur. Patellar dislocation indicates that the patella has been *completely* displaced from the femoral trochlea so that there is no longer any articular surface apposition. Dislocation frequently occurs as a sudden event, either related to trauma or to preexisting malalignment and torsional stress on the extensor mechanism, which causes complete displacement of the patella out of the trochlea. Hawkins et al (28) have pointed out that 30–50% of patients who have dislocated a patella will continue to have problems with pain and instability. In this landmark study, Hawkins emphasized that patients with predisposing factors, such as malalignment or structural abnormality, will be more prone to recurrent dislocation following an initial dislocation. He recommended that these predisposing factors be carefully considered in planning appropriate treatment following a dislocation. Releases and realignment make no sense when there is no structural malalignment. The clinician should also be aware that a "locked" patellar dislocation can occur that can preclude closed reduction, even under general anesthesia (29).

Clinical Picture

The patient who has experienced a complete acute dislocation of the patella is usually aware that the patella has gone out of place. Sometimes the patient has reduced the patella with or without someone else's help. Occasionally, a patient will say he/she has "dislocated his/her knee" when, in fact, only the patella has dislocated and then subsequently relocated. The examiner should be wary of such self diagnosis. It is apparent, nonetheless, that the experience of dislocating a patella is quite impressive to the patient, and usually the patient is aware that something terrible has occurred. The dislocation may occur as a result of vigorous activity, direct trauma, or some trivial movement. The typical patient is a short, young, obese woman with patellar malalignment and ligamentous laxity, but patellar dislocation also occurs fairly frequently in vigorous young athletes, male or female. The patient may have had some preexisting anterior knee pain, but this is not always the case. Sometimes the patient thinks that the patella has gone medially, when in fact they are feeling the medial femoral condyle that is medial relative to the patella.

When the patient is initially seen, the knee is generally swollen, and examination can be difficult. In fact, depending on the history, there may be some confusion as to whether there is other damage to the knee such as a torn cruciate ligament or meniscus. Limited range of motion is common because of pain, swelling, and loose articular fragments.

The careful clinician will examine the knee, first in extension, and assess the retinacular structures as well as ligament deficiency. The examiner should test for cruciate ligament insufficiency and joint line tenderness. At this point, it will often become apparent that there is tenderness in the medial retinaculum and apprehension on any attempt to displace the patella laterally. Integrity of the medial patellofemoral ligament should be checked. There may be swelling in the region of the vastus medialis obliquus. Flexion and extension of the knee may be limited because of pain, but if it is possible to flex the knee somewhat, there may be a sense of lateral displacement of the patella, as compared with the contralateral, unaffected knee. The lateral retinaculum may or may not be tender. The examining physician should also palpate and observe the entire extensor mechanism. In older patients, quadriceps muscle rupture can occur immediately above the patella, resulting in extreme extensor mechanism weakness and a defect that may be difficult to find in the presence of a hematoma. The patient should be encouraged to do a straight leg raise, and if this is not possible, the examiner should question again whether the extensor mechanism is intact. McMurray's test is usually not possible in these patients, but the examiner must be certain to examine the joint for localizable tenderness or instability. If possible, the patient should be examined standing also to observe the alignment of both lower extremities to assess rotation and valgus. Also, the examining physician should evaluate the patient's overall connective-tissue structure to determine if there is excessive laxity. In particular, the finger extension, elbow extension, thumb-to-wrist flexion, and knee recurvatum should be checked.

Radiologic Features

At the time of acute patellar dislocation, the diagnosis may be obscure. As part of the initial evaluation, radiographs should routinely include the standard standing anteroposterior (AP) view; the lateral view; a 30- to 45-degree knee flexion axial view; and a 30-degree knee flexion, 10-degree caudal posteroanterior standing view. These images may be completely unremarkable, but the trauma of dislocation may leave some residual lateral placement of the patella, either as an indication of baseline malalignment or as a result of medial retinacular disruption. The tangential radiograph, therefore, may indicate malalignment (primary or secondary). Any of the other views may reveal a small fleck of bone that will be attached to articular cartilage (sheared off the patella or lateral condyle at the time of dislocation and relocation). A defect in the medial patella or lateral trochlea may be detected on the tangential view in some patients. If there is no articular injury, or injury is limited to articular cartilage, radiographs may be completely normal. The notch view may be helpful if a loose fleck of bone with overlying articular cartilage has been displaced and dropped into the intercondylar notch.

Of course, the astute clinician will be looking for other findings on the radiograph that are suggestive of intraarticular lesions such as osteochondritis dissecans, calcified meniscus, avulsion of bone by the anterior cruciate ligament, or fracture.

The lateral radiograph is very sensitive for detecting tilt of the patella. A standing true lateral at 0 and 30 degrees of knee flexion, with posterior condyles overlapped, is extremely helpful for detecting malalignment in the patient who has experienced dislocation (see Chapter 4).

When the patient is first seen, CT, MRI, and arthrography are not usually necessary unless the clinician needs to know more about the extent of injury. Certainly, if meniscus or cruciate ligament damage is in question, MRI may be helpful. Serial transverse sections of the patellofemoral joint at 20 degrees of knee flexion should be done in every complete MRI study. Lance et al (30) noted that hemarthrosis, medial patellar and lateral femoral contusion, and retinacular disruption suggest patellar dislocation on MRI. Virolainen et al noted contusion of the lateral condyle, tear of the medial retinaculum, and joint effusion as the principal MRI findings following acute patella dislocation (31).

Pathoanatomy

Articular injury is common after acute patellar dislocation. The force necessary to dislocate a patella in most patients is substantial, particularly when one considers that the medial retinaculum must be substantially stretched and torn to permit the patella to drop off the lateral trochlea. Thomson (personal communication, 1988) has shown that most patients with acute patellar dislocation will have loose osteochondral fragments in the joint with injury to the medial patellar facet and lateral trochlea. Frequently, an unimpressive radiograph may accompany patellofemoral injury in which a large fragment of articular cartilage has been sheared away from the lateral femoral trochlea or medial patella (Fig. 10.4). Small bone flakes on radiograph sometimes accompany large sections of displaced articular cartilage. The arthroscopic evaluation of patients with acute patellar dislocation has revealed that this is not a benign condition. One must consider that preexisting malalignment has been aggravated by substantial articular injury, particularly to the medial patella and lateral trochlea, with medial retinacular disruption. For these reasons, acute patellar dislocation should be regarded not only as an extension of subluxation, but rather as a major traumatic event with implications of significant additional structural damage.

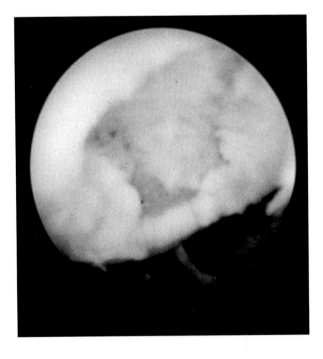

Figure 10.4. Medial facet articular injury is common after relocation of a dislocated patella. (Photo courtesy of David Burstein, Avon, Connecticut.)

Treatment

It has been customary to reduce the acutely dislocated patella and immobilize the extremity for a period of time to permit healing of the medial retinaculum, with presumed restabilization of the patella. Larsen and Lauridsen (32) have confirmed that conservative management is appropriate for many patients after a first-time patellar dislocation. Arthroscopic evaluation of such patients, however, by Neal Thomson (personal communication, 1988) and others has demonstrated that articular injury may be substantial, and arthroscopy, therefore, may be appropriate for many patients who have sustained an acute patellar dislocation. Hawkins et al (33) noted that those patients with a predisposing history of underlying malalignment may benefit from immediate arthroscopic intervention. Even in the face of unremarkable radiograms, articular injury may be substantial, and the best opportunity to restore significant displaced fragments is immediately following surgery. If the lateral retinaculum is particularly tight, lateral retinacular release at this time may be helpful in reestablishing a normal or near-normal tracking pattern. Vainion-paa et al (34) prospectively studied 55 patients treated surgically for acute patellar dislocation and noted a redislocation rate of 9%, with most patients returning to the preoperative level of athletic activity. More recently, Maenpaa and Lehto found even higher incidences of recurrent problems after patella dislocation (35), with unsatisfactory results most of the time following nonoperative treatment.

Although immobilization may be the treatment of choice by many orthopedic surgeons, we believe that an arthroscopy to evaluate these patients and surgery aimed at restoring major displaced fragments of articular cartilage or releasing major deforming forces, such as a tight lateral retinaculum, may improve the long-term prognosis for such patients. More extensive realignment surgery, however, should be avoided in the acute setting. Cofield and Bryan (36) noted a 42% failure rate after nonsurgical treatment for patellar dislocation. Certainly, the surgeon who undertakes arthroscopy of a patient with acute patellar dislocation must be prepared to correct the significant articular lesions identified.

If the treating physician is confident that there is no major articular fragment displacement, and if the patella can be reduced well into the trochlea and maintained there, a period of 6 weeks' immobilization may restore adequate stability. Nonoperative treatment will give satisfactory results, particularly when there is no preexisting congenital abnormality of the extensor mechanism (33, 37). With newer techniques and the availability of high-quality arthroscopy, however, the clinician should consider arthroscopy selectively. Diagnostic arthroscopy adds little risk and can add substantially to detecting serious damage to a patient's extensor mechanism. Simple replacement of osteochondral fragments and selective lateral retinacular release (particularly in patients with lateral tilt) may help avoid future problems when there is evidence of causative malalignment. Bigos and McBride (38) noted that there was no recurrence of dislocation in 23 knees at a mean follow-up time of 14.5 months after lateral release for dislocation. Dainer et al (39), however, noted less satisfactory results after lateral release for acute patellar dislocation, but their patients were not selected for preexisting malalignment. Major reconstruction, however, should generally be avoided immediately after an acute patellar dislocation.

Fulkerson's Approach to Acute Patellar Dislocation

When there is radiographic evidence of an osteochondral fragment in the knee, do an arthroscopy to locate the fragment and replace it if it is large enough. Pinning the fragment back to the trochlea generally requires a limited lateral arthrotomy, at which time a lateral release will normally be done if there is lateral patellar tilt. If there is a small fragment (<1 cm articular diameter), the fragment is usually removed arthroscopically. If the patient has evidence of significant lateral patellar tilt, a lateral release is done. We emphasize *tilt* because we agree with Christensen et al (40) that lateral release alone is not consistently helpful for patients with *subluxation* (41), and might make it worse.

However, if acute patellar dislocation has been a result of direct trauma *without underlying malalignment,* there is no reason to do a lateral release. Also, if there is no evidence of bone attached to a loose fragment, there is little reason to operate acutely inasmuch as replacement of cartilage alone will be destined to failure in the majority of cases. Nonetheless, when there are fragments of bone attached to a significant piece of articular cartilage, one should make an effort to restore the joint surface. At times, one may wish to use fine (6-0) suture to stabilize articular edges and allow fragment healing.

In short, then, we recommend a logical approach to these patients. Replace fragments that have been dislodged from the lateral trochlea or patella. Do a lateral release when there is evidence of a predisposing tilt. If disruption of the medial patellofemoral ligament has left a residual instability, acute repair of the medial patellofemoral ligament, isometrically and without undue tension, may be appropriate selectively, followed by early motion to avoid stiffness. When there is no major osteochondral fragment or clear malalignment, treat the patient with immobilization initially, followed by progressive quadriceps exercise emphasizing the vastus medialis obliquus. In such cases, any necessary reconstruction may be done later, electively.

RECURRENT PATELLAR DISLOCATION

The natural history of recurrent dislocation is quite variable, and there are multiple treatment options (42). The occasional patient is seen with only a single dislocation in his/her lifetime. This single presentation is unusual, estimated by Heywood (8) to be at 15%. Other patients are seen with simply two or three dislocations over a period of many years and generally escape surgical intervention as long as the knee remains stable in the interim. Some individuals are seen with frequent dislocation, even during benign activities such as walking, descending stairs, dancing, and so on. Even between dislocations, the knee is unstable and uncomfortable. Crosby and Insall (19) reported that the frequency of dislocation decreased with age in 26 patients who were treated nonoperatively. Nonetheless, one must remember that substantial articular injury occurs at the time of dislocation, and care must be taken to replace osteochondral fragments in the hope of avoiding recurrent dislocations. Arthroscopy becomes the cornerstone of decision making in this regard.

Loff and Friedebold (7) have associated the severity of a dislocation directly with poor long-term results. They found little correlation between the number of dislocations and subsequent degenerative changes. Those patients who had pain, swelling, and disability associated with each dislocation, even if the episodes were infrequent, fared much worse than those whose episodes were frequent but associated with little disability. These same authors reported the results of conservative treatment of 32 knees affected by recurrent dislocation. Only four stabilized. The remaining 28 continued to dislocate. Such reports raise the possibility that aggressive early treatment of certain patients (those with more severe malalignment and joint damage) may improve long-term results.

Clinical Features

History

Recurrent patellar dislocation is often a disorder of the second decade. In Ficat's series (43), the youngest patient was 10 years old and the oldest was 27, with a peak at 15 years. Baum and Bensahal (5) had similar findings, with a range from age 10 to 16 years and a peak at 14 years. Both studies noted peak incidents during puberty that may reflect both changes in axial alignment and length of the lower extremity as well as change in level of activity. Most series have reported a female predominance varying from 1.5:1 to as high as 5:1 (7, 44–46).

The initial dislocation most frequently occurs without any warning. It may occur simply as the result of twisting in one direction. In Baum and Bensahal's series (5), 38% experienced their initial dislocation during athletics in which external rotation and valgus stress were applied to the affected knee at the time of dislocation. The initial dislocation is acute and is generally associated with a fall and severe discomfort on the medial aspect of the knee. The patient is unable to arise alone, but this period of complete disability is generally short-lived because it is only necessary to extend the knee in order to achieve spontaneous relocation. It is, therefore, unusual for the patient to come to the emergency room with a completely dislocated patella.

While the anterior surface of the knee is uncovered, the prominence of the medial femoral condyle may attract the patient's attention. Particularly if the period of dislocation is short, therefore, the patient may not directly report that the patella has dislocated laterally. Once relocation has taken place by passive extension of the knee, the patient is generally able to walk unassisted. However, the knee is acutely tender, and each flexion causes not only discomfort but the apprehension of a recurrent episode. Therefore, gait is frequently characterized by holding the knee in fixed extension. The nature of the episode and symptoms are such that the patient frequently seeks immediate medical attention. Some, however, treat themselves with a compression bandage, believing that the knee has been sprained and do not come for evaluation until the second or third episode.

Examination

In the unusual circumstance that the patient presents with an acute unreduced dislocation, the diagnosis is evident, as the deformity is characteristic. The knee is painfully fixed in flexion by hamstring spasm. The anterior surface of the distal femur is not covered by the patella, and the outline of the condyles can be easily seen. The patella can be visualized as a prominence against the lateral surface of the lateral condyle. Passive extension of the extremity generally results in spontaneous relocation.

More commonly, the patient presents several hours after the accident. The clinical history will not always lead one directly to the correct diagnosis, particularly if the patient was involved in sports at the time of dislocation. However, the physical examination is characteristic. The hemarthrosis, although frequently considerable, is rarely under tension because the synovial membrane has been torn at the same time as the medial retinaculum. The patella is hypermobile laterally and could easily be redislocated if the patient would allow. The most pathognomonic sign is tenderness along the medial border of the patella, which testifies to the torn medial parapatellar structures, including the medial patellofemoral ligament.

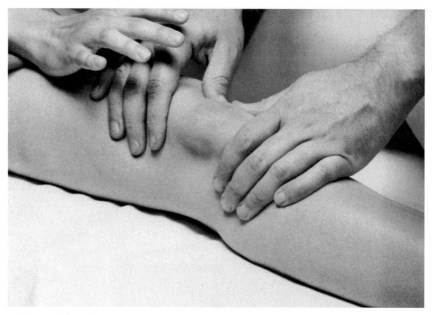

Figure 10.5. The apprehension sign is characteristic of recurrent dislocation.

Not infrequently, the patient presents for examination some time after the initial or subsequent episodes during a period when the knee is relatively, but not completely, asymptomatic. The characteristic reason for seeking an opinion is that the knee continues to feel insecure. In contrast with the acute presentation, the knee at this point is generally not very painful. The most important physical finding is the apprehension sign (Fig. 10.5) described by Fairbank (47) and Apley (48) and popularized by Smillie (49). With the patient supine, the knee extended, and the quadriceps relaxed, the examiner applies firm pressure to the medial border of the patella, subluxing it laterally while passively initiating flexion. The patient experiences acute apprehension that the patella is about to dislocate and contracts the quadriceps, which recenters the patella and prevents further flexion. This apprehension may or may not be associated with acute discomfort. The prominent finding is fear of dislocation. Although the sign is frequently present and very indicative of recurrent dislocation, it is not constant.

Under certain circumstances, when the diagnosis is in doubt, MRI may be helpful. Trillat and Dejour (50) have reported an associated meniscal tear 13 times in 91 operations for patella dislocation. Ficat (43) reported similar findings in only 1 of 18 operated cases. It is important to beware of a mistaken diagnosis in either direction.

Upon physical examination, it is important to look for a loose body. These are frequently cartilaginous and will not show up on routine radiography. Occasionally, loose bodies can be palpated in the suprapatellar pouch or along the medial or lateral recess (lateral is more common).

Radiologic Features

Radiologic evaluation of the patient with recurrent patellar dislocations can help establish the degree of traumatic articular injury, evidence of loose bodies, and predisposing malalignment.

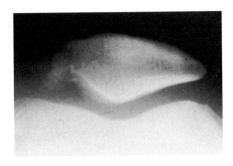

Figure 10.6. Marked medial retinacular soft-tissue calcification in a patient with a history of recurrent dislocations.

Standard anteroposterior, lateral, notch, and tangential (axial) radiographic views, as described in Chapter 4, will be adequate in many cases. If surgery is planned for recurrent dislocations that cannot be managed nonoperatively, CT of the patellofemoral joint will give the best overall view of patellar behavior through a range of motion. If a pattern of tilt with minimal or no subluxation is found, lateral release alone may be sufficient. However, the majority of these patients have substantial subluxation, and the CT data can be helpful in understanding trochlear morphology as well as the amount of malalignment and associated tilt. This may help the surgeon develop an appropriate operative plan.

In the patient with recurrent patellar dislocations, there may be soft-tissue calcification in the traumatized medial retinaculum (Fig. 10.6). Not infrequently, the medial border may show a defect where an osteochondral fracture has occurred during the dislocation (Fig. 10.7). Finally, the medial patellofemoral ligament may have pulled off a small fleck of bone at the time that it was torn. Sometimes this is visible on high-quality films (Fig. 10.8).

Osteochondral fracture with subsequent loose body formation is a frequent sequela of patellar dislocation. Ficat and Bizou (13) reported an incidence of 25%. This may not always be evident clinically if there is not the typical interference with mechanical function of the joint. A radiodense fleck seen in an unusual position should raise suspicion of a loose body. These loose bodies may be of four origins: (a) from the cartilaginous surface of the patella, in which case they are generally small and invisible on routine radiograms; (b) from an osteochondral fracture of the medial patella as it passes over the lateral trochlea at the time of *re*location; (c) pulled off by the medial patellofemoral ligament, in which case it is generally not free in the joint; or (d) from the lateral trochlea, sheared off at the time of patellar relocation.

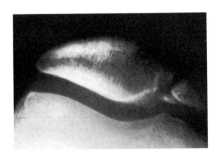

Figure 10.7. The subchondral outline of the medial facet is interrupted, suggesting an osteochondral fracture rather than soft-tissue calcification.

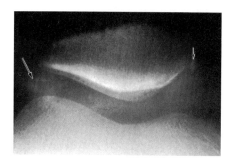

Figure 10.8. Patient with several episodes of recurrent dislocation. A small fragment of bone is pulled away from the medial patellar border (*small arrow*) at the level of attachment of the medial patellofemoral ligament. The density in the lateral joint line has the appearance of a loose body (*large arrow*).

Treatment

Treatment of this condition is similar to that in the patient with recurrent subluxation; also, the surgeon should be certain to replace major osteochondral fragments whenever possible as would be done in the patient with acute patellar dislocation. Results of surgical treatment are not always good at long-term follow-up, however (51).

In general, if the patient has had recurrent dislocations rather than subluxations, the degree of malalignment will be greater and there may be considerable damage to the medial patella and lateral trochlea such that more definitive surgical realignment may be necessary. Additionally, Cerullo et al (52) have noted that the best results of extensor mechanism realignment were in patients with greater preoperative instability.

In some cases, when there are symptoms related primarily to medial facet articular damage (Fig. 10.9), the loose articular fragments may be resected, and drilling, cautious abrasion, or microfracture can be used to induce bleeding from subchondral bone. One must assure patellar stability, however, to avoid further injury to the already compromised medial facet.

In our opinion, the Trillat procedure as described by Cox (53) and reviewed in Chapter 7 forms the basis of realigning a chronically dislocating extensor mechanism, particularly when the lateral trochlea is deficient. Riegler (54) also reported good results with the Trillat procedure, although other formal realignment procedures are available and may be preferred by some surgeons (55). Vastus medialis obliquus advancement may be necessary but carries the risk of overloading an already damaged medial facet. Placing "anchor" sutures in the distal aspect of the central quadriceps tendon avoids tethering the medial facet at the time of vastus medialis obliquus advancement. Lateral retinacular release alone is more appropriate to treat patients with recurrent dislocation with documented patellar tilt as a precipitating factor. Miller and Bartlett have reported satisfactory short-term results with lateral release for recurrent patellar dislocation (56). Aglietti et al (57), however, noted that results of surgical treatment for recurrent patellar dislocation were worse using lateral release alone. He recommended combining lateral release with proximal or distal realignment as necessary. In our opinion, lateral release is not adequate for all patients with patellar dislocation, and the surgeon should keep an open mind to medial imbrication or tibial tubercle transfer when necessary to fully correct patellar alignment. Also, as Gomes (58) noted, the surgeon must decide whether to do a medial patellofemoral ligament reconstruction following patellar dislocation. Another option is tenodesis of the distal adductor magnus tendon to the medial patella for recurrent dislocation (59), but we have no experience with this.

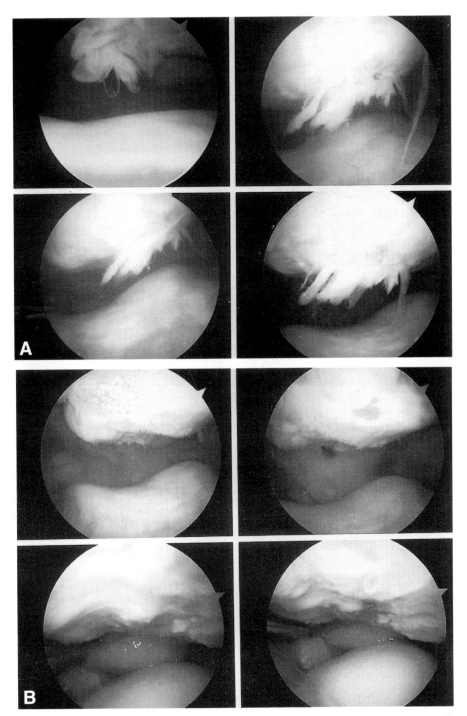

Figure 10.9. A, Patella dislocation can cause considerable medial facet damage. These arthroscopic views demonstrate medial facet chondral damage caused by patellar dislocation. **B,** After resection of cartilage flaps and microfracture of the exposed subchondral bone to induce fibrocartilage resurfacing, the patient experienced substantial relief. In this case, there was satisfactory patella alignment.

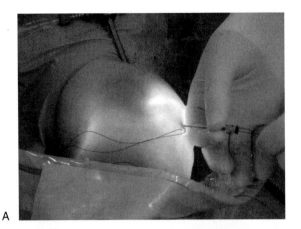

A

Figure 10.10. A, Placing initial 0 or #1 monofilament suture through an 18-gauge needle. **B,** Suture retrieved inside joint. **C,** Suture pulled out, then followed by #2 suture (we prefer fiber-wire [Arthrex, Naples, Florida]).

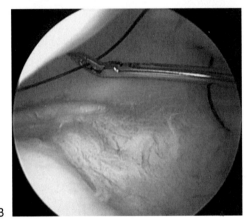

B

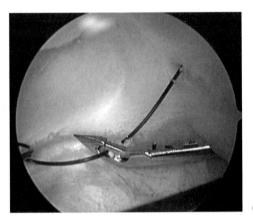

C

Some patients who have recurrent dislocation with Outerbridge Grades 3 to 4 arthrosis may benefit from anteromedial tibial tubercle transfer to unload a deficient patellar articular surface at the time of realignment.

When arthroscopic realignment can reconstitute the medial patellofemoral ligament without adding stress to deficient medial patella articular cartilage, this is a reasonable alternative (Fig. 10.10, A–E). In general, as the degree of patella instability increases, medial tibial tubercle transfer becomes increasingly attractive because there is increasing risk of medial repair disruption or adding excessive load to a damaged medial patella with imbrication. The option of viewing the imbrication arthroscopically has appeal and should add a measure of safety to an imbrication procedure. The final decision should be made to serve the patient's best long-term interest and avoid causing any added problem. As usual, surgical precision, both in decision making and execution, is most important.

PERMANENT PATELLAR DISLOCATION

As will be seen in other areas of pathology of the patellofemoral joint, there are some problems with semantics. The literature contains reference to permanent, congenital, habitual, and recurrent dislocations of the patella without, in many instances, defining what the author means by the term chosen. *By permanent dislocation of the patella, we*

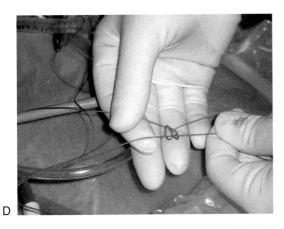

D

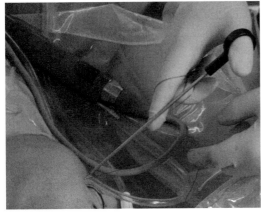

E

Figure 10.10. *Continued.* **D,** Sliding knot allows for titration of imbrication. **E,** Secure imbrication with knot tier.

choose to mean that the patella is no longer in contact with the articular cartilage of the distal femur throughout the full range of flexion. On extension, the patella may return toward, or nearly to, the midline, but on flexion, the patella always returns to the lateral surface of the lateral condyle. There are two clinical forms of permanent dislocation of the patella: congenital and acquired. These forms share certain aspects of their etiology, clinical and radiologic features, and treatment but remain distinct enough to be considered separately.

Congenital Form

Green and Waugh (60) believed that congenital dislocation of the patella occurs in utero or at birth. However, the diagnosis is seldom made until several years of age. Green and Waugh also presented a family tree suggesting hereditary predisposition.

Acquired Form

We select "acquired" form as a descriptive term to avoid the confusing term "habitual." Habitual has been used as a synonym for "recurrent" (61, 62). It has been defined by Benoist and Ramadier (63) and Rutt (64) to describe a form of dislocation that spontaneously dislocates by 90 degrees of flexion. The term "habitual dislocation" should be restricted to the form of permanent dislocation for which we prefer the term "acquired." On extension, the patella returns to near the midline while at each flexion it rolls over the lateral condyle to lie lateral to it. This form of dislocation is apparently not present at birth.

Etiology

Congenital Form

The cause of the congenital form of patellar dislocation may be an anomalous insertion of fibrous tissue into the lateral patella. In some patients, there is an abnormal band from the fascia lata to the patella (17, 65). In other patients, an abnormal fibrous band appears to arise from the vastus lateralis (66), which consists of a tendinous condensation inserting into the superolateral border of the patella. In either situation, the result is the same. The patella is drawn to the lateral side of the knee with the initiation of flexion.

Acquired Form

Hnevkovsky (67) awakened interest in progressive fibrosis of the quadriceps with his report of 12 cases in 1961. None of these were reported to involve patellar dislocation. However, since then, many more cases of progressive quadriceps fibrosis have been reported (60, 66–69). Twenty-eight of these cases involved permanent dislocation of the patella.

Some authors believe that quadriceps fibrosis is of congenital dysplastic origin similar to clubfoot, arthrogryposis, or congenital torticollis (8, 47, 69). However, in most cases one can obtain a history of multiple intramuscular injections (67, 68, 70, 71) into the thigh in infancy. This appears to have provoked a fibrous reaction that then becomes progressively manifest as the femur increases in length out of proportion to the fibrotic muscle. Whatever the origin, only the vastus lateralis, intermedius, and rarely the rectus femoris have been reported to be involved. The tethering then inevitably produces a lateral vector. Where the medial tissues hold, a progressive limitation of flexion occurs. When the medial soft-tissue structures give way, permanent dislocation of the patella results.

Clinical Features

The older the child, the more likely there is to be some secondary deformity such as genu valgum, external rotation of the tibia, flattening of the lateral condyle of the femur, and even shortening of the femur. The small size of the patella along with flattening of the articular surface also seem to be secondary deformities. There is, therefore, considerable interest in both early diagnosis and surgical correction before these early deformities become irreversible.

Although progressive extension contracture of the knee due to quadriceps fibrosis and the acquired form of permanent dislocation appear to have a common etiology, by and large, they tend to run separate clinical courses. No cases have been reported of a progressive extension contracture progressing to permanent dislocation. However, Williams (66) observed a case of permanent dislocation on one side and extension contracture on the other. As with the congenital form of permanent dislocation, the acquired form is also more likely to be associated with secondary deformities if allowed to continue untreated for significant periods of time.

The adult form presents with the signs and symptoms of patellofemoral arthrosis. The symptoms are generally mild in comparison to the radiologic and physical findings. Rapid clinical deterioration is not the usual pattern.

Congenital Form

It is unusual for the congenital form to be detected at birth. The patella is palpable in the infant only with the knee in full extension. It is not ossified until 4 to 5 years of age, so radiographs are of no help. The presence of fixed flexion contracture at birth is characteristic of both arthrogryposis and congenital dislocation of the patella. If the former can be excluded, the latter is likely. Even though the patella is dislocated throughout the full range of knee movement, extension is often quite good. Even though extension may not be complete, the patient is able to bear weight on the extremity. Flexion and lateral seating of the patella external to the lateral condyle is not accompanied by pain, but the children have difficulty arising from the squatting or sitting position.

The knee, particularly in the flexed position, lacks the normal contour. The condyles are uncovered anteriorly, giving an *apparent* predominance of the medial femoral condyle. Genu valgum is a frequent concomitant deformity (72–74) and is likely due to the lateral positioning of the entire extensor apparatus. The patella may be absent from its normal anterior position in extension as well as in flexion, or it may be nearly in the midline anteriorly in full extension, springing to the lateral side with the initiation of flexion. Because of the lateral position of the patella, the flexed knee presents a broader than usual appearance.

The range of movement of the knee may often be normal, although extensor power is diminished. Some authors have reported extensor lag (72), whereas others have reported fixed flexion contracture of the knee (66, 68, 74, 75). The quadriceps inevitably shows considerable atrophy, most notably in the vastus medialis. In addition, a fibrous band from either the fascia lata or the vastus lateralis can often be palpated inserting into the superolateral border of the patella. An attempt to prevent the lateral dislocation of the patella, while flexing the knee passively, will bring out this band of fibrous tissue, which plays a determining role in the dislocation.

Acquired Form

The usual age of presentation is between 5 and 7 years. The patient reports that the patella has been moving laterally on flexion for only a short time (months), sometimes as a result of injury. Often, this is not accompanied by functional disability or acute pain, giving way, and swelling, as are commonly associated with recurrent dislocation in the adolescent or adult.

Because age of presentation for the acquired form is older, the patella is easily palpable and visualized. It is usually more nearly in the midline with the leg fully extended. Neither fixed flexion contracture nor quadriceps lag is present. The remainder of the physical examination is nearly the same as for the congenital form.

Radiologic Features

Congenital Form

Before the appearance of the ossific nucleus of the patella at approximately age 4 years, the radiograph is of no help in establishing the diagnosis. Once the ossific nucleus

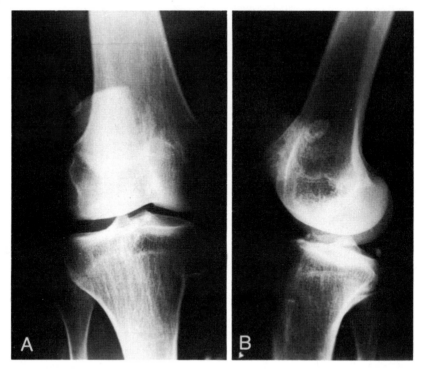

Figure 10.11. A, Anteroposterior radiographic view of patient with congenital dislocation of the patella. Note the lateral situation of the patella and particularly the medial tibial hypoplasia. **B,** Lateral radiographic view of same patient. Even with this slight degree of flexion, the patella is disappearing behind the condyles.

has formed, the patella will be seen (even on the AP view) to be lying lateral to its normal position (Fig. 10.11, A). The associated valgus may also be evident on the AP film. Ficat (43) has reported an associated hypoplasia of the medial tibial plateau and corresponding medial femoral condyle in his cases. Later, when the patella is more fully ossified, it may be seen to be smaller than normal and more proximally situated. An associated external torsion of the tibia may give the appearance of dissociation of the femoral and tibial outlines on the AP view.

The lateral radiograph (Fig. 10.11, B), when taken in a few degrees of flexion, suggests absence of the patella because it is hidden by the femoral condyles. In addition, the condyles themselves often appear flattened anteriorly, particularly the lateral condyle.

The axial view (Fig. 10.12) shows the lateral position of the patella, with its articular surface sitting against the lateral border of the lateral condyle. The patella itself is generally smaller than the contralateral side, and its articular surface is either flat or slightly convex. The sulcus of the trochlea appears shallow, particularly in the 30-degree flexion axial view, where a groove is sometimes barely evident and occasionally absent. CT or MRI study can be helpful in defining the trochlear morphology in detail. The shallow trochlea in these patients is presumably due to failure of modeling of the sulcus during growth due to lack of pressure from the patella in its normal anterior position. Brattstrom (2) has shown this to cause the shallow sulcus in recurrent dislocation of the patella, and it would seem logical that this same situation exists in permanent congenital dislocation.

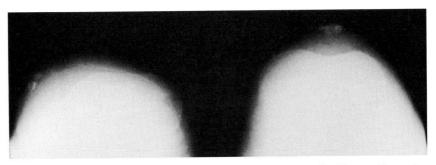

Figure 10.12. Axial view of congenital dislocation of the right patella. The ossific nucleus can be seen lying along the lateral condyle. Note also the difference in sulcus depth on the right compared with the left.

Acquired Form

Because the presentation of this form is later, the radiograph corroborates the physical findings. In this form, the AP view may be considered normal because the patella more frequently returns to near the normal position. There is usually only a relatively short period of time between the onset of the condition and the presentation of the patient for evaluation so that secondary deformities such as external tibial torsion and valgus deformities are much less common. The axial view will show the patella to be dislocated (Fig. 10.13), but both sulcus and patellar form are much more likely to be normal unless the condition has been neglected for a long time. The precise lateral will show the lateral facet edge posterior to the central ridge (Fig. 10.14) in milder cases. CT illustrates how chronic lateral dislocation will destroy the normal trochlea morphology (Fig. 10.15).

Treatment

Treatment of permanent patellar dislocation is difficult, and extensor mechanism realignment (proximal, distal, or both) may or may not work. Often, there is significant degenerative change that further complicates treatment, particularly in older patients (Fig. 10.16). Nonetheless, surgical centralization of the extensor mechanism using combined distal and proximal realignment is worthwhile selectively in patients who are substantially disabled and when there is appropriate articular cartilage to support this type of restoration.

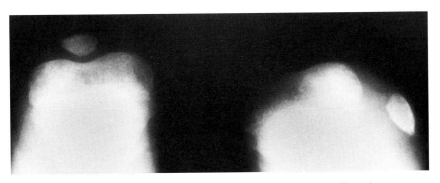

Figure 10.13. Acquired dislocation due to quadriceps fibrosis.

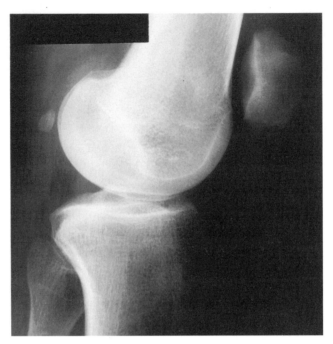

Figure 10.14. Lateral view showing lateral displacement of the patella in which the lateral facet is posterior to the central ridge.

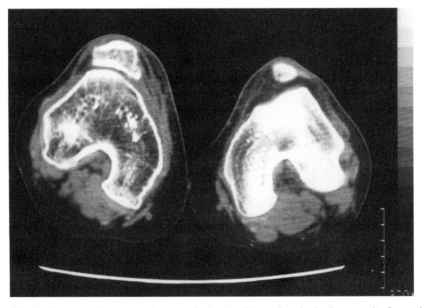

Figure 10.15. Computed tomography reveals the trochlear dysplasia that results from chronic patellar dislocation.

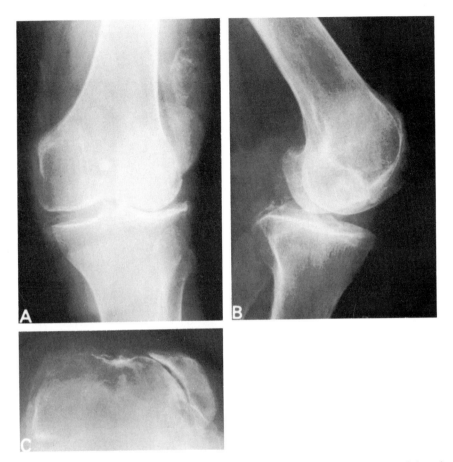

Figure 10.16. A, Anteroposterior view of a 56-year-old woman with permanent dislocation of the patella. The lateral compartment shows nearly complete loss of articular cartilage. **B,** Lateral radiograph of the same patient with the knee flexed 55 degrees. The patella is hidden lateral to the condyle and is not visualized on this projection. **C,** Axial view of the same patient showing complete lateral dislocation of the patella, which is half-moon in shape, conforming now to the lateral femoral condyle rather than to the trochlear sulcus.

In both the congenital and acquired forms of permanent dislocation, the main problem is an abnormal fibrotic band attaching to the superolateral aspect of the patella. The treatment for both of these conditions, when they involve dislocation of the patella, is rectus femoris lengthening, extensive lateral release, medial imbrication, and patellar tendon transfer. Gao et al (76) noted 87.8% satisfactory results in 35 children treated in this manner. Langenskiold and Ritsila (77) have also noted favorable results following operative treatment of this condition in young people. Surgery is most successful in children with minimal degenerative change.

Surgical Technique for Correction of Permanent Patella Dislocation

A long anterolateral, lateral, or midline incision is necessary to explore all the factors that may potentially be involved (Fig. 10.17). The incision should extend along the distal third of the thigh to the tibial tubercle, passing the patella at the level of the lateral

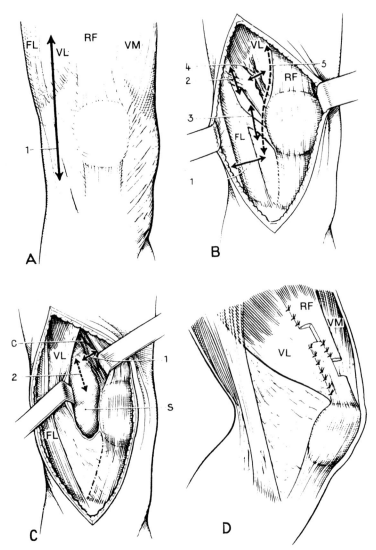

Figure 10.17. Technique for connecting severe habitual lateral dislocation. **A,** Lateral parapatellar skin incision. **B,** Systematic searching for and sectioning abnormal bands. *1,* Sectioning
of the fascia lata when necessary; *2,* division of any fascial slips from the fascia lata to the vastus lateralis; *3,* sectioning any insertion from the fascia lata into the patella; *4,* sectioning any
abnormal fibrous bands in the vastus lateralis; and *5,* separation of the vastus lateralis from the
rectus femoris. This division should extend down to and include separation of the vastus lateralis from the patella. **C,** Division of any fibrous tissue from the intermedius muscle. *S,* synovial
membrane; *2,* incision in the synovium in order to explore the joint. **D,** Z-plasty elongation of
the quadriceps tendon resutured with the knee in 90 degrees of flexion and reinforced by the
vastus lateralis. Reprinted with permission from Ficat P. Pathologie Fémoro-Patellaire. Paris:
Masson et Cie; 1970.

condyle. Avoid making the incision too far lateral so that any procedures to reinforce the medial patellar structures can be carried out through the same incision. A long midline incision may be used if desired. After the superficial fascia has been incised, the following structures are systematically explored.

Fascia Lata

Frequently, an abnormal band is encountered attached to the superolateral corner of the patella. In any event, the normal fibers attached to the inferior third of the patella and the patellar tendon will require release to allow reposition. Some authors (46, 61) also recommend sectioning the iliotibial tract, which is inevitably tight and seems to fix the tibia in external rotation. We have not found this to be necessary.

Vastus Lateralis

A thickened tendinous insertion into the superolateral corner of the patella may be concealed by overlying muscle fibers, in which case the insertion must be sought. It, too, is divided. Sometimes, the muscle itself appears diffusely fibrotic. In these cases, the vastus lateralis must be dissected free of the lateral and superior borders of the patella and the lateral border of the rectus femoris.

Rectus Femoris

Direct involvement is much less frequent, although secondary contracture frequently makes Z-plasty lengthening necessary. It should be sutured under some tension, with the knee flexed 90 degrees. The vastus lateralis insertion may be used to reinforce the repair.

Synovium

The synovium may also be contracted or fibrosed to the lateral condyle, in which case release or even limited synovectomy may be required.

Each level of the release is determined by restriction of passive knee flexion and, in many cases, only limited releases are necessary. It is possible that even after sufficient lateral and superior release, the patella will be unstable because of insufficient development of the lateral condyle or trochlear sulcus. In this case, a medial restraint must be constructed. Possibilities include imbricating the medial retinaculum, advancement of the vastus medialis along the medial patellar border, and reconstruction of the medial patellofemoral ligament with hamstring or quadriceps tendon. When the patient is skeletally mature, direct medial transfer of the tibial tubercle, using the Cox (53) modification of the Trillat procedure, is almost always necessary.

If the condition is due to fibrosis of the vastus lateralis and/or intermedius due to multiple intramuscular injections in childhood, the actual fibrotic element may be well proximal to the knee. This can usually be determined on physical examination, in which case the fibrotic area is approached through a middle and proximal thigh, midlateral longitudinal incision, releasing the vastus lateralis and intermedius where indicated from their femoral and intermuscular septum origins. The degree of release and progression of the exploration to involve factors previously reviewed depends upon the achievement of flexion and proper tracking of the patella. Reconstruction of the medial patellofemoral ligament may be necessary as well.

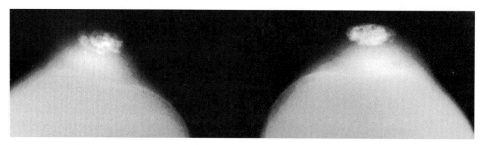

Figure 10.18. Same patient as seen in Fig. 10.11, 2 years after quadricepsplasty. Note that the patella is well centered and the trochlear groove is developing nicely.

Postoperative management is a crucial phase of the treatment. The leg is placed in a compressive wrap and knee immobilizer for the first week. When the leg becomes comfortable, this is changed to a hinged long leg knee brace with extension stop at 0 degrees and flexion stop at 90 degrees. Continuous passive motion may be used selectively, but all patients are instructed in passive range of motion exercise. Active quadriceps exercise should generally be started early, if the repair will tolerate it. Satisfactory results (Fig. 10.18) can be anticipated, but if the quadriceps is lengthened, 6 months may be required to achieve active extension (66).

REFERENCES

1. Markow RL, Soudry M, Insall JN. Patellar dislocation following total knee replacement. J Bone Joint Surg (Am) 1985;67(9):1321–1327.
2. Brattstrom H. Shape of the intercondylar groove normally and in recurrent dislocation of the patella. Acta Orthop Scand (suppl) 1964;68:134–148.
3. Vainionpaa S, Laasonen E, Patiala H, Rusanen M, Rokkannen P. Acute dislocation of the patella. Clinical, radiographic and operative findings in 64 consecutive cases. Acta Orthop Scand 1986;57(4):331–333.
4. Nietosvaara Y, Aalto K, Kallio PE. Acute patellar dislocation in children: Incidence and associated osteochondral fractures. J Pediatr Orthop 1994;14(4):513–515.
5. Baum C, Bensahal H. Luxation recidivante de la rotule chez l'enfant. Rev Chir Orthop 1973;59:583–592.
6. Rohlederer O. Atiologie and symptomatologie der praeluxio patellae. Zentralbl Chir 1951;76:103–115.
7. Loff P, Friedebold G. Die habituelle patellarluxation als praarthrotische deformitat. Ergeb Chir 1969;52:60.
8. Heywood A. Recurrent dislocation of the patella. J Bone Joint Surg 1961;43B:508–517.
9. Trillat A, Dejour HL, Coutette A. Diagnostic et traitement des subluxations recidivantes de la rotule. Rev Chir Orthop 1964;50:813–824.
10. Dupuis PV. La Torsion Tibiale. Paris: Masson et Cie; 1951.
11. Hughston JC. Recurrent Subluxation and Dislocation of the Patella. AOA: Thesis. December 1962.
12. Bizou H. Contribution a l'etude des desequilibres de l'appareil extenseur du genou dans le plan frontal. Thesis. Toulouse, France; 1966.
13. Ficat P, Bizou H. Luxations recidivantes de la rotule. Rev Orthop 1967;53:721.
14. Insall J, Falvo KA, Wise DW. Chondromalacia patellae. J Bone Joint Surg 1976;58A:1–8.
15. Fithian D. Meier S. The case for advancement and repair of the medial patellofemoral ligament in patients with recurrent patellar instability. Operative Tech Sports Med 1999;7:81–89.
16. Koskinen SK, Kujala UM. Patellofemoral relationships and distal insertion of the vastus medialis muscle: A magnetic resonance imaging study in nonsymptomatic subjects and in patients with patellar dislocation. Arthroscopy 1992;8(4):465–468.
17. Carter C, Sweetnam R. Familial joint laxity and recurrent dislocation of the patella. J Bone Joint Surg 1958;40B:664.
18. Jeffries TE. Recurrent dislocation of the patella due to abnormal attachment of the iliotibial tract. J Bone Joint Surg 1963;45B:740–743.
19. Bowker JHL, Thompson EB. Surgical treatment of recurrent dislocation of the patella. J Bone Joint Surg 1964;46A:1451–1461.
20. Crosby EB, Insall J. Recurrent dislocation of the patella. J Bone Joint Surg 1976;58A:9–13.

21. Dugdale TW, Renshaw TS. Instability of the patellofemoral joint in Down syndrome. J Bone Joint Surg (Am) 1986;68(3):405–413.
22. Diamond LS, Lynne D, Sigman B. Orthopedic disorders in patients with Down syndrome. Orthop Clin North Am 1981;12(1):57–71.
23. Mizuta H, Kubota K, Shiraishi M, Nakamura E, Takagi K, Iwatani N. Recurrent dislocation of the patella in Turner's syndrome. J Pediatr Orthop 1994;14(1):74.
24. Ikegawa S, Sakaguchi R, Kimizuka M, Yanagisako Y, Tokimura F. Recurrent dislocation of the patella in Kabuki make-up syndrome. J Pediatr Orthop 1993;13(2):265–267.
25. Weber W, Janek C, Mcleod P, Nelson C, Thompson J. Efficacy of various forms of fixation of transverse fractures of the patella. J Bone Joint Surg 1980;62A:215–220.
26. Mankin H. The response of articular cartilage to mechanical injury. J Bone Joint Surg 1982; 64A:460.
27. Maquet P, Simonet J, Marchin PD. Biomechanique du genou et gonarthrose. Rev Chir Orthop 1967;53:111.
28. Hawkins RJ, Bell RH, Anisette G. Acute patellar dislocations. The natural history. Am J Sports Med 1986;14(2): 117–120.
29. Corso SJ, Thal R, Forman D. Locked patellar dislocation with vertical axis rotation. A case report. Clin Orthop 1992;279:190–193.
30. Lance E, Deutsch AL, Mink JH. Prior lateral patellar dislocation: MR imaging findings. Radiology 1993;189(3): 905–907.
31. Virolainen H, Visuri T, Kuusela T. Acute dislocation of the patella: MR findings. Radiology 1993;189(1): 243–246.
32. Larsen E, Lauridsen F. Conservative treatment of patellar dislocations. Clin Orthop 1982;171:131–136.
33. Hawkins R, Bell R, Anisette G. Acute patellar dislocations. The natural history. Am J Sports Med 1986;14: 117–120.
34. Vainionpaa S, Laasonen E, Silvennoinen T, Vasenius J, Rokkanen P. Acute dislocation of the patella. A prospective review of operative treatment. J Bone Joint Surg (Br) 1990;72(3):366–369.
35. Maenpaa H, Lehto M. Patellar dislocation: the long-term results of nonoperative management in 100 patients. Am J Sports Med 1997;25:213–217.
36. Cofield R, Bryan R. Acute dislocation of the patella. Results of conservative treatment. J Trauma 1977;17: 526–531.
37. Cash J, Hughston J. Treatment of acute patellar dislocation. Am J Sports Med 1988;16(3):244–250.
38. Bigos SJ, McBride GG. The isolated lateral retinacular release in the treatment of patellofemoral disorders. Clin Orthop (June) 1984;(186):75–80.
39. Dainer R, Barrack R, Buckley S, Alexander A. Arthroscopic treatment of acute patellar dislocations. Arthroscopy 1988;4(4):267–271.
40. Christensen F, Soballa K, Snerum L. Treatment of chondromalacia patellae by lateral retinacular release of the patella. Clin Orthop 1988;234:145–147.
41. Fulkerson J, Schutzer S, Ramsby G, Bernstein R. Computerized tomography of the patellofemoral joint before and after lateral release or realignment. Arthroscopy 1987;(1):19–24.
42. Jackson AM. Recurrent dislocation of the patella (Editorial). J Bone Joint Surg (Br) 1992; 74(1):2–4.
43. Ficat P. Pathologic Femoro-Patellaire. Paris: Masson et Cie; 1970.
44. Andersen PT. Congenital deformities of the knee joint in dislocation of the patella and a chondrodysplasty. Acta Orthop Scand 1958;28:27–50.
45. Horwitz T. Recurrent or habitual dislocations of the patella. J Bone Joint Surg 1937;19A:1027.
46. Macnab I. Recurrent dislocation of the patella. J Bone Joint Surg 1952;34A:957.
47. Fairbank HAT. Internal derangement of the knee in children. Proc R Soc 1937;3:11.
48. Apley AG. The diagnosis of meniscus injuries. J Bone Joint Surg 1947;29:78.
49. Smillie IS. Injuries of the Knee Joint. Baltimore: Williams & Wilkins; 1962.
50. Trillat A, Dejour H. Les fractures chondro-osseuses du versant articulair interne de la rotule. Rev Chir Orthop 1967;53:331–342.
51. Arnbjornsson A, Egund N, Rydling O, Stockerup R, Ryd L. The natural history of recurrent dislocation of the patella. Long-term results of conservative and operative treatment. J Bone Joint Surg (Br) 1992;74(1):140–142.
52. Cerullo G, Puddu G, Conteduca A, Ferriti A, Mariani P. Evaluation of the results of extensor mechanism reconstruction. Am J Sports Med 1988;16(2):93–96.
53. Cox JS. Evaluation of the Roux-Elmslie-Trillat procedure for knee extensor realignment. Am J Sports Med 1982;10(5):303–313.
54. Riegler HF. Recurrent dislocations and subluxations of the patella. Clin Orthop 1988;227:201–209.
55. Turba J. Formal extensor mechanism reconstruction. Clin Sports Med 1989;8(2):297–317.
56. Miller R, Bartlett J. Recurrent patella dislocation treated by closed lateral retinacular release. Aust NZJ Surg 1993;63(3):200–202.
57. Aglietti P, Pisaneschi A, De Biase P. Recurrent dislocation of patella: Three kinds of surgical treatment. Ital J Orthop Traumatol 1992;18(1):25–36.
58. Gomes JL. Medial patellofemoral ligament reconstruction for recurrent dislocation of the patella: A preliminary report. Arthroscopy 1992;8(3):335–340.
59. Avikainen VJ, Nikko RK, Seppanen-Lehmonen TK. Adductor magnus tenodesis for patellar dislocation. Technique and preliminary results. Clin Orthop 1993;297:12–16.

60. Green JP, Waugh W. Congenital lateral dislocation of the patella. J Bone Joint Surg 1968;50B:285–289.
61. Malek R. Luxations de la rotule et retractions quadricipitales. Paris: Comm. 42nd Contres S.O.F.C.O.T.; November 8–11, 1967.
62. Roux D. Luxation habituelle de la rotule. Traitement operatoire. Rev Chir (Paris) 1888;8:682–689.
63. Benoist JP, Ramadier JO. Luxations et subluxations de la rotule. Rev Chir Orthop 1969;55: 1089-1099.
64. Rutt A. Die patellaluxation in ihren verschiedenen formen and deren pathomechnik. Z Orthop 1972;110: 235–241.
65. Ober RR. Recurrent dislocation of the patella. Am J Surg 1939;43:497.
66. Williams PF. Quadriceps contracture. J Bone Joint Surg 1968;50B:278–284.
67. Hnevkovsky O. Progressive fibrosis of the vastus intermedius in children. J Bone Joint Surg 1961;43B:318.
68. Gunn DR. Contracture of the quadriceps muscle. J Bone Joint Surg 1964;46B:492–497.
69. Karlen A. Congenital fibrosis of the vastus intermedius muscle. J Bone Joint Surg 1964;46B:488–491.
70. Lloyd-Roberts GC, Thomas TG. The etiology of quadriceps contracture in children. J Bone Joint Surg 1964; 46B:498–502.
71. Malek R. Retractions quadricipitales et injections intramusculaires chez l'enfant. Ann Chir Inf 1966;7:85-91.
72. Conn HR. A new method of operative reduction for congenital dislocation of the patella. J Bone Joint Surg 1925; 7:370.
73. Stern M. Persistent congenital dislocation of the patella. J Int Coll Surg 1964;41:654.
74. Storen H. Congenital complete dislocation of the patella causing serious disability in childhood: The operative treatment. Acta Orthop Scand 1965;36:301–313.
75. Goldthwait JE. Permanent dislocation of the patella. Ann Surg 1899;29:62.
76. Gao GX, Lee EH, Bose K. Surgical management of congenital and habitual dislocation of the patella. J Pediatr Orthop 1990;10(2):255–260.
77. Langenskiold A, Ritsila V. Congenital dislocation of the patella and its operative treatment. J Pediatr Orthop 1992;12(3):315–323.

11

Articular Cartilage Lesions in Patellofemoral Pain Patients

"And in the end, it's not the years in your life that count—it is the life in your years.

Abraham Lincoln

Budinger's (1) castigation of "internal derangement" as a diagnostic term has come to be true of "chondromalacia patellae" as well. The term has been used so widely with so little precision of meaning that much of its value has been lost. For the purposes of this book, however, the term "chondromalacia" will be defined very simply as *soft cartilage,* nothing more and nothing less!

The clinician sometimes finds it difficult to define accurately the *origin* of pain when dealing with documented *anatomic* and *histologic* lesions that do not coincide with the localization of pain on clinical examination. Such is the case with chondromalacia. On clinical examination, arthroscopy, and even at arthrotomy there may be *soft cartilage* on the patella of a patient with anterior knee pain. It is a mistake to assume that pain is *caused* by the chondromalacia. The astute clinician will recognize that chondromalacia is often a result of trauma or malalignment that causes multiple problems in the anterior knee—one of which is soft cartilage. Soft cartilage may be more clinically apparent, but in some patients the retinaculum or patellar tendon is more painful!

HISTORICAL REVIEW

In 1908, Budinger (1) drew attention to the importance of cartilage lesions on the undersurface of the patella, characterized by fissures and softening, with his report of 15 cases. Injury was involved in each of the case histories, and the etiology was interpreted to be traumatic rupture of articular cartilage. He reported treatment by excision with good results. In 1910, Ludloff (2) reported the single case history of a 15-year-old girl who likewise was cured by chondrectomy. Axhausen (3), in 1922, was the next to carry on the work of the German school in drawing attention to patellar lesions causing symptoms similar to meniscal lesions. All three of these authors indicated trauma to the patella, mostly in the form of a direct blow, as the cause of patellar cartilage lesions. In each case, their work was based upon both clinical symptoms and findings at operation. Laden (4) and Frund (5) used the term "chondropathy" in describing the articular surface of the patella to which they attributed symptoms. They, too, considered injury as the main cause and found good results after excision of damaged cartilage. The term chondropathy has been widely utilized in the European literature.

Koenig, in 1924, was the first to use the term chondromalacia patellae. According to Karlson (6), this term had been in use in Aleman's clinic since 1917, popularized with the reading of Aleman's classic paper (7) in Gutenberg in 1927. This term became widely used in Scandinavia and, subsequently, in the English literature (8, 9). Until that time, trauma in the production of cartilage lesions had been universally accepted and the cases reported were of patients with pain attributed to the pathologic articular lesion.

Owre (10) made the study of chondromalacia the subject of his doctoral thesis, examining 106 cadavers. He found an increasing incidence of cartilage lesions on the undersurface of the patella with age. Lesions were evident in a significant percentage, even in the teen years. Use of the term "chondromalacia" to associate these pathologic changes noted at autopsy with clinical symptoms has subsequently contributed to a great deal of confusion. Reports of clinical series began to appear more frequently with Silfverskiöld (11) adding his experience in 1938.

Wiberg (12), in his monumental work on the patellofemoral joint, defined the three main anatomic variations that carry his name and made important observations concerning the relationship between the medial and odd facets and loading during function. Although he suspected that the Type III patella was a form more associated with "chondromalacia," he was not able to prove this.

In 1944, Hirsch (13), in a comprehensive work, related loss of mucopolysaccharide in the ground substance to change in physical characteristics of articular cartilage. He hypothesized that the loss of mucopolysaccharides was on the basis of faulty cartilage nutrition, which then led to softening and, finally, to the formation of fissures. His original observation of the dependence of the physical characteristics of intact articular cartilage on the quality of ground substance has been confirmed by others.

Since these earlier reports, there has been considerable literature concerning chondromalacia patellae. However, rather than leading to a precise definition of chondromalacia, the term came to be used more loosely, not even requiring a description of the status of the articular cartilage by some authors. Darracott and Vernon-Roberts (14) published a report on the bone changes in chondromalacia. Furthermore, Robinson and Darracott (15) published criteria for establishing the diagnosis of chondromalacia patellae that are entirely clinical.

By the mid 1970s, there was growing awareness that soft-tissue surgery, particularly lateral retinacular release, could give relief for many patients with patellofemoral pain (16–18) suggesting that pain might originate somewhere aside from the softened articular cartilage. Meanwhile, Goodfellow et al (19), Radin (20), Abernathy et al (21), and others were emphasizing that soft cartilage on the patella is common and not necessarily a cause of pain. Casscells (22), Stougard (23), and others emphasized the frequency of chondromalacia at routine autopsy. Metcalf (24) and others noted that lateral retinacular release was effective in relieving anterior knee pain.

Lars Peterson introduced and popularized articular cartilage resurfacing with autogenous chondrocyte transplantation. Brittberg et al presented this concept in 1994 (25). Since that time, articular cartilage transplantation has been widely accepted. Tom Minas has experienced success with this technique, particularly in resurfacing the femoral condyle or trochlea (26).

NEUROTROPHINS AND PATELLOFEMORAL PAIN

We (27) noted in 1982 that the lateral retinaculum itself can be painful in patients with patellar malalignment and later substantiated these results with histologic studies (28), using Gomori's trichrome stain to show microscopic nerve injury in excised lateral retinaculum from patients with localized preoperative retinacular pain related to *malalignment.* This was the first report in the literature documenting histologically proven neural change associated with knee pain. This work, then, helps explain complaints of anterior knee pain in patients with no chondromalacia and in patients with no real correlation between arthroscopic quantification of chondromalacia and pain (24). The eccentrically aligned patella will inevitably cause abnormal stresses on its supporting retinaculum as well as on its articular cartilage. Pain producing cytokine neurotrophin excess may result from structural or iatrogenic patella imbalance. Such cytokines then may lead to elaboration of retinacular or osseous substance P and pain (29). These findings further explain our original observation of small nerve injury in the retinaculum of patients with patellofemoral imbalance (30).

The surgeon should recognize that, historically, operations to relieve the pain of chondromalacia have involved alteration of retinacular structures. Even the arthrotomy used by earlier surgeons to do patellar debridement would cause striking alteration of retinacular strains after closure and healing. Such *shifting* of retinacular strains may be significant in relieving neurotrophic pain of retinacular or bony origin. Certainly, patellectomy markedly reduces osseous and retinacular strains by removing the fulcrum (patella) tethering the retinaculum. Neurotrophin production related to abnormal subchondral bone pressure secondary to deficient cartilage must also be held accountable as a pain mechanism in patients with knee pain.

If chondromalacia patella is to have any meaning whatsoever in clinical–pathologic terms, then it must *not* be used as a synonym for patellofemoral pain (31) because the causes of this pain are complex.

PATELLAR ARTICULAR CARTILAGE BREAKDOWN

Patellar articular cartilage does not appear, from an anatomic or functional point of view, to be different from articular cartilage found in any other diarthrodial joint. Its function, nourishment, gross and microscopic anatomy, and relationship to synovium and subchondral bone is typical of articular cartilage in general. Staubli et al (32), however, have noted unique articular cartilage-subchondral bone relationships in the patellofemoral joint. One must be careful to understand that osseous and cartilaginous surfaces may vary among patients, and one should use magnetic resonance imaging (MRI) when necessary to fully appreciate apparent patellofemoral incongruities.

The terms *chondrosis,* to signify a disorder affecting only the articular cartilage, and *arthrosis,* a disorder affecting all three components of the patellofemoral joint (33) (cartilage, bone, and synovial membrane), may be helpful. For ease of understanding, we use the term arthrosis when there is *exposed* bone in the joint.

Patellar articular cartilage undergoes different modes of degeneration. Cartilage softening (chondromalacia) of the lateral facet appears to be secondary in most cases to prolonged patellar tilt and secondary compression with eventual arthrosis. Seedholm et al (34) noted that this breakdown occurs on areas of the patella corresponding to what articulates in the 40- to 80-degree knee flexion range. Increased density of subchondral bone appears early in the disorder, after the initial cartilage changes. Initial cartilage softening often progresses to fissure formation, ulceration, and arthrosis.

Chondromalacia of the medial facet appears to be somewhat different. It may be secondary to deficient contact or to a combination of compression and shearing forces, particularly in knee flexion. Iatrogenic medial facet chondromalacia or arthrosis may be a consequence of overzealous medial imbrication (Fig. 11.1) or excessive medial transfer of the tibial tubercle. Müller (35) pointed out that relatively little is known about nutritional factors that lead to medial facet articular cartilage breakdown. Goodfellow et al (19) differentiated between "age-dependent surface degeneration" on the medial facet and "basal degeneration" on the ridge separating the medial and odd facets. Radin (20), Abernathy et al (21), and others believe that central medial facet chondromalacia is *not* a significant entity causing pain in most patients. Nonetheless, a chronically *unloaded* medial facet will deny its articular cartilage an appropriate mechanism of synovial fluid nutrition (36), and in patients with malalignment or trauma, this may lead to eventual extension of medial facet degeneration and symptomatic arthrosis. If changes in bone are present, the radiograph more often shows decreased density rather than an increase in the subchondral bone of the region affected. The surgeon must consider the specific alignment pattern and how it might affect patellar (and trochlear) contact (Fig. 11.2) in different degrees of knee flexion.

A review of patellofemoral joint contact patterns reveals that the secondary ridge marks the medial edge of the contact zone from 20 to 90 degrees. Progression to full flexion involves sliding across the convex secondary ridge that may bring it briefly into high

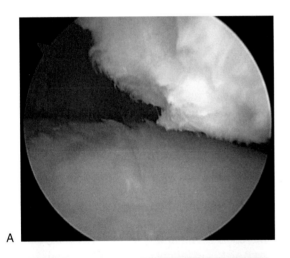

A

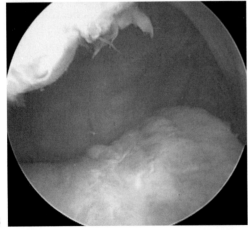

B

Figure 11.1. A, Medial facet damage from iatrogenic overload. **B,** Medial osteophytes from medial imbrication overload.

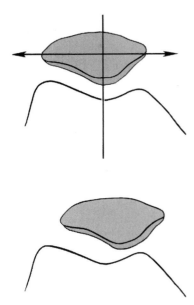

Figure 11.2. The specific pattern of patellofemoral alignment will determine the nature, location, and extent of cartilage breakdown.

pressure contact with the convex femoral condyle. It is also likely that considerable shear forces are developed as the contact area traverses the ridge, as suggested by Goodfellow et al (19).

Several authors (19, 37–39) have pointed out the tendency for cartilage that is habitually out of contact with other articular cartilage to undergo surface fibrillation. This age-dependent, nonprogressive, surface change does not usually tend to develop into an advanced cartilage lesion (20) with eventual full-thickness cartilage loss and bony eburnation. Autopsy series have shown these lesions to increase in frequency with age. The odd facet represents an area of habitual noncontact. Akizuki et al (40) noted that cartilage from low weight-bearing areas is *stiffer* than that from high weight-bearing areas. It is, therefore, not surprising that the medial facet is also a site for nonprogressive age-related surface changes. The lack of recognition of this form of cartilage abnormality may explain the predominance of medial facet chondromalacia described in many series. Of particular interest, along these lines, is the report of Marar and Pillay (41) on the low incidence of chondromalacia of the patella in a series of autopsies in people of Chinese descent. In Asian people, the odd facet is not a habitual noncontact area because of the frequent squatting, characteristic of this population. The observation of Hoaglund et al (42) on the low incidence of osteoarthritis of the hip in South Cantonese Chinese and its relation to movement and, therefore, also to decreasing habitual noncontact cartilage may have some bearing on this subject. One must, however, consider other factors also, including the overall smaller stature of many Asians.

There would seem, under normal circumstances, to be a *possible* conflict between the secondary ridge and the femoral condyle. Because not everyone has chondromalacia of the medial facet, other factors must play an important role. There is considerable variation in the prominence of the secondary ridge. Several authors (43, 44) have called attention to a prominence of the medial ridge separating the medial trochlear facet from the femoral metaphysis. This has been called the Outerbridge ridge, after the surgeon who first drew attention to its significance. There is no clear evidence, however, that this ridge is important in patients with patellofemoral pain.

Finally, it is important to remember that articular cartilage injury may occur at the time of arthroscopy (45) or other knee surgery. Antiinflammatory agents (46), hemarthrosis (47), immobilization (48–50), irrigating solutions (51, 52), iatrogenic trauma, local anesthesia (52), and corticosteroids (53) can have profound effects on patellar articular cartilage. We have found evidence of considerable articular cartilage loss and subchondral bone damage (resulting in osteochondral loose body formation) after overzealous laser chondroplasty. After arthroscopic or open surgical intervention, a suitable period of time should be allowed before returning to vigorous athletics (45) so that articular cartilage metabolism and function can stabilize. Most important, when operating on patients with patellofemoral pain, *the surgeon must avoid articular cartilage damage as a result of excessive patella realignment or posterior imbrication.*

ANATOMIC ASPECTS OF PATELLAR CARTILAGE BREAKDOWN

The clinical expression of the principal forms of patellar cartilage degeneration does not always allow their differentiation. The arthroscope now permits much more accurate evaluation of patellar articular cartilage lesions.

Closed Chondromalacia

Closed chondromalacia is common and may or may not be symptomatic. How and when this causes pain remains unclear, although the arthroscopic surgeon frequently sees soft patellar cartilage as an incidental finding in patients with pain elsewhere. It consists of simple softening of articular cartilage, which begins in a very localized area and then extends progressively in all directions. The initial appearance may be that of a small blister. Macroscopically, the surface is intact (Fig. 11.3). It appears that this blister phenomenon is the fundamental and initial lesion of patellar articular cartilage degeneration.

Because the surface is intact in this earliest of all cartilage lesions, it may pass unrecognized. It is important to emphasize that articular cartilage always be palpated with a blunt instrument at arthroscopy because there is not always a difference in surface color or appearance to draw attention to abnormality. Softening, which may at times appear fluctuant, may be present in varying degrees of severity, from simple softening to a more advanced form in which a type of "pitting edema" can be observed after digital or blunt instrument pressure.

The loss of elasticity, which this softening represents, decreases the function capacity of cartilage and explains the reaction of adjacent subchondral bone to which the compression forces are transferred abnormally. One can even wonder how these abnormal areas can stand up against the pressures developed in the patellofemoral joint. Biedert and Kernan (54) have given a wonderful review of pain origin around the patella and cite several authors who have indicated the importance of neural factors in the origin of patellofemoral pain. It is possible that excessive pressure on subchondral bone after cartilage softening might cause *relative ischemia* and elaboration of neural growth factor, which then causes release of neuroceptive mediators such as substance P, which can cause pain. This alteration of the physical properties of cartilage helps us to understand better the mechanical destruction of cartilage by fissure formation, fragmentation, and eventual ulceration, as well as certain symptoms (catching, giving way). The discovery of this localized area of softening also explains the computed tomographic (CT) or MRI finding of localized loss of cartilage, whereas the standard axial radiograph shows a normal joint space. Surrounding normal cartilage maintains the overall normal appearance of the

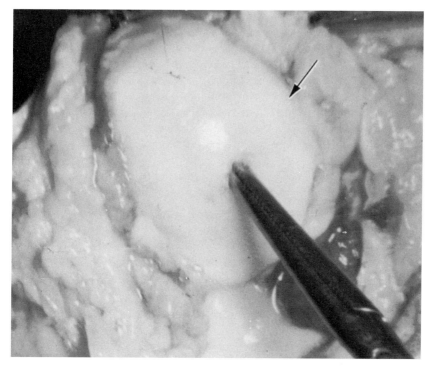

Figure 11.3. Operative photo of closed chondromalacia. The reflection of light is off a rounded "blister" lesion, which projects above the surface. Arrow marks proximal border at median ridge; lateral facet superior.

joint, whereas a tomographic study with progressive knee flexion will pick up specific narrowing on a localized surface of the patella.

The techniques of MRI and CT make possible the early diagnosis of this minimal lesion but are not usually necessary in clinical practice unless the clinician needs to evaluate patellar tracking preoperatively. Extension of the initial malacic lesion, which leads to overall joint narrowing, will be evident eventually on the standard axial radiograph. The finding of this lesion in a radiographically "normal" joint gives significance to the slightly narrowed "joint line," which tends to be underestimated. This incipient lesion will pass completely unobserved in most patients until the time of arthroscopy.

Open Chondromalacia

Fissures

Fissures may be multiple or single, relatively superficial or extending down to subchondral bone (Fig. 11.4). They are nearly always associated with adjacent softening and represent the second stage in the evolution of chondrosis. Once the surface layer has been interrupted, the cartilage lesion would appear to be irreversible because surface lesions do not heal. The clinician might recall, however, the teachings of Goodfellow et al (19) that "surface degeneration changes do not cause patellofemoral pain until they have progressed to exposure of bone upon an area of habitual patellofemoral contact." Today, however, it is clear that patients can have substantial, even severe, pain caused by closed

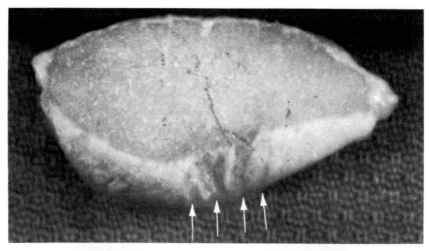

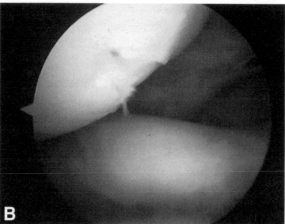

Figure 11.4. A, Cross-section of a patella removed at autopsy through the 40-degree flexion zone shows deep fissured cartilage localized to the critical zone with fissures extending to the subchondral bone. **B,** Arthroscopic view of a critical zone lesion similar to that noted in 11.4, **A.**

articular lesions that are under stress. Because there are no nerves in cartilage itself, the pain must emanate from subchondral bone, which is experiencing deficient conduction of stress through mechanically inadequate cartilage. Exactly how this occurs remains unknown, although the work by Biedert suggests that this pain may involve ischemic elaboration of neurotrophic factors.

Fibrillation of articular cartilage usually follows fissuring with progression to ulceration in some cases. When fibrillation progresses to a larger area of the patella (greater than ½ inch in diameter), bone may begin to experience abnormal pressure increases or irritation from flaps of cartilage that are placed under pressure, much as a flap of meniscus can cause pain. Presumably these flaps create tugging and irritation at the subchondral bone level similar to the pain created by pulling on a "hangnail."

Ulceration

By this stage, there is localized loss of cartilage substance, more or less extensive, which eventually exposes the dense subchondral bone. When it is extensive, the bone has a polished appearance and is said to be eburnated. This is the final stage in cartilage destruction.

Chondrosclerosis

With chondrosclerosis the process seems reversed. Instead of finding softened cartilage, the surgeon finds cartilage that appears to be abnormally hard; not depressible; and presenting a translucent, yellowish, glazed appearance. We believe that the term chondrosclerosis is applicable to this condition because it seems to be the opposite of chondromalacia. At the same time, the histology would seem to support this definition. Even though this abnormality appears to be the opposite of chondromalacia, it has similar significance in that it represents a complete loss of the normal qualities of articular cartilage, which implies a considerable diminution in its functional capacity in transferring load to subchondral bone.

Tuft Formation

Tuft formation is a particular lesion both in terms of localization and appearance. It is nearly always localized to the medial facet. In its well-developed form it has the appearance of a sea anemone and consists of multiple deep fronds of cartilage separated from one another by deep clefts that extend to subchondral bone. The base of attachment of these fronds is usually well limited, but the surgeon is struck by the quantity of cartilage that hangs over the facet, which suggests that the lesion may be proliferative as well as destructive. It is possible that this particular pathologic appearance is due to the special conditions affecting the medial patella, namely, incongruence, intermittent excessive pressure, shearing forces, and the possibility of reduced compression. This tufting has also been noted at the time of arthroscopy following cartilage cell implantation, presumably a type of overgrowth.

Superficial Surface Changes

Damage to the lamina splendens may be considered superficial. Other superficial lesions include surface fibrillation that may be overt or detectable only by India ink (55). Longitudinal striations may be present in the axis of movement of the joint, which, in more severe form, may give the appearance of scoring of the articular cartilage. Some areas of the surface may take on a dull appearance without any other significant abnormalities. These surface changes are frequent findings both at arthrotomy and at autopsy. Little is known about long-term consequences of superficial articular cartilage injuries.

Global Chondromalacia

In addition to the previously described lesions localized to either facet, there are other, more diffuse forms of patellar articular cartilage degeneration. Fracture of the patella may cause malacic changes on both facets. Also, when there has been significant periarticular fibrosis, the surgeon may observe extensive malacic changes involving the entire patella. Sometimes, if cartilage destruction is diffuse on the patella, it is difficult to be certain as to the site of the original lesion.

There are patients with a typical malacic lesion, with or without fissures, centered perfectly on the median ridge. This may then extend in both directions but appears to have a tendency toward medial extension. Some of these cases, at least, have the typical findings of excessive pressure on the lateral facet, and release of a tight lateral retinaculum may give some symptomatic relief. One must remember, however, that lateral release may result in increased medial contact and the potential for aggravation of a medial articular lesion.

Minor alterations of patellar alignment (particularly lateral tilt) may cause accentuation of lateral facet loads and diminished medial facet loads such that minor insults, or even obesity, can result in diffuse patellar cartilage destruction in some unfortunate patients.

Outerbridge Classification (56)

It is important that surgeons accurately describe their findings on open or arthroscopic examination of the patellar or trochlear articular surfaces. Overall, in the arthroscopic or macroscopic assessment of patellar articular cartilage lesions, we have found the Outerbridge classification most helpful.

In essence, the Outerbridge classification is as follows:

Grade 1—Articular cartilage softening (closed chondromalacia) only (Fig. 11.3).
Grade 2—Fibrillation of less than ½ inch in diameter (Fig. 11.5).
Grade 3—Fibrillation of more than ½ inch in diameter (Fig. 11.6).
Grade 4—Erosion to bone (Figs. 11.7, B and 11.8).

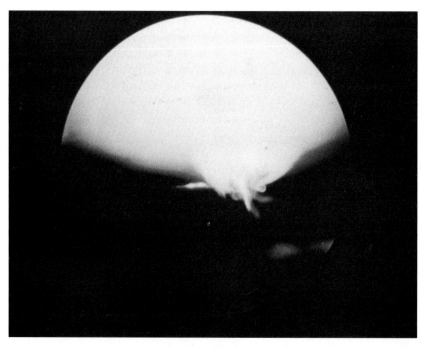

Figure 11.5. Patellar articular cartilage fibrillation less than ½ inch in diameter (Outerbridge Grade 2 changes) as viewed with an arthroscope. Photo courtesy of Dandy D. *Arthroscopy of the Knee* slide collection, Gower Medical Publishing.

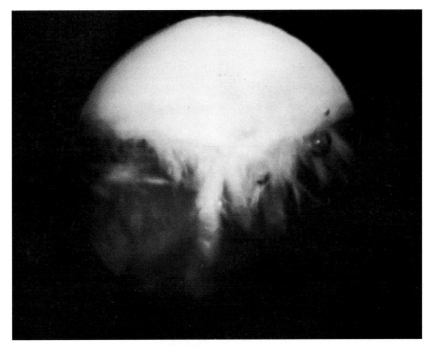

Figure 11.6. Patellar articular cartilage fibrillation greater than ½ inch in diameter (Outerbridge Grade 3 changes) as viewed with an arthroscope. Photo courtesy of Dandy D. *Arthroscopy of the Knee* slide collection, Gower Medical Publishing.

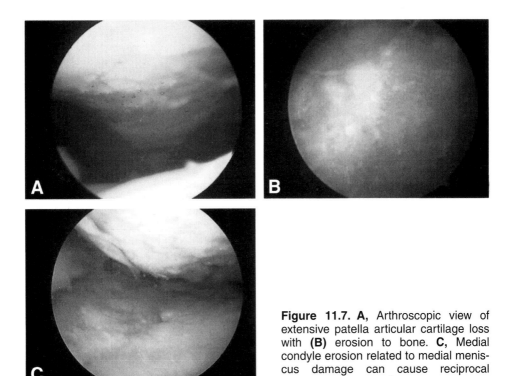

Figure 11.7. A, Arthroscopic view of extensive patella articular cartilage loss with **(B)** erosion to bone. **C,** Medial condyle erosion related to medial meniscus damage can cause reciprocal changes on the patella.

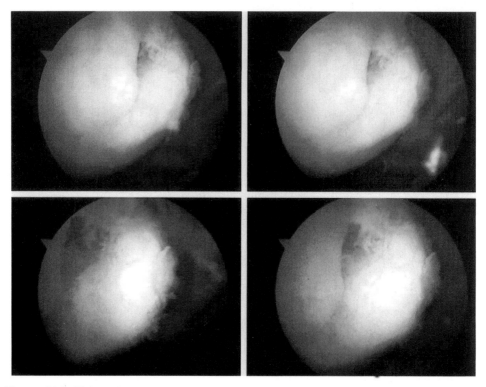

Figure 11.8. This patient sustained a proximal pole crush, which resulted in full-thickness (Grade 4) articular cartilage loss to bone when viewed with an arthroscope.

This classification system has been useful because it allows the clinician to quantitate operative or arthroscopic findings in a simple and accurate yet reproducible manner.

LOCATION OF LESIONS

The author has noted that articular cartilage breakdown will occur on different portions of the patellar articular surface, depending on the nature of the malalignment or trauma. Figure 11.6 shows the regions to be considered.

When there is recurrent shear stress and habitual noncontact, the distal central portion of the patella may break down. This area corresponds to Ficat's critical zone (57). Consequently, this area frequently deteriorates in patients with patellar malalignment but would *not* be expected to degenerate as a result of direct trauma in the majority of cases if the knee is flexed. Trauma with the knee in *extension,* however, could result in articular cartilage damage to the distal central portion of the patella. This is less common because the majority of injuries occur with the knee flexed.

The *lateral facet,* as described by Ficat (57), is a site of articular cartilage breakdown as a result of increased contact stress in the excessive lateral pressure syndrome (ELPS). Concentration of load on this portion of the patella has been well recognized to occur with chronic patellar lateralization and tilt.

The *medial facet* is more commonly damaged at the time of patellar dislocation and *relocation.* At this time, a shear fracture of the central medial facet can occur. Sometimes,

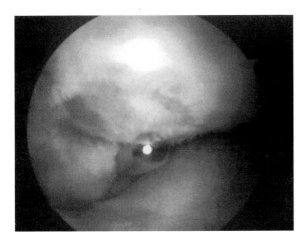

Figure 11.9. Overzealous medial imbrication, medial tubercle transfer, or posteromedial tibial tubercle transfer (Hauser) can cause erosion of distal medial patella cartilage to bone. This patient needed anterolateral transfer of the tibial tubercle.

extensive damage to the entire patellar medial facet can occur as the patella relocates. Unfortunately, this cartilage damage can be severe, leaving little or no articular cartilage on the medial patella, in some cases. This is particularly important to note because the medial facet shear fracture occurs in patients with lateral instability. Consequently, *medialization* of the patella is necessary to provide stability of the patella, but at the same time this medialization may cause loading onto the damaged medial facet. A skillful surgeon will recognize this and move the patella only enough to provide stability, probably with some anteriorization of the tibial tubercle (anteromedial tibial tubercle transfer), and will avoid imbrication of the medial structures that tilts the patella down onto the damaged medial cartilage. Repair or reconstruction of the medial patellofemoral ligament carries particularly great risk of medial overload and must be done with care and skill and only when indicated.

Another cause of medial patella articular breakdown is previous medial tibial tubercle transfer with *posterior* placement of the tibial tubercle (Hauser procedure). This can result in severe pain related to exposed bone on the distal medial facet (Fig. 11.10). Often there is a reciprocal lesion on the trochlea.

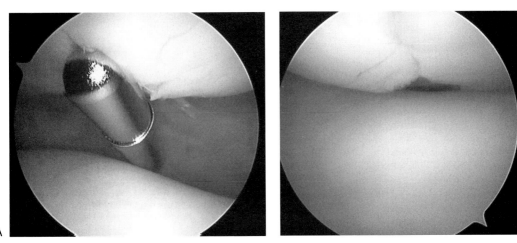

A   B

Figure 11.10. A, Debridement of articular crush with local fragmentation. **B,** Following debridement.

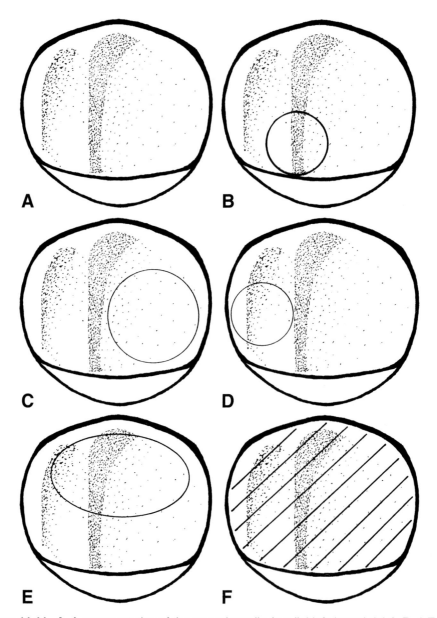

Figure 11.11. A, A representation of the normal patella (medial left; lateral right). **B,** A Type I lesion (Ficat critical zone) at the distal central ridge. **C,** A Type II lesion of the lateral facet is usually related to excessive lateral pressure with tilt. This lesion is often associated with a Type I lesion, and the two lesions may connect, particularly in a patient with longstanding lateral patellar tilt and subluxation. **D,** A Type III lesion will occur related to relocation of a patella following dislocation, with shearing off of the medial facet. Lesions of the medial facet also occur from excessive medial overload (overzealous medial imbrication or Hauser transfer of the tibial tubercle). **E,** The proximal patellar lesion (Type IV) that spans the facets is most often related to a crush, knee flexion injury (dashboard type) in which the proximal patella is articulating (knee flexed) at the time of impact. **F,** End-stage diffuse patella articular cartilage degeneration. Illustrations by Phoebe Fulkerson.

The *proximal patella* is more commonly damaged as a result of a dashboard or crush type of injury in which the knee is flexed at the time of impact. The patella will be articulating on more proximal cartilage with the knee flexed. This is the lesion that often occurs in litigation-related and worker's compensation-related injury. Unfortunately, it is also an injury that frequently defies adequate treatment and responds poorly to tibial tubercle anteriorization procedures because these procedures will cause load shift onto the more proximal patella that is injured in these patients. Simple arthroscopic debridement may give some relief (Fig. 11.10).

Diffuse articular cartilage damage more frequently occurs as a result of generalized arthritis or extensive damage following malalignment and recurrent dislocation.

The different patella cartilage breakdown location patterns are shown in Figure 11.11.

MICROSCOPIC ASPECTS OF PATELLAR ARTICULAR CARTILAGE DEGENERATION

Closed Chondromalacia

To better understand the degenerative process, it is necessary to approach, insofar as possible, the earliest lesion. In this case, the localized nodule with intact surface (Outerbridge Grade 1) characterizes the first phase of chondromalacia.

Optical Microscopy

The surface of the cartilage, in general, shows regressive fibrous metaplasia (57–59) of the surface cells that appear to be more flattened than normal. Some superficial fissures may be evident. The deeper layer of cartilage shows what can best be described as edema with apparent increase in the quantity of ground substance. There is an unmasking of collagen fibers and a diminution of ground substance staining with Alcian blue, toluidine blue, and safranin O. However, the ground substance remains periodic acid Schiff (PAS)-positive. The chondrocyte lacunae retain a normal appearance. Hirsch (13) has shown that these histochemical changes represent a diminution in the glycosaminoglycan content, which accounts for the softening of the cartilage and its decrease in resistance to compression.

Electron Microscopy

The percentage of strictly intact surfaces steadily decreases as one progresses from naked eye appearance through optical, scanning electron, and transmission electron microscopy (Fig. 11.12). With this progression, the criteria for surface integrity become increasingly strict. With the light microscope, one is measuring defects in tens of microns, whereas with the electron microscope, defects of a few angstroms are apparent. The absence of fissures, however, does not exclude other alterations such as edema, in which the superficial fibers are separated. This might explain the decrease in tensile strength over the entire zone of softening. The superficial microfibrillar covering has frequently disappeared and collagen fibers running parallel to the surface are often separated by electron transparent lacuna zones. These zones are bordered by microfibrillar condensation, which may foreshadow fissures running parallel to the surface. At other times there may be areas of more or less irregular osmiophilic microfibrils.

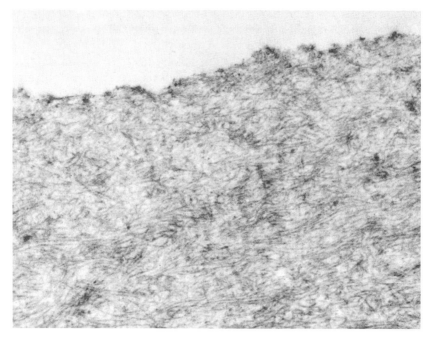

Figure 11.12. Transmission electron micrograph of a Stage I lesion; superficial layer showing the surface to be intact.

The area of softening is situated between the superficial zone (C1), more or less normal but always macroscopically intact, and the deep layer (C3), which is also normal to electron microscopic examination. The area of abnormality then is localized in the intermediate zone (C2) and, at least in the beginning, in the superficial portion of this zone. Initially the lesion is relatively well defined. This localized focal picture appears to be consistent in degenerating cartilage. All three constituents of cartilage (chondrocytes, collagen fibers, and ground substance) demonstrate abnormalities.

Chondrocytes

In these earliest lesions, signs of cellular hyperactivity abound. These are expressed primarily at the cytoplasmic level. There are the following cytoplasmic alterations that may demonstrate increased cellular activity:

1. Increase in pinocytosis (Fig. 11.13).
2. Increase in the number of cytoplasmic villi and fine filaments (Fig. 11.14).
3. An abundance of glycogen or ribosomal granulation (Fig. 11.15).
4. Development of the Golgi apparatus (Fig. 11.15).
5. Encirclement of the cell by proteoglycans, which, in turn, are ringed by granular or amorphous microfibrillar material (Fig. 11.16).
6. Cellular multiplication and cloning (Fig. 11.17).
7. Increase in the number of dense bodies of all sizes and character (lipid, lysosomal) (Fig. 11.18).

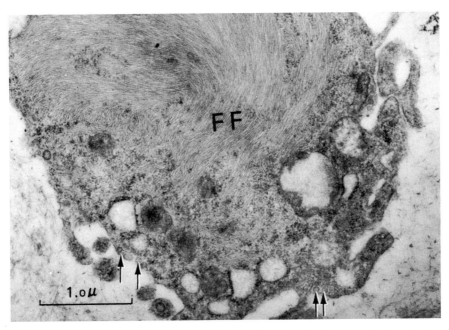

Figure 11.13. Chondrocyte from intermediate zone (C2) showing increased pinocytosis. *FF* = fine filaments.

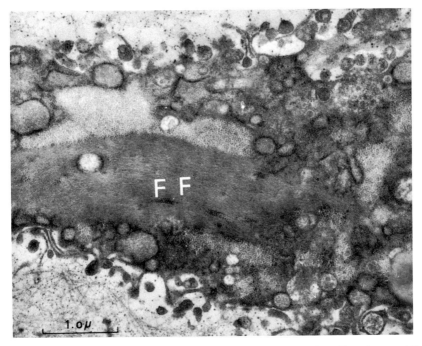

Figure 11.14. Chondrocyte from superficial layer at the median ridge. Abundance of fine filaments (*FF*) and cytoplasmic villi abound.

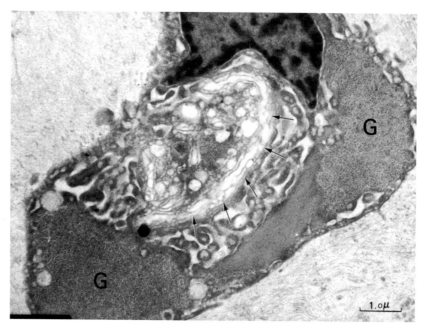

Figure 11.15. Deep portion superficial layer, median ridge, Stage I lesion. Abundant glycogen (*G*), well-developed Golgi apparatus (*arrows*).

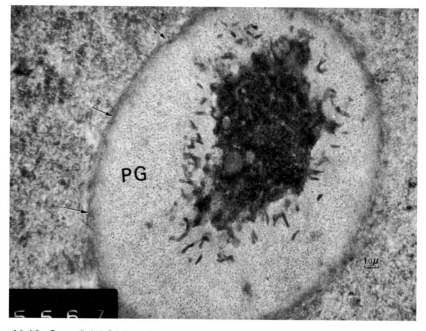

Figure 11.16. Superficial C2 layer. The cell is surrounded by a ring of proteoglycans (*PG*) and an amorphous microfibrillar ring (*arrows*).

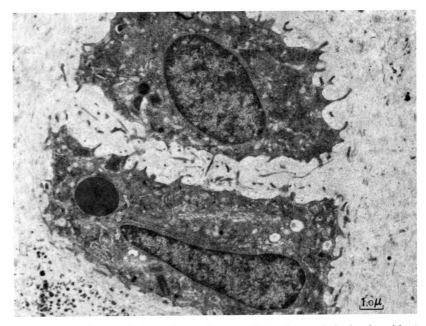

Figure 11.17. Deeper in layer C2. Cellular multiplication and cloning is evident.

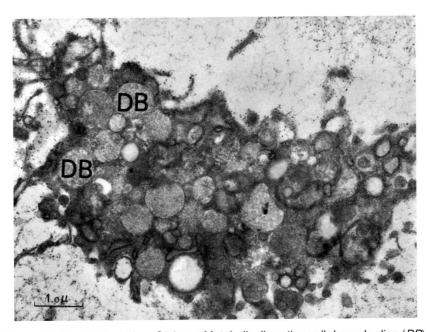

Figure 11.18. Median ridge, C1 layer. Metabolically active cell dense bodies (*DB*).

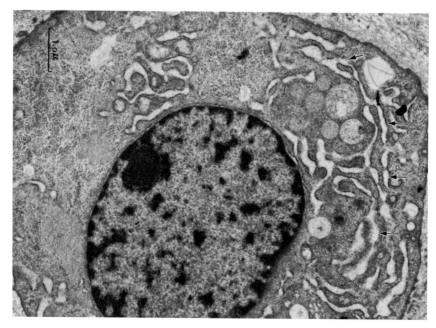

Figure 11.19. Layer C2 at median ridge, closed chondromalacia. Marked dilatation of the endoplasmic reticulum (*arrows*).

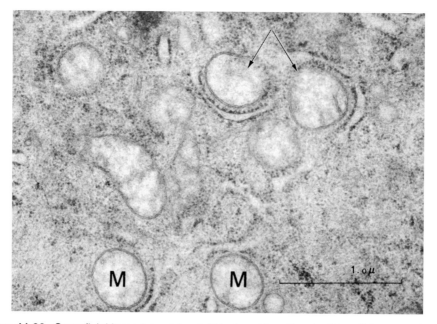

Figure 11.20. Superficial layer, lateral facet. Mitochondria without cristae (*M*)–some with rupture (*arrows*).

8. Dilatation of the endoplasmic reticulum (Fig. 11.19).
9. Mitochondrial distention, with disappearance of cristae and, occasionally, rupture (Fig. 11.20).

The last four signs imply the tendency toward degeneration. However, cells that are typically degenerating or, more important, necrotic occur infrequently in these earliest lesions. It would, therefore, appear that the initial phase of cartilage disorder is characterized by a proliferative reaction manifest by increased cellular activity. Stimulated by increased load, the chondrocytes lose their quiescent appearance and increase metabolism and secretion, as if this defensive reaction would reinforce those structures that are endangered.

Collagen Fibers

The collagen component of the cartilage matrix shows a variety of abnormalities. Those encountered in the earliest lesions include the following:

1. Angulation and abrupt change of direction, sometimes more than 90 degrees, of a whole series of fibers, which suggests a process of compression and disorganization (Fig. 11.21).
2. Inequality of fiber diameter (Fig. 11.22).
3. Anomalies in both diameter and orientation of fibers that are involved in a disorganized process (Fig. 11.23).
4. Loss of the usual functional orientation, loss of striation and fragmentation, and dissociation of fibers by edema (Fig. 11.24).
5. Fiber disintegration (Fig. 11.25).

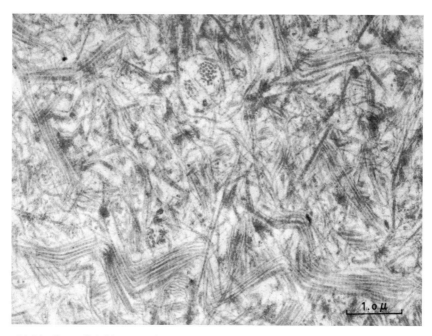

Figure 11.21. Superficial layer at the "critical zone" showing markedly irregular fiber direction.

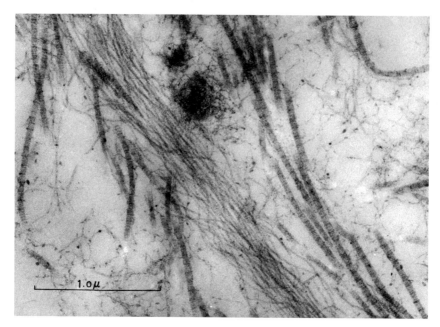

Figure 11.22. Marked variation in fiber diameter from 100 to 500 angstroms. There is also considerable separation of fibers for this layer.

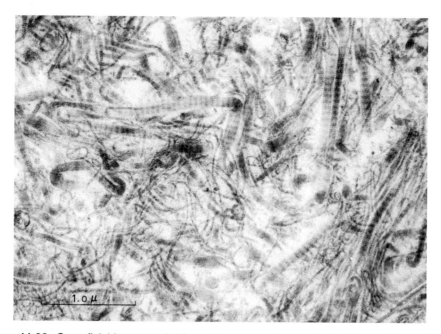

Figure 11.23. Superficial layer, medial facet. Fibers are disorganized, disoriented, and separated by abundant ground substance. Tremendous variation in fiber thickness from 220 to 1100 angstroms.

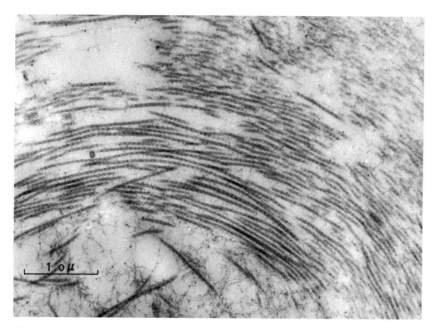

Figure 11.24. Superficial layer. Fiber fragmentation and dissociation by edema.

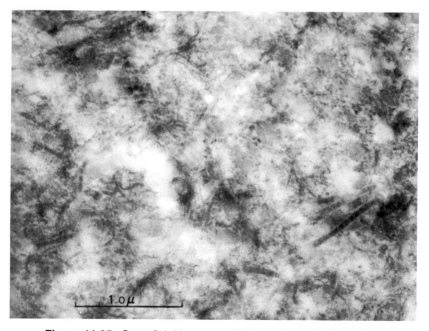

Figure 11.25. Superficial layer, medial facet. Fiber disintegration.

Ground Substance

Ground substance seems to increase in volume and appears more abundant. Mankin and Thrasher (60) have noted a 9% increase in the water content of osteoarthritic articular cartilage, and this may constitute the basis for cartilage edema (Fig. 11.26), which is characteristic of chondromalacia. Occasionally, the surgeon can find crevices or small fissures, particularly in those cases that are clinically more developed. Some of these fissures may be interpreted as artifacts (Fig. 11.27), but others are lined by material that is electron dense and amorphous (Fig. 11.28). Other fissures show margins that have a different aspect, a fibrillar border with random orientation (Fig. 11.29). The authenticity of these fissures is without doubt because some of them have a cystic appearance, even with parietal proliferation protruding into the cavity. All these matrix lesions are relatively discrete, particularly in the early cases. This must not be forgotten in the interpretation of the ultramicroscopic photographs. The clinician must not expect profound and spectacular changes in incipient lesions. These lesions are characterized more by their repetitive nature than their intensity, which makes interpretation potentially controversial.

Open Chondromalacia

Electron Microscopy

When the surgeon biopsies an area of malacic cartilage with the surface apparently intact just adjacent to chondromalacia with the surface fissured, he/she is struck by two facts. First, changes affecting each of the constituents of the articular cartilage are more exaggerated, and second, the distribution of the kinds of lesions has shifted to a predominance of degenerative lesions. This increase in severity of the abnormality affects each of the constituents of the cartilage.

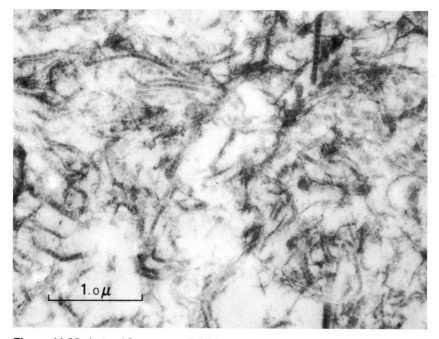

Figure 11.26. Lateral facet, superficial layer. Marked fiber separation by edema.

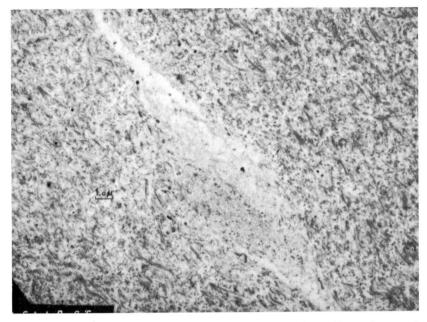

Figure 11.27. C2 layer. Fissures are evident, which may be artifactual but only seem to occur in advanced cases.

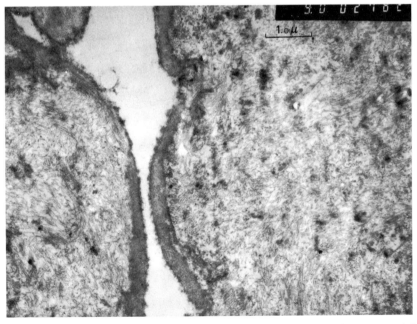

Figure 11.28. Deep portion, superficial layer. Fissure lined by electron-dense material is certainly not artifactual.

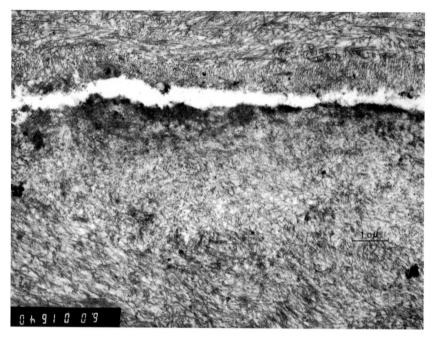

Figure 11.29. Superficial portion of C2; fissure with a randomly oriented fibrillar border.

Chondrocytes

Next to cells showing hyperactivity, as described in the previous section, there is an increase in degenerating and even necrotic cells. Degeneration now exceeds proliferation. At the cytoplasmic level there is the following:

1. A tendency toward disappearance of organelles (Fig. 11.30).
2. A granular microfibrillar or amorphous homogenization and dilatation of endoplasmic reticulum (Fig. 11.31).
3. A more or less extensive degeneration of the cytoplasmic membrane (Fig. 11.32).
4. At the extreme, a disintegration of the cytoplasm, with rupture and fragmentation (Fig. 11.33).

At the level of the nucleus, important changes are evident, which include the following:

1. Alteration of the chromatin (Fig. 11.34).
2. A thickened and greatly invaginated nuclear membrane (Fig. 11.35).
3. Pyknosis.
4. Disappearance of the nuclear membrane–the principal sign that allows confirmation of necrosis.
5. Finally, fragmentation and rupture of the nucleus, which may involve entire clones (Fig. 11.36).

Collagen Fibers

In general, the clinician sees both a quantitative and qualitative increase in the early changes previously described. The collagen fibers are more dissociated and fragmented,

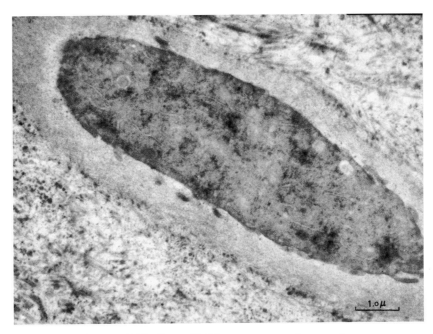

Figure 11.30. Zone C2. Disappearance of organelles.

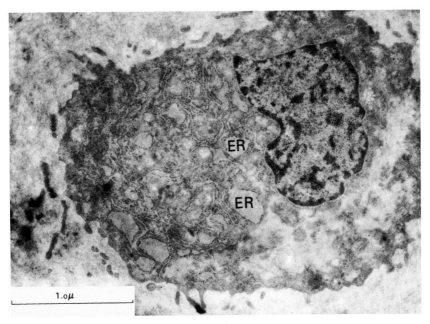

Figure 11.31. Chondrocyte from zone C2 showing homogenization of a portion of the cyto-plasm and dilatation of the endoplasmic reticulum (*ER*).

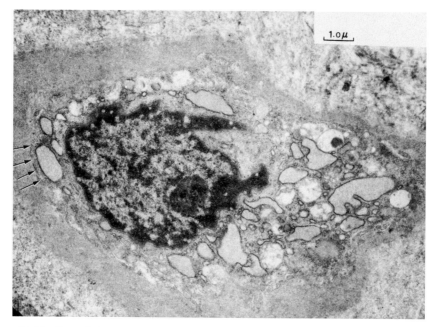

Figure 11.32. Superficial layer, medial facet in Stage II lesion showing a more or less extensive degeneration of the cytoplasmic membrane (intact membrane seen at *arrows*).

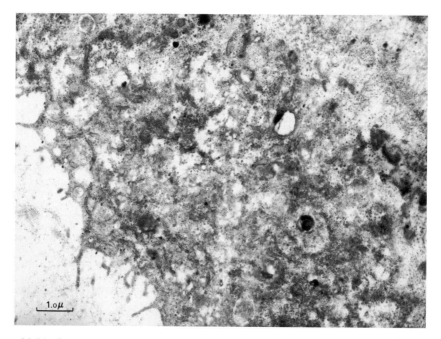

Figure 11.33. Deep layer in an advanced cartilage lesion showing rupture and fragmentation of the cytoplasm.

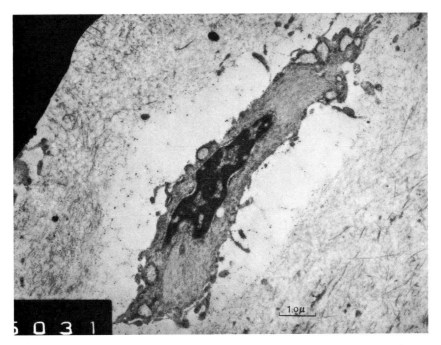

Figure 11.34. Chondrocyte of the superficial layer showing alteration of chromatin patterns.

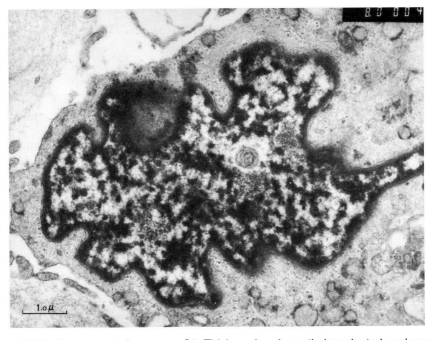

Figure 11.35. Chondrocyte from zone C1. Thickened and greatly invaginated nuclear membrane.

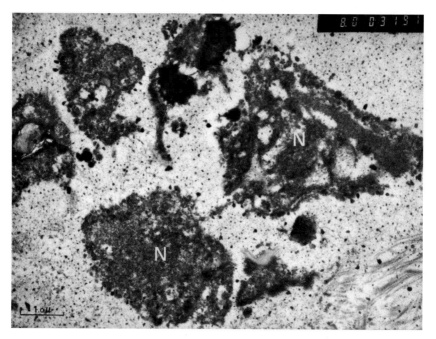

Figure 11.36. Zone C3. This could represent several nuclei undergoing fragmentation and rupture. *N* = nuclear fragment.

the degree of severity paralleling the severity of edema. These changes are maximal in the exuberant lesion of the medial facet where the intermittent pressure and excessive shearing forces do not seem to exercise the same degree of restraint evoked by the more constant aggressive pressure on the lateral facet.

Ground Substance

The edema is more marked, with its development paralleling the clinical importance. The change is one of degree rather than character. One exception should be noted. There are some cases of considerable edema involving the medial facet, particularly the region between the medial and odd facet. The cartilage remains closed and the ultramicroscopic examination shows little or no chondrocyte necrosis, even though the cells themselves show degenerative changes. It is probable that the chondrocytes are protected from necrosis because of the anatomic situation that prevents the excessive forces from being continuous.

As the cartilage lesion progresses from the incipient stage into the well-developed stage, the distribution of changes of all three elements is modified. Early, the middle of the edematous nodule that is the site of our biopsy is characterized by a mixture of changes where proliferative lesions predominate. Cellular necrosis is very rare. Fibril separation by edematous ground substance remains discrete as long as the lesion is small and not particularly soft. By Stage II, and particularly where softening is important, the surgeon sees involvement of the entire intermediate zone with the beginning of proliferative changes affecting the C3 layer as well. The necrotic and degenerative lesions become more apparent and affect more chondrocytes. These lesions are more concentrated in the center of the softened area where one might suppose the zone of compression is maximum. Surrounding this central zone of predominant degenerative lesions is a circle of proliferative abnormalities. Finally, all of this reactional regenerative peripheral activity disappears and is replaced by a massive collar of cartilage necrosis surrounding the ulcerative lesion.

1. Initially, the excessive pressure elicits a response on the part of the cartilage in the sense of increased chondrocyte activity that appears to be an attempt to counter the increase in mechanical load. This increase is manifested by increased metabolism, increased proteoglycan synthesis, accumulation of filaments, cellular multiplication (mitoses), and formation of clusters and clones. These lesions appear essentially proliferative and reconstructive. The quiescent cells are stimulated and resume activity. This would correspond to an initial reactional and proliferative phase. It is even conceivable that this might be successful if the inciting cause is minimal or if the excessive pressure is terminated.

2. Later, there will be failure of increasing numbers of chondrocytes and fatigue rupture of the fiber network of the matrix. Initially, the central, predominantly degenerative and necrotic zone is surrounded by a proliferative reaction that is progressively pushed toward the periphery and the depth of the articular cartilage. This is the phase of degeneration and necrosis characterized by increasing numbers of cellular necroses, increase in softening of the cartilage, and destruction of the collagen network. It is, of course, possible that this degenerative phase proceeds directly from a severe injury without passing through the initial proliferative phase. It might also be evident early in the disorder if the cause is overwhelming or the proliferative response is insufficient.

3. Finally, there is fragmentation of the matrix. Eventually, the subchondral bone becomes exposed and eburnated. This is the terminal destructive phase of arthrosis. Even the cartilage that borders the ulceration dies progressively, leading to expansion of the defect by means of mechanical pressure.

There is one additional observation that has some bearing on this process. The surgeon can see dead yellow cartilage, with reduced elasticity but apparently preserved when it is situated in an area that is not submitted to mechanical constraint. We see this on the medial facet in patients with lateral subluxation and excessive lateral pressure as well as the superior third of the patella in patients who have limitation of flexion to less than 90 degrees, and therefore, this area does not come into contact (Fig. 11.37). This observa-

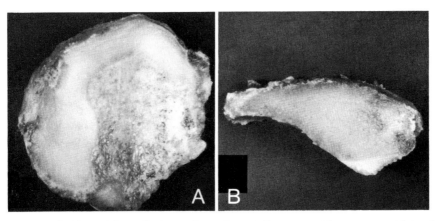

Figure 11.37. A, View of the articular surface of a patella removed for permanent lateral subluxation. Note the preservation of a superior and medial cartilage. The patient had only 80 degrees of flexion. **B,** Tangential view through the midportion of the patella.

tion accents the necessity of the mechanical factor for the complete destruction of carti-lage.

Chondrosclerosis

There is a lesion essentially the reverse of chondromalacia but much less common. The cartilage becomes extraordinarily firm under the effect of mechanical pressure. There-fore, chondrosclerosis may represent one route of progression instead of the more com-mon route of fissuring, fragmentation, and ulceration. The electron microscope shows that the surface is intact and, in general, is covered by a thin amorphous or microfibril electron dense material. The network of parallel fibers in C1 is very tight and very dense (Fig. 11.38). Ground substance is scarce, and there is no trace of edema. The collagen fibers form a dense network intermingled but frequently with a general preferential direc-tion (Figs. 11.39, 11.40). The lesion is, with regard to the relative distributions of colla-gen and proteoglycan, not fibrocartilage.

The chondrocytes in all cases of chondrosclerosis have certain characteristics in com-mon. They take on an aspect of storage cells with an excess of microfibrils (Fig. 11.41) and diverse vacuoles, some containing dense black globules (Fig. 11.42) and others con-taining myelin-like bodies. Frequently, glycogen-forming granules are heaped up in thick layers spread throughout the whole cytoplasm (Fig. 11.43). These cells often have an aspect of hyperactive secretory activity and secrete quantities of proteoglycan, which is found as a crown surrounding the cell. This crown is itself limited by dense thick microfibrillar or amorphous layer (Fig. 11.44). Finally, there is a great deal of cellular multiplication with double cells and grouping of more numerous cells that show the same

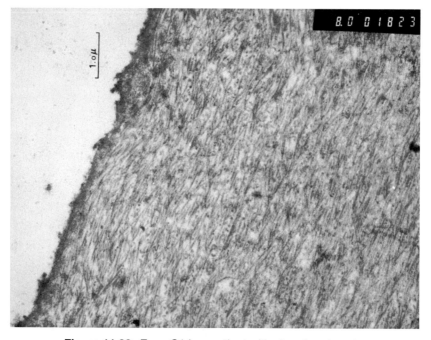

Figure 11.38. Zone C1 in a patient with chondrosclerosis.

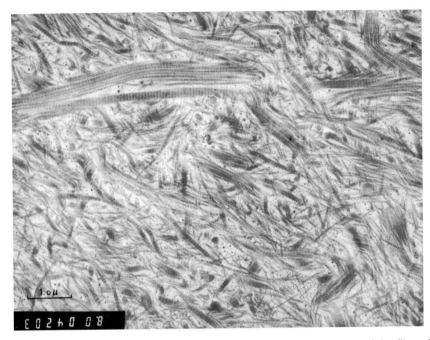

Figure 11.39. Superficial layer, middle portion. Contrast the compactness of the fibers in this condition to Figure 11.22.

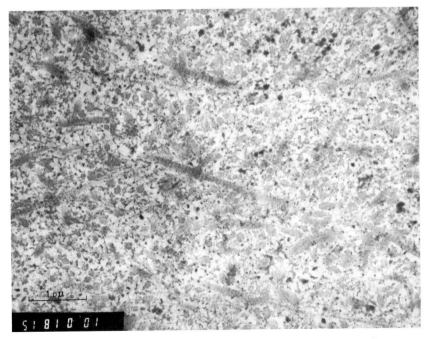

Figure 11.40. Same patient as in Figure 11.39. Deep in zone C2.

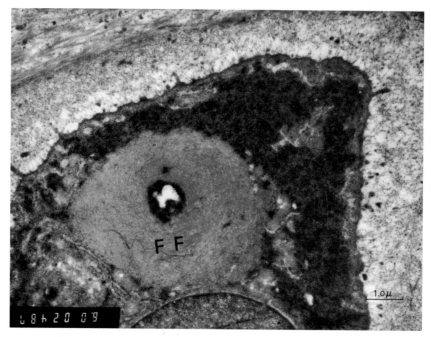

Figure 11.41. Superficial aspect, zone C2. *FF* = fine filaments.

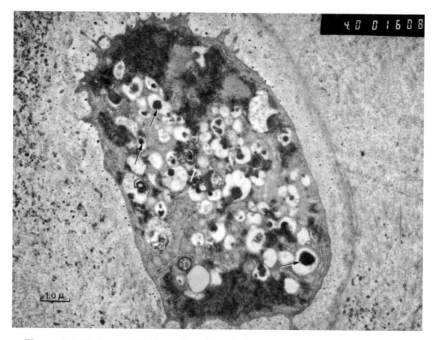

Figure 11.42. Zone C2. Chondrosclerosis (dense black globules—*arrows*).

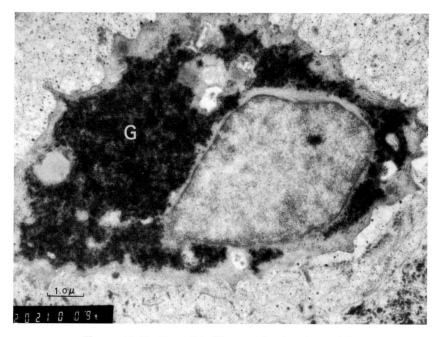

Figure 11.43. Zone C1. Glycogen in abundance (*G*).

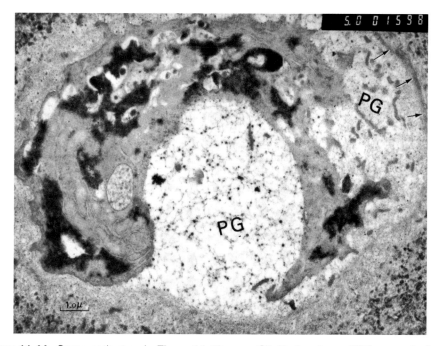

Figure 11.44. Same patient as in Figure 11.43, zone C2. Proteoglycan (*PG*) crown limited by a microfibrillar layer (*arrows*).

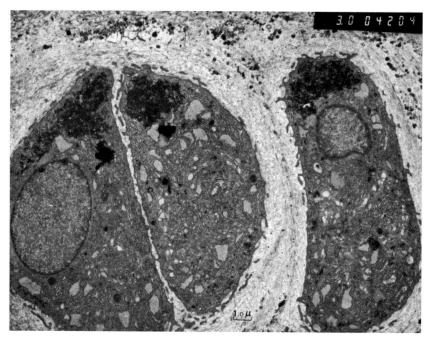

Figure 11.45. Deep C2 layer. Multiple cell groupings.

characteristic of excess secretory activity (Fig. 11.45). However, there is little evidence of necrosis. Chondrosclerosis seems to be very different from chondromalacia, not only as to the anatomic and clinical appearance but also at the ultramicroscopic level.

MECHANICAL PATHOGENESIS OF ARTHROSIS

There is generally a mechanical reason for patellar cartilage breakdown, as has been demonstrated in earlier chapters. This often consists of excessive pressure from trauma or abnormal alignment. Aging facilitates either of these processes. The initial lesion is perfectly isolated and localized in the superficial half of the intermediate zone. It is detectable both clinically and radiologically from its beginning and is accessible by biopsy. This cartilage lesion is characterized by nodular edema, which is the beginning of the degenerative process that leads to arthrosis. Microscopic studies have demonstrated that clinically apparent softening is due to a change in the ground substance and disorganization of the collagen network. The superficial layer (C1) is undergoing fibrous dedifferentiation. Even if the surface has a normal appearance, it is qualitatively not less changed than the deeper layer and participates in the softening effect, which explains the blister appearance. The intermediate zone (C2) shows alterations in collagen, cells, and ground substance, with perhaps some evidence of the chondrocytes themselves changing earliest.

Origin of Arthrosis: Its Mechanical Nature

It is likely that excessive pressure from tilt/compression bears the primary responsibility for the more severe lateral facet lesions encountered (61). Trauma, dysplasias with diminution of load-bearing surfaces, incongruence of load-bearing surfaces, and static disorders (genu varum, genu valgum, and so on) all enter into a group in which joint breakdown relates to excessive articular cartilage compression. Abnormal articular cartilage loading may eventually cross the threshold of cartilage resistance and lead to the failure of healthy cartilage under conditions of mechanical overload. Deficient medial cartilage contact pressure created by abnormal alignment also leads to cartilage breakdown. This is frequently less severe (although common) than the lateral facet lesions created by overload and probably requires intermittent shear or compression to cause breakdown (61). Certain occupations and activities also increase the risk of patellofemoral degeneration. Kivimaki et al (62) found that kneeling activities (such as carpet and floor laying) increase the risk of patellar osteophytosis.

Breakdown of articular cartilage of the femoral trochlea occurs commonly as a result of direct trauma. Dislocation of the patella leads to an articular cartilage defect on the lateral trochlea, probably as a result of patella relocation in most cases. Trochlear degeneration can occur in other ways also. Butler-Manuel et al (63) noted that there is increased scintigraphic uptake in the femoral trochlea of patients following patellectomy.

Lesions created in this manner often lead to arthrosis. This group of disorders symbolizes the pathologic action of excessive pressure on cartilage, whatever form that may take, whether a single severe traumatic overload, moderately excessive and repetitive microtraumatic episodes, continuous pressure of abnormal tilt, excessive pressure associated with facet incongruity, or the excessive pressure of high unit load on reduced surface area (as in a dysplasia). Areas of chronically deficient load (at the central and medial patella) may soften from cartilage malnutrition and eventually break down spontaneously in areas that experience only intermittent normal loads.

Another unfortunate cause of patellofemoral breakdown is excessive or poorly performed patellofemoral surgery. Because of the considerable motion and shifting contact on the patella, imbricating and tightening procedures, including medial patellofemoral ligament reconstruction, carry substantial risks of focal cartilage overload unless very well done.

Initiation of Arthrosis

The evolution of cartilage breakdown demonstrates two distinct phases. The primary lesion is often in cartilage (chondrosis) without any radiologic evidence of bone reaction. The patella occupies a unique position in presenting us the opportunity to investigate fully joint breakdown from its inception. For all practical purposes, this phase passes undetected at the level of other joints because the clinician normally waits for the second phase (arthrosis) before making the diagnosis. The arthrosis phase is characterized by the appearance of bone remodeling with a triad of reaction: osteophytosis, cyst formation, and sclerosis. These are finally associated with "joint space narrowing" (articular cartilage loss). Even minimal "joint space narrowing" takes on added significance because there may be fissures and even ulcerations with a normal joint space on radiograph.

If we return to the very beginning of articular cartilage breakdown and to the true initiating lesion of the process, two questions should be asked: (1) Does the beginning involve the surface layer or the deep layer of cartilage? and (2) Which of the three substances of cartilage is first affected, ground substance, collagen, or chondrocytes? We do not intend to carry out a general review of these questions but limit ourselves to pointing out the contribution that this study of patellar pathology has brought to these problems.

Surface or Deep Layer?

The deep layer of cartilage (C3) has consistently appeared normal. The intermediate zone is the site of a focal lesion where the surgeon sees evidence of abnormalities in all three of the cartilage constituents. At the cellular level there is a mixture of cellular hyperactivity and necrosis. The more advanced the lesion the more numerous the number of necrotic cells. However, degenerative-type cells with overloading of the cytoplasmic matrix appear frequently. The fibers are of unequal diameter and, occasionally, lose their striation. They become fragmented and separated by amorphous lakes. They sometimes appear tortuous and disorganized. The ground substance appears increased in volume by homogeneous material, which shows little electron density. This disruption of the equilibrium between fibrillar material and ground substance, which predominates, recalls the concept of cartilage edema.

The C1 layer is macroscopically intact but, as Meachim (55) has pointed out, that which is intact to the naked eye may be fissured under the light microscope. It remains that we can see some cases in which the integrity of the superficial layer has been verified by both transmission and scanning electron microscopy. However, this integrity may be purely morphologic, and the several layers of fibrillar material that appear normal may be functionally quite different. The cells of the superficial layer may appear to be involuting and take on a fibroblastic appearance. The fibers may be separated by lacunar zones or microfibrillar lakes of osmiophilic material, having a fibrinoid appearance. Any of these alterations could cause this layer to lose its mechanical role of containment, which may explain the blister or nodule formation at the surface in the early stage.

These observations make an answer to the question concerning the initial lesion, surface or deep layer, particularly difficult. It is possible that the first manifestations of cartilage alterations apply to both the superficial and intermediate layers (C1 and C2) at the contact zone of excessive pressure. It may be that the C1 lesion is more subtle and more difficult to substantiate.

Which Is the First Element Affected?

Ficat (57) obtained cartilage biopsy specimens as early as possible in the disease process in order to approach the initial lesion of the disease. He always found abnormalities in collagen fibers, chondrocytes, and ground substance and felt that the surgeon should not separate one of these elements from the whole and hold it responsible for everything that followed. Anything that affects one of these elements inevitably affects the others. One can say the same for the relationship between matrix and chondrocyte. What affects the matrix must affect the cell and vice versa. The fact that there is evidence of abnormality in all three elements of articular cartilage at the very earliest stage argues for simultaneous involvement from the beginning. No one of these elements appears to be more affected than the other. The failure of any one can, in fact, lead to the eventual degradation of cartilage as a whole. Rupture of the collagen network allows abnormal compression of the cartilage and chondrocytes. This facilitates loss of ground substance and depletion of glycosaminoglycan, which, in turn, weakens support for the collagen fiber network. Disturbance of function of chondrocytes leads to diminution or complete cessation of production of both collagen and proteoglycans matrix, weakening each in its turn and leading to destruction of the whole. The whole process revolves around three fundamental interdependent poles: depletion of proteoglycans, rupture of the collagen network, and disturbance or suppression of chondrocyte function. It is likely that excessive pressure reacts in each of these spheres, upsetting the tissue as a whole and unleashing a vicious cycle that ultimately leads to diffuse cartilage destruction. Chrisman et al (64) hypothesized that initial release of arachidonic acid in traumatized articular cartilage might initiate a series of events leading to catheptic enzyme release and subsequent progressive articular cartilage degradation, presumably mediated by prostaglandins (65, 66).

Subchondral bone undoubtedly plays an important, and early, role in the production of patellofemoral arthrosis. Radin's work (67–69) points out the importance of this layer in understanding patellar cartilage breakdown. Microfractures in subchondral bone lead to increased stiffness of this layer after healing, and, therefore, the surgeon might expect diminished resiliency of this subchondral support layer. Stiffening of subchondral bone may lead ultimately to overloading of articular cartilage because of inadequate subchondral impact resistance.

The diarthrodial joint is a functional entity (33), comprised of articular cartilage, subchondral bone, and synovium held together by ligaments and capsule. What affects any of these components usually affects all.

Patellar Articular Cartilage Healing

A healing response occurs after articular cartilage injury (70). In the case of superficial injury, the initial death of chondrocytes at the margin of injury is followed by increased metabolic activity of surrounding chondrocytes but no significant change in appearance of the superficial injury (71).

Once full-thickness loss of articular cartilage occurs, a more dramatic response occurs. There is predominantly Type I collagen formed initially, followed by a predominance of Type II (articular cartilage) collagen formation at 6 to 8 weeks (72) in rabbit knees. By 1 year, however, the defects in articular cartilage are comprised of fibrocartilage because of collagen predominance and loss of proteoglycan.

The patella will respond in a similar fashion. Once an Outerbridge Grade 3 to 4 lesion occurs, the defect will never fill again with the true articular cartilage. Therefore, the smart clinician will recognize that isolated shaving of an area of patellar articular cartilage, which is chronically overloaded, will not stop the progression of surface degradation. The concept in patient treatment, therefore, is to remove loose flakes of cartilage and perform abrasion drilling, or microfracture (Fig. 11.46), *after adequate relief of focal articular loading.* In severe cases, autologous or allograft osteochondral transfer may be necessary (Figs. 11.47 and 11.48). In the case of chronic patellar tilt, lateral release alone may be sufficient to alter patellar tracking, but more extensive alteration of patellar alignment may be required to provide relief of articular overload when there is widespread patellar articular cartilage loss. Anteromedial tibial tubercle transfer (73) is the procedure of choice to unload areas of excessive lateral and distal patellar overload and cartilage destruction, thereby providing an environment for resulting fibrocartilage healing that will not necessarily lead to further erosion. When there is *proximal medial* cartilage deficiency, however, this procedure is not appropriate.

It is possible that relieving intraosseous hypertension may facilitate articular healing. Intraosseous pressure, as measured in the metaphysis, has been shown to be in direct correlation to rest pain in arthrosis of the knee (74). Intraosseous hypertension has been demonstrated in both osteonecrosis of bone (75, 76) and reflex sympathetic dystrophy of bone (77). Drilling or abrasion of an Outerbridge Grade 3 to 4 defect may both relieve pain and enhance the healing response by reducing intraosseous hypertension as in

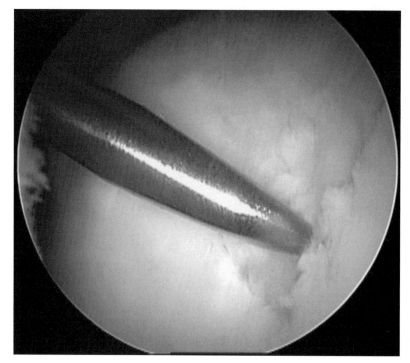

Figure 11.46. Microfracture arthroplasty of the trochlea.

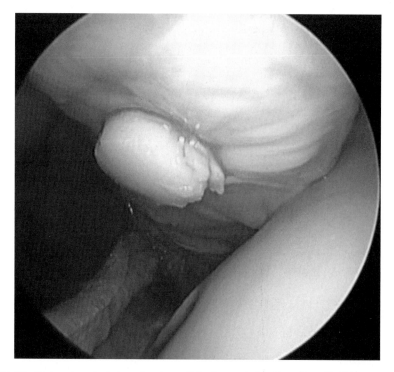

Figure 11.47. Osteochondral dowel autograft to the patella. Results with this procedure are very inconsistent, and it is not currently recommended unless an unloading procedure is done at the same time.

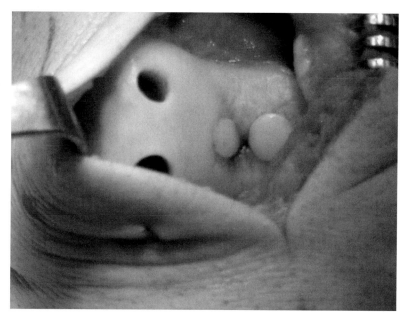

Figure 11.48. Osteochondral autograft from lateral to central trochlea—lateral approach.

osteoarthritis. This, however, is not commonly effective unless the damaged surface is unloaded as well as drilled.

Osteotomy of the proximal femur causes an immediate fall in intraosseous pressure (78) as well as relief of rest pain in patients with arthrosis of the hip (78–81). It may be that biomechanical failure of articular cartilage results in alteration of load transfer to subchondral bone and secondary intraosseous hypertension. It is certainly possible that articular cartilage degeneration may lead to pain in this way. Pressure on softened, but intact, articular cartilage can cause pain in some patients, whereas pressure on normal articular cartilage will not. However, many patients with focal articular cartilage degradation and fibrillation (noted incidentally at the time of arthroscopy for another problem) have little or no pain referable to the anterior knee.

In clinical practice, it is most important to determine where pain is coming from and then try to identify and modify the pathomechanics leading to the painful disorder. Specific articular lesions must be considered and treated individually and collectively. It is clear that softened articular cartilage alone does not always cause pain.

ARTICULAR CARTILAGE LESIONS IN THE PATIENT WITH CHRONIC PATELLAR TILT

The articular cartilage of a chronically tilted patella will usually experience focal overloading. Chronic lateral tilt, related to malalignment with adaptive shortening of the lateral retinaculum, will concentrate loads on a lateral facet contact area that is substantially less than the usual contact area across the medial and lateral facets of a normally articulating patellofemoral joint. These loads may be further accentuated by a tight lateral retinaculum, which exerts posteriorly directed force on the patella with knee flexion as the iliotibial band moves posteriorly. This combination of mechanical load concentration on

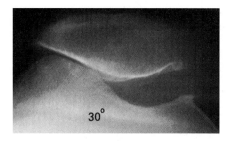

30°

Figure 11.49. Chronic patellar tilt with subluxation will eventually lead to lateral facet breakdown.

the lateral facet and accentuation of the load by adaptively shortened retinaculum can have devastating effects on the patellofemoral joint and lead ultimately to the excessive lateral pressure syndrome, as described by Ficat (57). Medial facet breakdown may also evolve, either by extension across the midpatella or because of chronically deficient medial facet contact pressure and excessive shear.

Tilt with subluxation (Type II malalignment) poses a slightly different problem in which lateral movement of the patella may actually permit better adaption to retinacular strain such that a patella is drawn laterally by tight lateral retinaculum rather than driven into the lateral trochlear facet. The combination of tilt and subluxation still leads to patellar cartilage degeneration in many patients (Fig. 11.49), and such patients generally experience more instability of the extensor mechanism than the patient with tilt alone.

Medial tilt, created by overzealous medial imbrication, can cause severe medial breakdown (see Fig. 11.1).

ARTICULAR CARTILAGE LESIONS RELATED TO PATELLAR SUBLUXATION

The patient with connective tissue laxity and subluxation of the patella *without* tilt will be less prone to articular degeneration than the patient with tilt. Subluxation in the absence of tilt will most commonly cause apprehension and a feeling of instability, but arthrosis may not occur. It is not uncommon to operate on a patient for patellar instability with documented subluxation (*without* tilt or a history of dislocation on CT) and find minimal or no evidence whatsoever of articular cartilage softening or breakdown on arthroscopic or open evaluation.

Subluxation will predispose a patient, however, to dislocation, and dislocation itself can cause substantial injury both to the medial patellar facet and the lateral femoral trochlea in many patients (Fig. 11.50). Such injuries will increase the risk of articular cartilage injury substantially.

Subluxation of the patella, *as an isolated entity,* is less destructive of the patella than other mechanical disorders. It is the *association of tilt or dislocation* with subluxation that creates a more worrisome picture of traumatic articular cartilage injury, lateral facet overload, or progressive arthrosis. In short, then, the clinician should look most critically at the presence of tilt as a harbinger of arthrosis and treat subluxation as it limits function or is associated with recurrent patellar instability. Iwano et al (61) have reported that 28% of patients with isolated patellofemoral osteoarthritis have a history of patellar subluxation or dislocation.

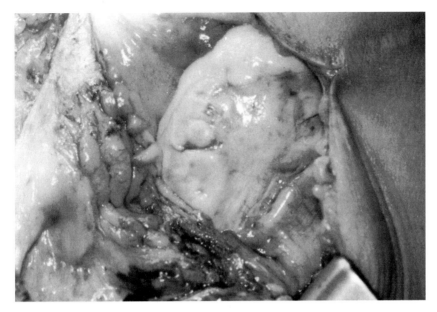

Figure 11.50. The lateral trochlea of this 16-year-old girl with recurrent patellar dislocation shows ample evidence of chronic injury.

CLINICAL FEATURES—CHONDROMALACIA RELATED TO MALALIGNMENT

As already noted, chondromalacia may cause no problems whatsoever in some patients. Consequently, it behooves the clinician to identify the cause or causes of *pain* by careful clinical evaluation.

Often, the patient will describe rather nonspecific pain around the anterior knee, and clinical evaluation will reveal a *subluxation-instability syndrome, a tilt-compression syndrome,* or a combination of the two. The majority of patients will fall into one of these categories. Nonetheless, there is an occasional patient who may enter the office with complaints of anterior knee pain that *can* be localized only to the patellar articular surface and attributed to articular cartilage breakdown.

Trauma and Infrapatellar Contracture

Some patients will give a history of trauma causing the onset of this pain. The infrapatellar contracture syndrome described by Paulos et al (82) following cruciate ligament surgery can also cause isolated patellar arthrosis. On clinical examination, such patients will often have pain on compression of the patella. The clinician should demonstrate that pain may be reproduced only by maneuvers that accentuate loading of the patella in varying degrees of flexion. The clinical history may be similar to that in the patient with malalignment and retinacular pain—that is, discomfort with activities, difficulty with stairs, sharp or aching pain in the anterior knee, limitation of physical activities, crepitation, and/or difficulty squatting. The physical examination, however, will be different in most patients with articular versus retinacular pain. The careful clinician will develop a clear picture of pain localization, either in the patella itself or in the surrounding retinacular structures, including the patellar tendon. Sometimes both will be present, particularly if a tilt compression syndrome has progressed from initial retinacular strain and fibroneuropathy to central lateral facet breakdown and progressive arthrosis.

SYMPTOMS AND PHYSICAL FINDINGS IN PATIENTS WITH CHONDROMALACIA-ARTHROSIS

Symptoms and findings in patients with chondromalacia-arthrosis are similar to those of other patellofemoral pain problems but generally are more severe, more persistent, and sometimes more disabling. Swelling and stiffness are more common. Pain is referred to the anterior knee, medial or lateral joint line, or anterior tibia. Stair climbing and descending may have become extremely difficult. Giving way while walking is less frequent only because use of the knee has become guarded. Sudden giving way while arising from a chair or descending stairs, associated with sharp pain, is common. It is, however, quite different from the giving way associated with an unstable patella in which there is a sudden movement of the patella. In arthrosis, the issue is *pain* and sometimes "catching" of irregular joint surfaces. This "catching" can cause the sensation of instability and must be differentiated.

The gait may have lost its spontaneity and become more cautious or stiff-legged. Seeing the patient rise slowly with pain from a chair, with the aid of his arms, raises clinical suspicion. Crepitus may be audible. The patella may be chronically tilted with or without subluxation.

Osteophytes may widen all margins, and patella magna may become apparent (Fig. 11.51). Transverse passive movement is usually limited. *Compression against the sulcus causes acute pain, as does extension against resistance.* Crepitus may be easily felt in many cases. Flexion is frequently limited. When tibiofemoral arthrosis is present, exten-

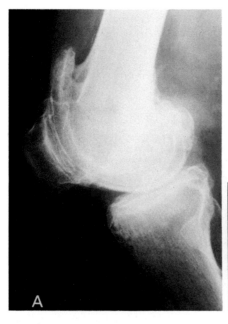

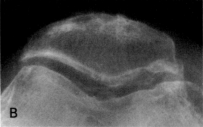

Figure 11.51. A, Massive osteophytosis had nearly doubled the patellar height and extended the trochlear margins proximally. **B,** Medial and lateral osteophytes have created a secondary patella magna.

sion may also lack 5 to 10 degrees. Quadriceps atrophy is inevitably present and proportional to severity of symptoms and disease. *The clinician should always look for pain that evolves from a single prominent osteophyte. Arthroscopic resection of such an osteophyte can give great relief even when there is general radiologic evidence of osteoarthrosis.* One must wonder how many knee joints have been replaced in patients with joint narrowing who really were experiencing pain from a snapping osteophyte that might have been resected using an arthroscope. Hence the importance of *careful* clinical examination.

Clinical Forms

Lateral Patellofemoral Arthrosis

Lateral patellofemoral arthrosis is by far the most common form. It is predictable, given the lateral predominance of the patellofemoral joint, the lateral vector of force resulting from the physiologic valgus, and the prevalence of lateral tilt in patients with chronic malalignment. Chronic lateral tilt, with or without subluxation, often leads to lateral facet erosion. The lateral facet shows the greatest incidence of wear both clinically and in autopsy series (22, 37, 57, 83). Such patients respond very well, in most cases, to anteromedial tibial tubercle transfer.

Lateral Bicompartment Arthrosis

The patella contact area extends on to the portion of the femoral condyle that articulates with the tibia in full extension, particularly the lateral compartment. It is not uncommon to see a combination of lateral arthrosis affecting both the tibiofemoral and patellofemoral compartments. This is particularly true if there is associated valgus of the knee. The combination of lateral bicompartment arthrosis is more common in women, likely due to their greater frequency of clinical valgus (Fig. 11.52).

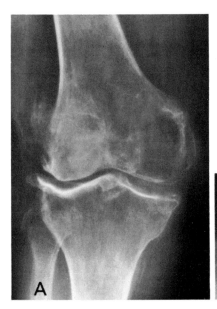

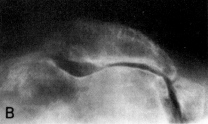

Figure 11.52. A, Standing anteroposterior (AP) view—the knee shows moderate valgus with lateral joint line narrowing. **B,** Axial view shows significant lateral patellofemoral arthrosis.

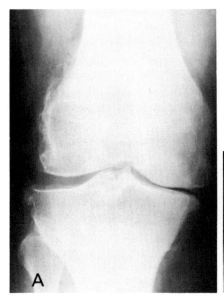

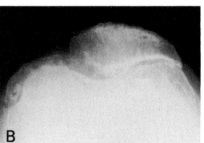

Figure 11.53. The combination of medial joint line narrowing on the standing anteroposterior (AP) radiograph of the knee *(A)* and significant lateral patellofemoral arthrosis *(B)* is quite common. It is important that the patellofemoral joint be radiologically evaluated when tibiofemoral arthrosis is suspected.

Crossed Bicompartment Arthrosis

Lateral patellofemoral and medial tibiofemoral compartment arthrosis (Fig. 11.53) are commonly associated. Chronic medial meniscus pathology may cause chronic effusions and diffuse softening of articular cartilage resulting in earlier breakdown of an overloaded lateral facet, particularly in the obese, elderly patient. It is important in such patients to determine if pain is most troublesome in the patellofemoral or medial compartment, so that treatment can be appropriately planned. Often one compartment is the source of pain despite radiographic breakdown of both compartments. The careful clinician will establish the primary source of pain.

Medial Patellar Arthrosis

Severe medial patellofemoral arthrosis is less common than its lateral counterpart. When it does occur, however, it is accompanied by all the radiologic signs that are so common laterally: joint line narrowing, subchondral sclerosis, and cysts (Fig. 11.54).

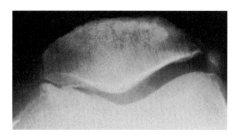

Figure 11.54. Medial patellofemoral arthrosis with joint line irregularity, osteophytes, and subchondral thickening.

This is in marked contradistinction to the radiographic picture associated with the florid type of chondromalacia encountered in the second and third decades. Medial bicompartment arthrosis is often associated with significant varus deformity. Excessive imbrication of the medial retinaculum at the time of proximal realignment can lead to progressive medial patellar arthrosis (see Figs. 11.1 and 11.9).

When dealing with symptomatic arthrosis of the knee, with or without deformity, an axial patellofemoral view is essential. When performing a high tibial osteotomy, this knowledge of the status of the patellofemoral joint may indicate including lateral retinacular release or anterior placement of the distal tibia, after osteotomy, to anteriorize the tibial tubercle.

Radiologic Features

Patients with simple, medial facet "chondromalacia," in addition to being asymptomatic in most cases, will generally have normal radiographs. If there is associated malalignment, *differentiation between tilt and subluxation* is most important, and the clinician, using criteria described in Chapter 4, should determine the specific malalignment patterns. In short, radiographic studies should enable the clinician to determine whether or not the patient has chondromalacia or arthrosis related to abnormal patellar alignment. Radiographic findings of osteophytes and patellofemoral arthritis with subchondral sclerosis may be found independent of malalignment but will most often be related to earlier trauma and articular cartilage injury or generalized knee arthritis. A superolateral osteolytic lesion in the patella, particularly if there is peripatellar calcified soft tissue, may indicate gout (84). Metastasis of adenocarcinoma to the patella is another rare cause of anterior knee pain (85).

The simple tangential/axial radiograph will give some idea about articular cartilage integrity and patellar alignment. The lateral knee radiograph will also give an indication if there is significant subchondral sclerosis or other evidence of arthrosis. In the patient who is a candidate for reconstructive surgery because of patellar arthritis, however, it is most important to recognize if there is significant malalignment because treatment will thereby be determined more accurately. Advanced chondromalacia or arthritis (Outerbridge Grades 3 to 4) without evidence of malalignment on standard radiographs and CT may be handled differently than arthritis in the patient with clear lateral tilt/compression. Traditional axial radiographs may not always demonstrate the extent of abnormal alignment. Bentley and Dowd (86) have commented specifically on the limited usefulness of traditional radiologic measurements in evaluating patients with chondromalacia.

If subluxation and tilt were present when the joint still had cartilage, when the cartilage is gone, both tilt and subluxation may be greater, with osteophyte production even more prominent.

A tilt/compression syndrome is the most common cause of lateral patellofemoral arthrosis. CT may show mild lateral tilt (Fig. 11.55) due to articular cartilage softening and loss of normal articular cartilage mechanical properties (87) (Fig. 11.56). If the patella starts out subluxated and tilted and then loses articular cartilage, subluxation and tilt will often progress (Fig. 11.56). The extent of this progression can be best determined using either CT or MRI.

In evaluating tomographic images, the clinician may note changes on the trochlear side that correlate with pain and require surgical correction (Fig. 11.57).

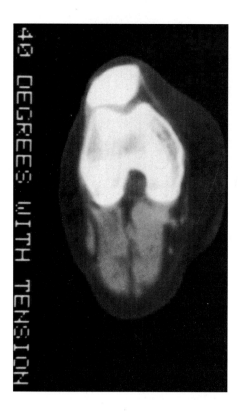

Figure 11.55. Computed tomography reveals early lateral facet collapse secondary to chronic tilt.

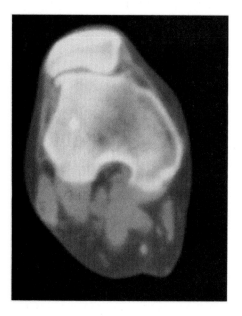

Figure 11.56. As the lateral facet collapses, osteophytes form along the trochlea, and there may be some evidence of increasing tilt or subluxation.

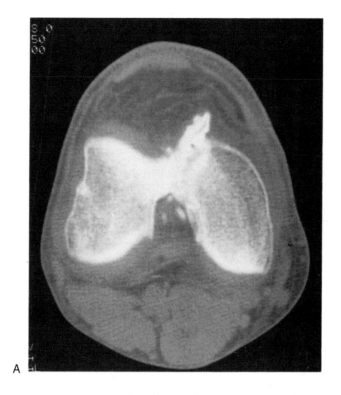

A

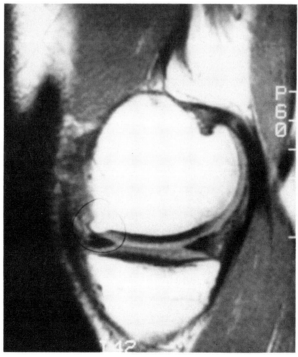

B

Figure 11.57. Trochlear osteophytes, either from the degenerative process or from trauma, can cause mechanical symptoms and pain that may warrant debridement. **A and B,** Posttraumatic. *Continued on next page.*

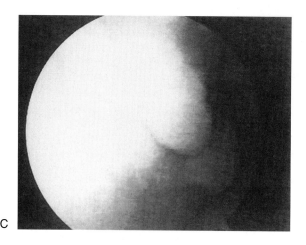

C

Figure 11.57. *Continued.* **C,** Degenerative.

OSTEOCHONDRITIS DISSECANS AND OSTEONECROSIS

Patellar osteochondritis is a rare cause of anterior knee pain (88). Occasionally, the clinician may notice an *osteochondritis dissecans* of the patella or trochlea. Although uncommon, such lesions can cause persistent pain, particularly in the athlete. As in osteochondritis dissecans of the medial femoral condyle, there is some possibility that the lesion may heal in a skeletally immature patient, so a period of immobilization (approximately 6 weeks) is appropriate in these patients. In adults, healing of the osteochondritis dissecans fragment is unlikely, and removal of the fragment may become necessary if it will not compromise articular surface congruity. If the osteochondritis dissecans fragment is so large that patellofemoral congruence or stability might be compromised, fixation with screws or wires will result in healing in most cases. Following fixation, a period of immobilization is wise, particularly if the fragment will undergo significant pressure during knee motion. Immobilization of the knee in full extension will minimize contact pressure on the healing fragment.

Removal of a small fragment can give satisfactory results when immobilization, modification of activity, and symptomatic treatment fail. In the author's experience, however, it is not uncommon to have some residual symptoms, even after removal of the fragment. Although patients are improved, a perfect result seems difficult to achieve following removal of small osteochondritis dissecans fragments from the patella. In the author's opinion, this procedure is best done open to permit thorough debridement of the defect.

Osteonecrosis may occur in patients following laser debridement of articular cartilage fragments. The author is aware of several cases in which patients underwent laser debridement of loose articular cartilage fragments and later experienced subchondral bone fragmentation with resulting loose body. Surgeons should be alert to subchondral fragmentation, presumably related to thermal necrosis of bone, following laser or radiofrequency thermal debridement of articular cartilage.

Osteonecrosis of the patella is also possible following steroid therapy. Mizuta et al (89) report a case of bilateral patellar osteonecrosis during steroid therapy. Hodge et al (90) have pointed out that CT arthrography is a very accurate and helpful technique for identifying significant synovial plicae and therefore recommend this technique as a way of differentiating thick from thin plicae. Galloway and Noyes (91) reported cystic degeneration of the patella following arthroscopic debridement and subchondral bone perforation. Thermal ablation of articular cartilage using any energy source other than straightforward shaving carries risks of chondrocyte modulation or death, but risk is less now with limited depth penetration radiofrequency ablation. Absolute minimal cartilage removal is required. Only loose fragments should be taken.

REFERENCES

1. Budinger K. Ueber traumatische knorpelrisse im Kniegelenk. Dtsch. Z Chir 1908;92:510.
2. Ludloff G. Zur pathologie der Kniegelenks. Verb Dtsch Ges Chir 1910;223.
3. Axhausen G. Zur pathogenese der arthritis deformans. Arch Orthop Unfallchir 1922;20:1.
4. Laden H. Knorpelresektion bet fissuraler knorpel degeneration der patella. Beitr Kling Chir 1925;134:265; Ueber knorpelresektion bet traumatisher gelenkstorung. Arch Klin Chir 1925;138:222.
5. Frund H. Traumatische chondropathie der patella, ein selbstandiges krankheitsbild. Zentrlbl Chir 1926;53: 707–710.
6. Karlson S. Chondromalacia patellae. Acta Chir Scand 1940;83:347–381.
7. Aleman O. Chondromalacia post-traumatica patellae. Acta Chir Scand 1928;63:194.
8. Chaklin VD. Injuries to the cartilages of the patella and the femoral condyle. J Bone Joint Surg 1939;37:133.
9. Slowick FA. Traumatic chondromalacia of the patella. N Engl J Med 1935;213:160–161.
10. Owre AA. Chondromalacia patellae. Acta Chir Scand 1936;77 (suppl 41).
11. Silfverskiöld N. Chondromalacia patellae. Acta Orthop Scand 1938;9:214.
12. Wiberg G. Roentgenographic and anatomic studies on the femoro-patellar joint. Acta Orthop Scand 1941;12: 319–410.
13. Hirsch C. A contribution to the pathogenesis of chondromalacia of the patella. A physical, histologic, and chemical study. Acta Chir Scand 1944;90(suppl):83.
14. Darracott J, Vernon-Roberts B. The bone changes in "chondromalacia patellae." Rheumatol Phys Med 1971;11: 175.
15. Robinson AR, Darracott J. Chondromalacia patellae. A survey conducted at the Army Medical Rehabilitation Unit, Chester. Ann Phys Med 1970;10:286–290.
16. Merchant A, Mercer R. Lateral release of the patella. A preliminary report. Clin Orthop 1974; 103:40–45.
17. Dandy D, Poirier H. Chondromalacia and the unstable patella. Acta Orthop Scand 1975;46:695.
18. Larson RL, Cabaud HE, Slocum DB, James SL, Keenan T, Hutchinson T. The patellar compression syndrome: surgical treatment by lateral retinacular release. Clin Orthop 1978;134:158–167.
19. Goodfellow JW, Hungerford DS, Woods C. Patello-femoral mechanics and pathology. II. Chondromalacia patellae. J Bone Joint Surg 1976;58B:291.
20. Radin E. Anterior knee pain: The need for a specific diagnosis. Orthop Rev 1985;14:128–134.
21. Abernathy PJ, Townsend P, Rose R, et al. Is chondromalacia patella a separate clinical entity? J Bone Joint Surg 1978;60B:205.
22. Casscells SW. Gross pathological changes in the knee joint of the aged individual. Clin Orthop 1978;132:225.
23. Stougard J. Chondromalacia of the patella. Physical signs in relation to operative findings. Acta Orthop Scand 1975;46:685–694.
24. Metcalf RW. An arthroscopic method for lateral release of the subluxating or dislocating patella. Clin Orthop 1982;167:11–18.
25. Brittberg M, Lindahl A, Nilsson A, Ohlsson C, Isaksson O, Peterson L. Treatment of deep cartilage defects in the knee with autogenous chondrocyte transplantation. New Engl J Med 1994;331:889–895.
26. Minas T. A practical algorithm for cartilage repair. Op Tech Sports Med 2000;8(2):141–143.
27. Fulkerson J. Awareness of the retinaculum in evaluating patellofemoral pain. Am J Sports Med 1982;10(3): 147–149.
28. Fulkerson J, Tennant R, Jarvin J, Grunnet M. Histologic evidence of retinacular nerve injury associated with patellofemoral malalignment. Clin Orthop 1985;197:196.
29. Witonski D, Wagrowska-Danielewicz M. Distribution of substance P nerve fibers in the knee joint of patients with anterior knee pain syndrome. Knee Surg Sports Traumatol Arthrosc 1999;7:177–183.
30. Sanchis-Alfonso V, Rosello-Sastre E. Immunohistochemical analysis for neural markers of the lateral retinaculum in patients with isolated symptomatic patellofemoral malalignment. Am J Sports Med 2000;28:725–731.
31. Kelly MA, Insall JN. Historical perspectives of chondromalacia patellae (review). Orthop Clin North Am 1992;23(4):517–521.
32. Staubli H, Durrenmatt U, Porcellini B, Rauschning W. Anatomy and surface geometry of the patellofemoral joint in the axial plane. 1999;81:452–458.
33. Ficat P. L'articulation, entite fonctionnelle. Rev Med Toulouse 1966;2:719–723; Rev Med Toulouse 1967;3: 373–378.
34. Seedholm BB, Takeda T, Tsubuku M, Wright V. Mechanical factors and patellofemoral osteoarthrosis. Ann Rheum Dis 1979;38:307–316.
35. Müller W. The knee: Form, function and ligament reconstruction. New York: Springer-Verlag; 1983.

36. Fulkerson J, Edwards C, Chrisman OD. Articular cartilage. In: Albright J, Brand R, eds. The Scientific Basis of Orthopaedics. Appleton and Lange: East Norwalk, Conn; 1987.
37. Emery I, Meachim G. Surface morphology and topography of patellofemoral cartilage fibrillation in Liverpool necropores. J Anat 1973;116:103–120.
38. Goodfellow J, Bullough P. The pattern of aging of the articular cartilage of the elbow joint. J. Bone Joint Surg 1967;49B:175–181.
39. Harrison MHM, Schajowicz F, Trueta J. Osteoarthritis of the hips: A study of the nature and evolution of the disease. J Bone Joint Surg 1953;35B:598–626.
40. Akizuki S, Mow VC, Muller F, Pita JC, Howell DS, Manicourt DH. Tensile properties of human knee joint cartilage. I. Influence of ionic conditions, weight bearing, and fibrillation on the tensile modulus. J Orthop Res 1986;4:379–392.
41. Marar BC, Pillay VK. Chondromalacia of the patella in Chinese. A postmortem study. J Bone Joint Surg 1975;57A:342–345.
42. Hoaglund FT, Yau ALMC, Wong INL. Osteoarthritis of the hip and other joints in Southern Chinese in Hong Kong. Incidence and related factors. J Bone Joint Surg 1973;55A:545.
43. Crooks LM. Chondromalacia patellae. J Bone Joint Surg 1967;49B:495–501.
44. Outerbridge RE. The etiology of chondromalacia patellae. J Bone Joint Surg 1961;43B:752–757.
45. Fulkerson JP, Winters TF. Articular cartilage response to arthroscopic surgery: A review of current knowledge. Arthroscopy, J Arthroscop Rel Surg 1988;2:184–189.
46. Palmoski MJ, Brandt KD. Effects of some nonsteroidal anti-inflammatory drugs on proteoglycan metabolism and organization in canine articular cartilage. Arthritis Rheum 1980;23:1010–1020.
47. Hoaglund FT. Experimental hemarthrosis: The response of canine knees to injections of autologous blood. J Bone Joint Surg 1967;49A:285–298.
48. Enneking WF, Horowitz M. The intra-articular effects of immobilization on the human knee. J Bone Joint Surg 1972;54A:973–985.
49. Langenskiold A, Michelsson JE, Videman T. Osteoarthritis of the knee in the rabbit produced by immobilization. Acta Orthop Scand 1979;50:1–14.
50. Trojer H. The effect of short-term immobilization on the rabbit knee joint cartilage. Clin Orthop 1975;107: 249–257.
51. Reagan BF, McInerny VK, Treadwell BV, Zarins B, Mankin JJ. Irrigating solutions for arthroscopy. J Bone Joint Surg 1983;65A:629–631.
52. Nole R, Munson N, Fulkerson JP. Bupivacaine and saline effects on articular cartilage. Arthroscopy, J Arthroscop Rel Surg 1985;1:123–127.
53. Mankin JJ, Conger KA. The acute effects of intra-articular hydrocortisone on articular cartilage in rabbits. J Bone Joint Surg 1966;48A:1383–1388.
54. Biedert R, Kernan V. Neurosensory characteristics of the patellofemoral joint: what is the genesis of patellofemoral pain? Sports Med Arthrosc Rev 2001;9:295–300.
55. Meachim G, Ghadially FN, Collins DH. Regressive changes in the superficial layer of human articular cartilage. Ann Rheum Dis 1965;24:23.
56. Outerbridge R. The etiology of chondromalacia patellae. J Bone Joint Surg 1961;43B:752–757.
57. Ficat C. La degenerescence du cartilage de la rotule, de la chondromalcre a l'Arthrose. Semin Hosp Paris 1974;50:3210–3219.
58. Durroux R, Ficat P. Etude optique et ultrastructurale du cartilage rotulien dans la chondromalacie. Rev Chir Orthop 1969;543–546.
59. Zimny M, Redler I. An ultrastructural study of patellar chondromalacia in humans. J Bone Joint Surg 1969;51A:1179–1190.
60. Mankin H, Thrasher A. Water content and binding in normal and osteoarthrotic human cartilage. J Bone Joint Surg 1975;57A:76–80.
61. Iwano T, Kurosawa H, Tokuyama H, Hoshikawa Y. Roentgenographic and clinical findings of patellofemoral osteoarthrosis. With special reference to its relationship to femorotibial osteoarthrosis and etiologic factors. Clin Orthop 1990;252:190–197.
62. Kivimaki J, Riihimaki H, Hanninen K. Knee disorders in carpet and floor layers and painters. Scand J Work Environ Health 1992;18(5):310–316.
63. Butler-Manuel PA, Guy RL, Heatley FW, Nunan TO. Scintigraphy in the assessment of anterior knee pain. Acta Orthop Scand 1990;61(5):438–442.
64. Chrisman OD, Ladenbauer-Bellis IM, Fulkerson J. The osteoarthritic cascade and associated drug actions. Osteoarthritis Symposium Arthritis Rheum (suppl) 1981;145.
65. Fulkerson JP, Damiano P. Effect of prostaglandin E2 on adult pig articular cartilage slices in culture. Clin Orthop 1983;179:266–269.
66. Fulkerson JP, Ladenbauer-Bellis I-M, Chrisman OD. In vitro hexosamine depletion of intact articular cartilage by E prostaglandins. Arthritis Rheum 1979;22:1117–1121.
67. Pugh JW, Rose RM, Radin EL. Elastic and viscoelastic properties of trabecular bone: Dependence on structure. J Biomech 1973;6:475–485.
68. Radin EL, Paul IL. Response of joints to impact loading. Arthritis Rheum 1971;14:3.

69. Radin EL, Parker HG, Pugh JW, Steinberg RS, Paul IL, Rose RM. Response of joints to impact loading. III. J Biomech 1963;6:51–57.
70. Mankin H. Current Concepts Review: The response of articular cartilage to mechanical injury. J Bone Joint Surg 1982;64A:460–466.
71. Ghadially F, Thomas I, Oryschak A, LaRonde J. Long term results of superficial defects in articular cartilage. J Pathol 1977;121:213.
72. Furukawa T, Eyre D, Korde S, Glimcher M. Biochemical studies on repair cartilage resurfacing experimental defects in the rabbit knee. J Bone Joint Surg 1980;62A:79.
73. Fulkerson J. Anteromedialization of the tibial tuberosity for patellofemoral malalignment. Clin Orthop 1983;177:176–181.
74. Lynch J. Venous abnormalities and intraosseous hypertension associated with osteoarthritis of the knee. In: Ingwersen M, ed. The Knee Joint. New York: American Elsevier Publishing–Excerpta Medica; 1974.
75. Ficat P, Arlet J, Vidal R, Ricci A, Forniala J. Resultats therapeutiques du forage biopsie dans les osteonecroses femoro-capitales primitive (100 cas). Rev Rhum Mal Osteoartic 1971;38:269.
76. Hungerford DS. Early diagnosis of ischemic necrosis of the femoral head. Johns Hopkins Med J 1975; 137:270–275.
77. Ficat P, Arlet J, Lartigue G, Pujol M, Tran MA. Algo-dystrophies reflexes post-traumatiques. Rev Chir Orthop 1973;59:401–414.
78. Arnoldi C, Lemperg R, Linderhoml H. Immediate effect of osteotomy on the intramedullary pressure of the femoral head and neck in patients with degenerative osteoarthritis. Acta Orthop Scand 1971;42:357–365.
79. Nissen K. The arrest of early primary osteoarthritis of the hip by osteotomy. Proc R Soc Med 1963;56:1051.
80. Osborne G, Fahrni W. Oblique displacement osteotomy for osteoarthritis of the hip joint. J Bone Surg 1950; 32B:148.
81. Phillips R, Bulmer J, Hoyle G, Davies W. Venous drainage in osteoarthritis of the hip. A study after osteotomy. J Bone Joint Surg 1967;49B:301.
82. Paulos L, Rosenberg T, Drawbert J, Manning J, Abbot P. Infrapatellar contracture syndrome. Am J Sports Med 1987;15(4):331–341.
83. Bennett GA, Waine H, Bauer W. Changes in the knee joint at various ages with particular reference to the nature and development of degenerative joint disease. New York: The Commonwealth Fund; 1942.
84. Recht MP, Seragini F, Kramer J, Dalinka MK, Hurtgen K, Resnick D. Isolated or dominant lesions of the patella in gout: A report of seven patients. Skeletal Radiol 1994;23(2):113–116.
85. Cavaciocchi A, Fusi M, Rigutti E. A solitary metastasis of the patella. Ital J Orthop Traumatol 1992;18(4):7–560.
86. Bentley G, Dowd G. Current concepts of etiology and treatment of chondromalacia patellae. Clin Orthop 1984;189:209–228.
87. Mow V, Holmes M, Lai W. Fluid transport and mechanical properties of articular cartilage. A Review. J Biomech 1984;17:377–394.
88. Pfeiffer WH, Gross ML, Seeger LL. Osteochondritis dissecans of the patella. MRI evaluation and a case report. Clin Orthop 1991;271:207–211.
89. Mizuta H, Kubota K, Shiraishi M, Kai K, Nakamura E, Takagi K. Steroid-related bilateral osteonecrosis of the patella. Arthroscopy 1993;9(1):114-116.
90. Hodge J, Gehlman B, O'Brien S, Wickiewiez T. Synovial plicae and chondromalacia patellae. Radiology 1993;186(3):827–831.
91. Galloway MT, Noyes FR. Cystic degeneration of the patella after arthroscopic chondroplasty and subchondral bone perforation. Arthroscopy 1992;(3):366–369.

12

Nonoperative Treatment

*"The winner has an answer for every problem; the loser has a
problem for every answer."*

One thing remains clear in the minds of orthopedic surgeons, physical therapists, and
other health care providers: *nonoperative treatment provides satisfactory results in most
patients with anterior knee pain* (1–9). In fact, Jensen and Albrektsen (10) have shown
that 81% of patients treated for patellofemoral pain without malalignment had mild or no
pain at 12-year follow-up. In a randomized, double-blind placebo-controlled study,
Crossley et al (11) proved the worth of physical therapy in the treatment of patellofemoral
pain.

In years past, nonoperative treatment for the patient with patellofemoral pain was standardized, usually involving aspirin, quadriceps strengthening, and limited activity. Today
the therapist designs a much more specific program tailored to the unique physical findings of the patient. The goal of patellofemoral rehabilitation will be to define the specific
problem(s) causing pain or instability and organize treatment accordingly (12).

PLANNING TREATMENT

Having examined the patient closely after obtaining a detailed history, the clinician can
develop a treatment plan. In particular, the therapist should observe the patient (Fig.
12.1); evaluate patellar position, tilt, and alignment (Fig. 12.2, A and B); determine if
there is retinacular, patellar tendon, or quadriceps tendon tenderness (Fig. 12.3); identify
tightness of the quadriceps, hamstrings, or iliotibial band (Fig. 12.4, A to C); and gain
some insight into the patient's motivation. The goal will be to match a treatment plan with
the specific findings (13). One must define the (a) patellar malposition, (b) degree and
location of chondrosis-arthrosis, (c) retinacular–soft tissue causes of pain, (d) referred
pain, and (e) compensation-related problems.

Malposition

Short of surgery, it is unlikely that patellar tracking can be changed much. Tight structures can be stretched. Tape and braces can apply some mild support. One can strengthen
muscles to give dynamic support. Structural alignment is maintained by dense retinacular structures that are not likely to elongate significantly with stretching. Whereas it is
possible to reduce stiffness and increase mobility, stretching, bracing, and taping probably will not make a malaligned patella track normally in most patients.

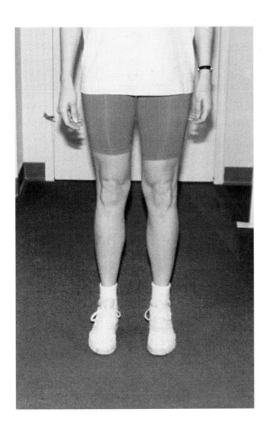

Figure 12.1. Looking at the patient will reveal alignment problems, muscle atrophy, skin changes, and gait alteration. Observe the patient standing and walking, with and without sneakers.

Consider the quadriceps-patellar tendon mechanism. One can mobilize the muscle with strengthening, but one will not elongate the patellar tendon itself. However, if the patellar tendon is tethered by bands of scar, as in an infrapatellar contracture syndrome (IPCS) (14), the patient and therapist may be able to stretch out some of the abnormal scar tissue and allow the tendon to come back to length if the scar has not become fixed. This concept is important because there is a difference between releasing abnormal tissues that have formed in the short term (adhesions related to immobility) and changing the structural alignment of the extensor mechanism that is genetically or developmentally determined. One must consider also, however, that it may be possible to compensate for abnormal alignment by developing strength in muscles that will selectively counteract tight, deforming forces around the anterior knee. Doucette and Goble (5) have suggested that proper rehabilitation will improve iliotibial band flexibility and radiographic alignment but not the Q angle, patellofemoral index, or hamstring flexibility. This issue, however, is more complicated. Witvrouw et al (15) have introduced the importance of altered vastus medialis obliquus (VMO) response time, quadriceps shortening, reduced explosive strength, and patella hypermobility.

A tilting patella will not come to sit normally in the femoral trochlea by nonoperative treatment alone. After identifying structural tilt, however, the therapist will be able to mobilize those structures that have dynamic components (iliotibial band and quadriceps muscle) while reducing stiffness and discomfort in a tight retinaculum (Fig. 12.5, A and

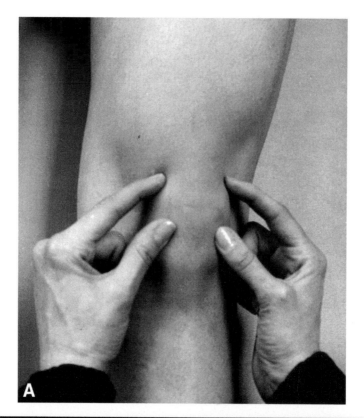

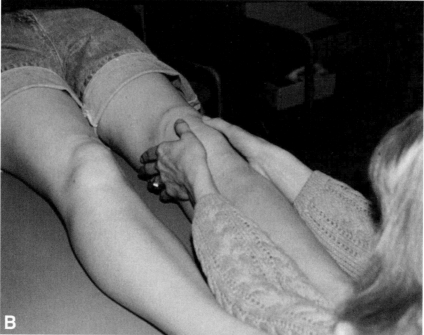

Figure 12.2. A, Look critically to see if the patella is tilted or just displaced on the trochlea. This is also an ideal time to palpate muscle and retinacular structure around the patella. **B,** Look at the patella from above and below. This is particularly helpful in identifying tilt.

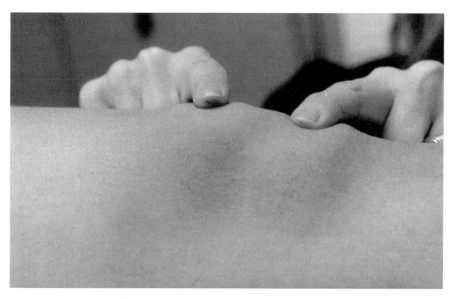

Figure 12.3. Palpate carefully above and below the patella to detect tenderness of the patellar tendon or quadriceps tendon.

B), mostly on the lateral side of the patella. Quadriceps strengthening with emphasis on the VMO will add to the subjective feeling of support and will improve functional capability in many patients (Fig. 12.6). Prone stretching of the quadriceps (see Fig. 12.4, B) becomes particularly important in the patient with a tilting patella in order to further mobilize stiff retinacular or muscular structures around the anterior knee. Local modalities may provide symptomatic relief during the rehabilitation process (Fig. 12.7). Ultimately, the patient should work into an aerobic conditioning program (Fig. 12.8) for improved confidence and self-esteem as well as to maintain supple connective tissue around the front of the knee.

A patient with recurrent subluxation and feelings of instability, however, will need emphasis predominantly on *support* of the patella, including emphasis on the VMO (Fig. 12.9). These patients may have little or no connective-tissue stiffness but generally have an abnormal extensor mechanism vector that is not likely to become normal with nonoperative treatment alone. Orthotics may give enough support to alter this vector somewhat and should be included when there is need to balance the kinetic chain, particularly in the patient with excessive pronation. Bracing and taping may be helpful in giving *proprioceptive feedback* and improved dynamic support for the extensor mechanism thereby.

In the patient with patella baja (however severe or mild), the emphasis will be on prone stretching of the extensor mechanism and strengthening of the hamstrings and quadriceps (see Fig. 12.3). Such patients need a lot of assurance and may need surgical intervention if there is a true IPCS. Following release of an IPCS surgically, such patients may be undergoing continuous passive motion and a regular regimen of stretching-extensor mechanism mobilization. Aquatic therapy can be particularly helpful in these patients as they regain motion and confidence.

Physical therapy will not correct a patella alta because the patella cannot be brought distally by nonoperative means. Often, however, there is malalignment or soft-tissue strain associated with patella alta that will respond to physical therapy.

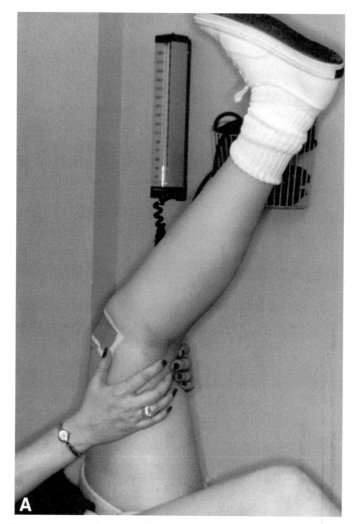

Figure 12.4. Evaluate the patient for tightness of the hamstrings (*A*), quadriceps (*B*), or iliotibial band (*C*). The prone position is particularly useful for stretching the quadriceps (*B*).

The patient with recurrent patellar *dislocation* needs particularly close attention because he/she is at high risk for articular damage to the patella and may need to have surgical correction of the extensor mechanism vector. In the rehabilitation program, VMO support for the patella is extremely important, along with mobilization of tight, deforming lateral structures. Following acute dislocation, there may be a significant hemarthrosis. Removal of this by aspiration is usually helpful to reduce tension of the medial soft tissues that need to heal in as shortened a position as possible. Fortunately, following a single patellar dislocation, many patients will have adequate healing, and rehabilitation may enable these patients to return to normal activities without surgery. The patient who experiences recurrent dislocations, however, should seek surgical intervention. Each dislocation carries a significant risk of damaging the joint further.

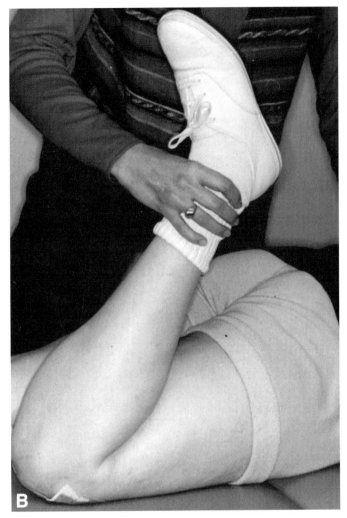

Figure 12.4. *Continued on next page.*

Chondrosis-Arthrosis

The physical examination has yielded some concept of the extent and location of artic-ular lesions. The goal of rehabilitation is to reduce contact on these lesions when possi-ble, mobilize sensitive and stiff retinacular structures around the degenerating patella, reduce effusion when possible, and control structural factors that may have led to this problem in the first place (e.g., infrapatellar contracture, tilt, subluxation).

Throughout the rehabilitation of patients with patellar chondrosis-arthrosis, it is important to avoid excessive contact stress on a lesion. Consequently, exercises should be individualized to avoid loading the lesion. When the articular lesion is distal on the patella, quadriceps exercise will be best done with the knee more flexed. If the lesion is proximal on the patella (as in a dashboard-type injury), exercise will be better accom-plished closer to full knee extension (see Chapter 2 on Biomechanics). Taping and brac-

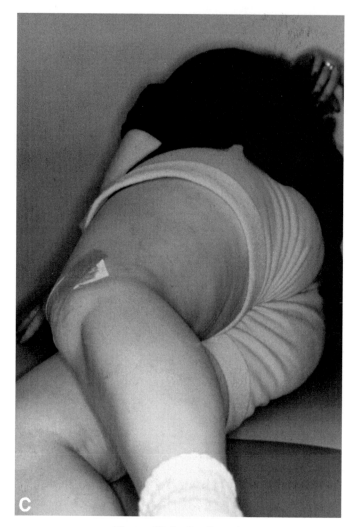

Figure 12.4. *Continued.*

ing as well as nonsteroidal antiinflammatory medication may facilitate the exercise program and improve muscle reactivity by providing proprioceptive feedback.

Most important in the patient with an articular lesion is to mobilize the retinaculum and extensor mechanism. *Prone stretching of the quadriceps* is the cornerstone of this mobilization process.

Retinacular Pain

Surgery, blunt trauma, or chronic stress of any sort around the anterior knee can lead to retinacular damage, small neuromata in the peripatellar retinaculum, or painful scar tissue in the structure around the patellofemoral joint. Retinacular pain, related to soft-tissue trauma or stress, will respond only to strengthening, stretching, or surgery that is

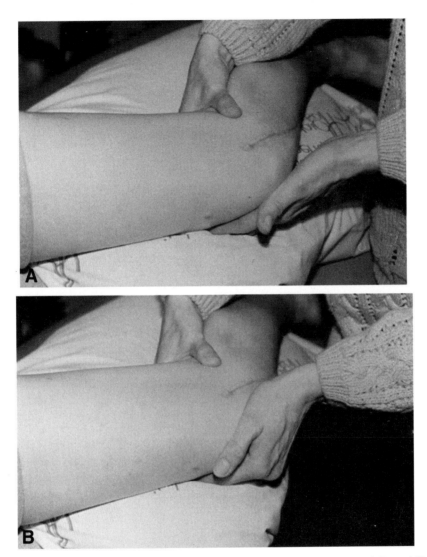

Figure 12.5. A and B, The therapist should stabilize the knee and then carefully mobilize the lateral retinacular structure with continuous firm pressure. This may be accomplished best with the patient lateral and the affected side up. By relaxing the extensor mechanism in this manner, the therapist may stretch the lateral retinaculum more effectively in varying degrees of knee flexion.

specifically designed to treat the affected area. Only a careful correlation of clinical examination with the patient's history will uncover the specific source of pain.

Once identified, a retinacular source of pain may be treated by stretching, mobilization, modalities, injection, nonsteroidal antiinflammatory medication, or skillful neglect (the more acute strains may get better with time alone). Reassurance is particularly helpful in these patients, who may feel that the joint itself is deteriorating and that previous activities (sports, work, and so on) may no longer be possible. When therapy directed to the affected area of retinaculum fails, surgical exploration, selective release, and/or excision may be curative in carefully selected patients.

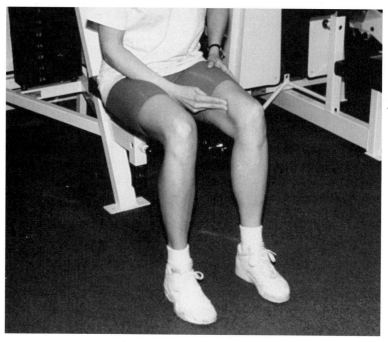

Figure 12.6. The patient should learn to contract the vastus medialis and exercise it regularly.

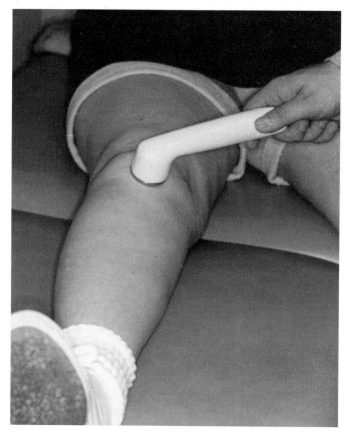

Figure 12.7. Ultrasound, iontophoresis, and other modalities may be used to facilitate stretching and also to relieve pain.

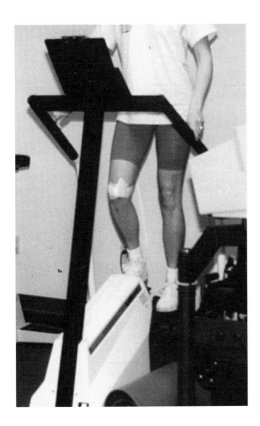

Figure 12.8. An aerobic conditioning program is important for every patient. Pain-free exercise is possible for almost all patients, but the therapist may have to improvise and supervise an exercise program initially to assure that the patient did not aggravate his/her condition.

Plica

Nonoperative treatment may be fruitless in the patient with a painful, mechanically irritable plica. Stretching the quadriceps with the patient prone, local modalities, and selective injection of a painful plica with corticosteroid may bring the problem under control; however, arthroscopic excision of a painful, snapping plica will often be necessary.

Synovitis

In most patients with inflamed synovium, nonsteroidal antiinflammatory medication and/or corticosteroid injection will be helpful. In the patient with rheumatoid disease or more prolific synovitis, arthroscopic synovectomy may become necessary. Physical therapy alone is less helpful in these patients, although maintaining or improving strength in the patient with rheumatoid disease may bring functional improvement while the inflammatory disease is coming under control. Reduction or elimination of effusion is necessary in order to restore quadriceps function (16).

Muscle-Tendon Pain

When pain is identified in the distal quadriceps muscle immediately around the patellofemoral joint, the physician or therapist should remember the possibility of skeletal muscle hemangioma or referred pain. In muscle or tendon pain related to chronic overuse and strain, stretching, local modalities, antiinflammatory medication, and selective local

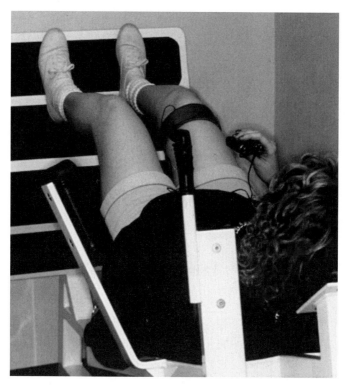

Figure 12.9. Awareness and control of vastus medialis obliquus contraction will help the patient gain confidence and control of extensor mechanism function.

anesthetic with corticosteroid injection will often bring relief. Again, it is most important to identify a very specific pain focus so that treatment may be directed appropriately. Nonspecific treatment, including strengthening, may be ineffective and, when pushed excessively, may actually make the patient worse when muscle or tendon is the source of pain.

Referred Pain

One of the great dangers of applying nonspecific treatment to patients with anterior knee pain without a specific awareness of the source of pain is treating a patient's knee when the pain is coming from another area, usually the back or hip. Problems in the hip joint are particularly likely to refer pain to the anterior knee region. By obtaining a careful history, watching how the patient localizes pain in the anterior knee, and doing a thorough physical examination (including evaluation of hip rotation with the patient prone), the examiner is far less likely to mistake a degenerative hip for patellofemoral pain. Before starting nonoperative treatment for anterior knee pain, every patient should be placed prone both for examination of quadriceps tightness and evaluation of hip rotation. If internal rotation of the hip is limited, a radiograph of the hip should rule out degenerative change or slipped capital femoral epiphysis. Missing the latter diagnosis in a young patient can be catastrophic.

Back problems can also cause pain in the anterior knee region. A herniated disk, particularly at the L3 to L4 level, can cause pain in the anterior aspect of the knee. Before initiating treatment in a patient with anterior knee pain, the physician or therapist should consider the possibility of discogenic pain, perform a straight leg raising test to rule out radicular pain, and check for neurologic signs such as numbness or weakness. Even worse, one might risk missing a spinal cord tumor in nonspecific treatment of anterior knee pain.

FORMS OF TREATMENT

Injection

Once a specific focus of pain is identified in the physician's office, a single appropriate injection can be diagnostic. Intraarticular local anesthetic should temporarily eliminate intraarticular pain in the majority of patients. If the patient identifies a specific retinacular, tendon, or muscular pain site, injecting the focus of pain, possibly with a small amount of corticosteroid, will confirm or disprove this source of pain. Of course, one should warn the patient that there can be a temporary increase of pain when corticosteroid is injected into a retinacular area. If there is a noninflammatory source of pain, there may be temporary relief from local anesthetic but return of pain once it wears off, despite corticosteroid. Neuroma pain may subside temporarily after corticosteroid injection, but the pain often returns. This is equally true of surgically created neuromata and microneuromata related to chronic patellar malalignment and retinacular nerve strain.

Compartment Syndrome Treatment

Particularly in the high-demand athlete, the clinician should consider a compartment syndrome of the quadriceps compartment or the anterior compartment of the lower leg. Bicyclists, in particular, are prone to quadriceps compartment syndrome. Runners and other high-demand athletes can develop anterior compartment syndrome in the lower leg. Quadriceps compartment syndrome is particularly notable in the anterior knee region and should be considered in any athlete who points to the distal quadriceps when asked to localize his pain. In such patients, modification of activity, quadriceps stretching, ice application after activity, and reduced emphasis on quadriceps strengthening may help, particularly after a period of rest. It is very important to differentiate this problem from other sources of anterior knee pain because treatment will generally be quite different and there will be less emphasis on quadriceps strength. In more extreme cases, compartment pressure manometry may be necessary. Straight leg raising with a 5- to 10-pound weight on the ankle is the method of choice for gaining quadriceps strength after resolution of the compartment syndrome. This form of isometric strengthening, however, takes considerable self-discipline, and patient compliance is probably less than with the exercise bicycle or another form of quadriceps exercise that gives aerobic benefit as well. Such exercise, however, must wait until complete resolution of the original compartment syndrome. In some patients, fasciotomy of the involved compartment may be necessary.

Home Therapy

Many patients, following the initial diagnosis, will respond to a home treatment program. Tailoring the home program to the specific diagnosis, as noted earlier in this chapter, is most important. Nonsteroidal antiinflammatory medication will usually help with pain control, incorporating exercise and stretching with the patient's day-to-day activities. When quadriceps or hamstring strengthening is advisable, a program that allows strengthening through a pain-free range of motion, without stressing articular lesions, must be created. The seat of an exercise bicycle, or even a regular bicycle, can be adjusted for the desired knee range of motion. The seat will generally be lowered when there is an articular lesion on the distal articular surface, such that exercise is accomplished in a more flexed-knee position. Similarly, for a lesion on the more proximal patella (such as dashboard injury), the seat may be set very high, such that there is more exercise toward full extension of the knee. Ankle weights, theraband, or surgical tubing may be used in a similar fashion.

A simple elastic knee sleeve with patella cut-out or a patellar tendon strap may be used for pain control in the patient with patellofemoral pain. Beware of using a patellar tendon strap in the patient with a distal patella articular lesion, however, because there is risk of increasing load on the distal patella articular lesion with one of these straps.

Stretching at home is advisable in most patients with anterior knee pain. The prone quadriceps stretch (lying on the stomach, grasping the ankle, and pulling the knee into flexion gradually over a period of 20 to 30 seconds) will reduce adhesions, stiffness, and muscle tightness. There is substantial benefit with minimal cost and effort doing stretching at home. The patient can also stretch the hamstrings by doing simple toe-touching exercises with the legs straight.

Simple orthotics may be extremely helpful in the home management of patients with pronation. We recommend simple off-the-shelf orthotics initially, at considerable cost savings, when orthotics seem to be necessary to balance the kinetic chain. When effective, these may be replaced selectively with custom orthotics for more long-term use at a later time. Also, some patients prefer a soft off-the-shelf type of orthotic, or cork-and-leather orthotic, to the more rigid plastic custom orthotic.

Aerobic Exercise

Aerobic exercise should be a goal in most patients with anterior knee pain. Once there is pain control using antiinflammatory medication, strengthening, stretching, and bracing, a program of gradual aerobic conditioning will help to enhance self-esteem and confidence while further mobilizing retinacular structures around the patella. Water exercise, such as bobbing or swimming laps, may be available to some patients, whereas the more vigorous exercise bicycle using high repetition and lower resistance training may be best for other patients. Still others may progress into a running program when articular disease is absent or less pronounced. The specific form of exercise will vary depending upon the severity of articular disease, the amount of pain, the patient's preference, and the success of other home therapy management techniques.

Physical Therapy

When home therapy fails, skilled physical therapy can be of great help in patients with anterior knee pain, depending upon the specific diagnosis. The physical therapist can help implement the exercise program by controlling pain and introducing stretches and exercises that the patient can tolerate, thereby making progress without causing aggravation of the problem. Often, this takes considerable creativity on the part of the physical therapist.

Taping the patellofemoral joint can be particularly effective in the hands of a skilled physical therapist. A therapist's taping can provide proprioceptive feedback to the patient, thereby facilitating strengthening. Appropriate taping can also reduce pain to allow more effective exercise. Most patients can learn how to tape their own patella once the therapist has found the most appropriate taping configuration.

Although some patients are able to stretch effectively in a home program, many patients benefit from structured physical therapy to maximize stretching. The physical therapist may implement reflex inhibition techniques, modalities, heat, and other modalities to maximize the benefits of stretching.

Although *isokinetic exercise* is less important in the patient with patellofemoral pain generally, high-speed exercise in a pain-free range of motion concentrically may be helpful in selected patients. Also, *isokinetic testing* at higher speeds will help to objectify the patient's strength gain. This type of feedback is very important in many patients. Eccentric isokinetic exercise, when carefully monitored, may be particularly beneficial to the patient with patellar tendinitis and retinacular pain *as opposed to* true articular disease. When there is articular cartilage breakdown, particularly as a source of pain, the therapist should avoid isokinetic eccentric exercise in most cases. In fact, isokinetic exercise, at lower speeds in particular, can be dangerous in such patients and can cause more pain or trouble.

A knowledgeable physical therapist can *evaluate the entire kinetic chain.* By equalizing leg lengths, balancing foot posture, restoring normal gait, doing appropriate stretching and strengthening, and restoring normal posture and balance, patellofemoral joint function may be improved and, in most patients, pain will be reduced or eliminated (Fig. 12.10).

Structured aquatic therapy is generally forgiving and often helpful in the patient with resistant patellofemoral pain. In the water, these patients can exercise more effectively using fluid resistance. The water also provides compression around the joint to reduce swelling. Some patients can progress more rapidly into an aerobic exercise plan in a pool program.

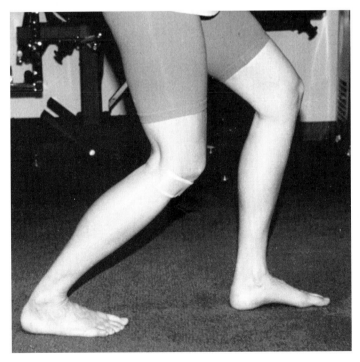

Figure 12.10. Mobilization of the kinetic chain above and below the knee is usually helpful. Stretching the gastrocnemius-soleus, balancing the foot, and working on balance-proprioception should be part of most patellofemoral rehabilitation programs.

The therapist can use *creative techniques* to help the patient. Training the patient to respond to household stimuli such as a doorbell or phone ringing, a dog barking, or visual cues in the home by contracting the quadriceps muscle (with particular emphasis on the VMO) can help a patient to develop patellar control.

In more severe cases, a *transcutaneous nerve stimulator* may be helpful for pain control. An electric muscle stimulator can also be helpful in initiating strength gain, but an active program of quadriceps and hamstring strengthening will be far more desirable in the majority of patients. Ultrasound and other modalities are useful, particularly for soft-tissue mobilization and pain control, to facilitate exercise.

REHABILITATION

Kinetic Chain Mobilization, Alignment, and Proprioception

Look at the patient standing, sitting, and moving. There are many variables from the ground up that will affect patellar tracking.

Starting at ground level, excessive pronation can lead to accentuation of valgus at the knee, external rotation of the foot and tibia, and resulting accentuation of lateral patellar alignment.

Simple, off-the-shelf orthotics can provide immediate reduction of this pronation and improvement of this component of the kinetic chain. Careful examination of the foot may reveal more pronation in the hindfoot or forefoot, so custom orthotics may be desirable in selected patients to address more severe functional deficits in these areas. One *exception* to medial posting or reduction of pronation is the patient with medial knee arthrosis (varus gonarthrosis). In such pronating patients, reduction of pronation may actually increase medial knee pain. Fortunately, such patients are relatively rare.

It is most helpful in the rehabilitation process to have a variety of antipronation orthotics available on the shelf. "Off-the-shelf" arch supports are surprisingly comfortable and may suffice for many patients at much less cost than custom-molded orthotics.

In addition to kinetic chain balancing structurally, a well-structured patellofemoral rehabilitation program will emphasize proprioceptive balance. Wilk and Reinold (17) recommend weight shifting side to side and diagonally as well as minisquats on an unstable surface (such as a tilt board). Activities on an unstable surface progress from double leg to single leg with added perturbations (tapping the balance board).

Stretching the Kinetic Chain

Excessive tightness above or below the patellofemoral joint can create elevated stress around the patella by limiting the normal progression of impact absorption through the kinetic chain. An unyielding gastrocnemius muscle, for instance, may give an abrupt pronation moment at the foot during the "foot flat" component of gait.

The gastrocnemius will stretch most effectively with the knee extended because the gastrocnemius crosses the knee joint. Stretching the heel cords at home on a step after warm-up exercises is important.

Stretching the hamstrings following warm-up will help reduce elevated patellofemoral contact stress during knee extension. Toe-touch exercises or standing hamstring stretches usually suffice if these are conducted on a regular basis. Doucette and Goble (5) noted that hamstring flexibility was not always increased during a minimum 6-week rehabilitation program. We have observed, however, that rigorous hamstring stretches following warm-up exercises frequently will increase hamstring flexibility in the motivated patient.

Quadriceps flexibility should be examined with the patient prone, and stretching the quadriceps is also accomplished best in this position. The patient may need to use a towel or sheet around the ankle to stretch the quadriceps in the prone position initially, until the knee can be flexed to bring the ankle to the hand of the patient for manual stretching. It is surprising how often patients come to our office for evaluation of anterior knee pain having never been examined or stretched in the prone position! Prone quadriceps stretching is useful (see Fig. 12.3), particularly because it enables the patient to see his/her progress and reduces stiffness around the anterior knee. This is, in our opinion, the most important component of extensor mechanism rehabilitation. Prone stretching also helps to mobilize any minor infrapatellar contracture, postoperative scar from arthroscopy, stiffness of the patellar tendon, hematoma, and some plicae.

Prone stretching also helps to mobilize the *lateral retinaculum*. Patients should learn manual stretching of the lateral retinaculum (see Fig. 12.5), with emphasis both on reducing patellar tilt and improving medial mobility of the patella. Deep friction massage may help in this area, and modalities such as ultrasound may help in mobilizing the lateral retinaculum. Patellar taping also facilitates mobilization of the lateral patellofemoral support structures.

Mobilization of the *iliotibial band* adds to compliance of the lateral retinaculum. In any patient with lateral tightness, the therapist should incorporate iliotibial band stretches with the pelvis neutralized, patient lateral, hip extended, and preferably with the ankle held by the patient (knee flexed) while bringing the hip into adduction. Again, modalities may be helpful, at least in initiating these exercises.

If *hip internal rotators* are tight, preventing adequate external rotation at the hip, stretches should start at the hip level. Tight hip internal rotators or tight anterior hip capsule may diminish normal hip external rotation, which can be important in maintaining patellofemoral congruence.

Patellofemoral Taping

Jennie McConnell (18) revolutionized rehabilitation of patellofemoral patients with the introduction of taping concepts. Use of special tape to counteract patellar tilt, subluxation, and rotation may be enormously helpful in the rehabilitation process (Fig. 12.11, A to C). Studies and opinions have differed with regard to how these taping techniques work. There seems little doubt that patients benefit from tape around the front of the knee. Cushnaghan et al (19) have shown that patellofemoral taping is helpful in relieving pain in patients with patellofemoral osteoarthritis. Bockrath et al (20) have shown similar benefits of taping in patients with anterior knee pain. Some patients express immediate relief of pain that has gone unrelieved for a year or more. What is happening?

There is undoubtedly great psychological benefit to the patient who becomes involved in his/her own treatment. Tape application brings a sense of "doing something" that is tangible and logical. Taping often brings a new sense of hope and a positive approach to the problem.

Application of tape to the skin around the patellofemoral joint undoubtedly moves skin more than patella (Fig. 12.12). Application of tape, however, may provide additional position sense and improve proprioceptive function around the anterior knee. Increased sense in this area may actually provide improved reflex inhibition of deforming muscle forces while improving reflex and functional support for the patella. Ernst et al (21) have shown improved knee extensor function after taping.

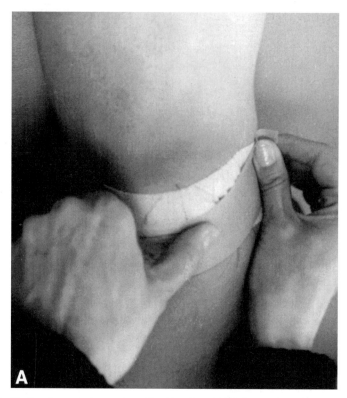

Figure 12.11. Taping the patella as described by Jennie McConnell involves the application of tape to control tilt (*A*), subluxation (*B*), and rotation of the patella (*C*). New devices and braces to control the patella are also available using modified taping and brace combination techniques.

Is it possible that tape anterior to the knee may actually improve alignment? Some studies have indicated that minor changes of patellar alignment may result from patellar taping. In one study, Tom Murray at the University of Connecticut School of Medicine (unpublished data, 1996) demonstrated actual improvement of patellar malalignment immediately following the tape application, doing computed tomography before and after taping. The changes were noted, however, only with the knee in *full extension*. Upon flexion of the knee to 15 or 30 degrees, changes effected by the tape were promptly eliminated and preexisting subluxation or tilt returned. Nonetheless, this study raised the possibility that taping may, to a minor degree, alter patellar entry into the trochlea.

In any case, major changes of patellar alignment are unlikely using tape. What is clear, however, is that taping is beneficial. The minor changes in alignment, together with patient involvement in the process and improved sensation-proprioception around the front of the knee, can explain the efficacy of patellar taping for control of patellofemoral pain and the resulting improved rehabilitation after taping in many patients. Newer brace techniques, particularly the DJOrtho Tru-Pull wrap or Tru-Pull Advanced System (DJOrtho, Vista, California), offer important alternatives to taping.

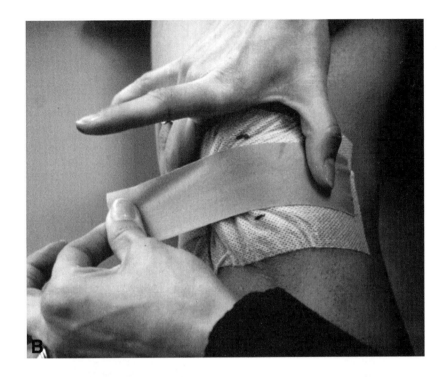

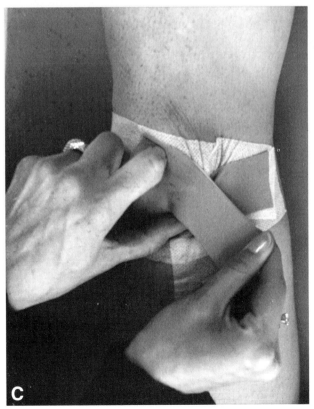

Figure 12.11. *Continued.*

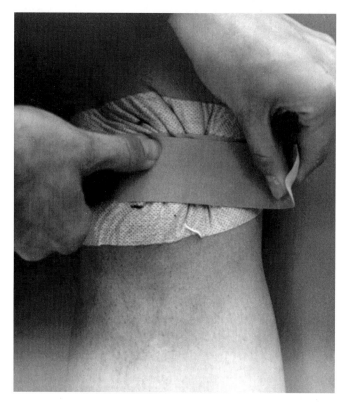

Figure 12.12. One must be particularly aware of the skin when applying tape.

Strengthening

Strengthening the entire kinetic chain will benefit the patient with anterior knee pain. Although specific emphasis on quadriceps strength, particularly the VMO (Fig. 12.13), is important in improving support for the patella (22), balance of strength is equally important (23). Therefore, isolated quadriceps strengthening is less effective than balanced strengthening of both lower extremities (Fig. 12.14). Steinkamp et al (24) have noted that *leg press exercise* (Fig. 12.15) from 0 to 30 degrees of knee flexion will diminish the knee moment and patellofemoral joint reaction force as well as patellofemoral stress when compared with knee extension exercise (Fig. 12.16). Therefore, leg press exercise, emphasizing high repetition and reduced weight, is most logical in the 0- to 30-degree range of motion.

Nonetheless, at 60 to 90 degrees of knee flexion, patellofemoral joint stress is *greater* using leg-press exercise, according to Steinkamp. Consequently, the therapist must adapt the strengthening program depending on the degree of knee flexion at which exercise is accomplished. The rule is as follows: leg press exercise in early knee flexion and leg extension exercise past 60 degrees of knee flexion. This is particularly important because patients with lesions more distal on the patella will need to exercise in more knee flexion to reduce contact stress on the distal patella (which occurs predominantly in early knee flexion; see Chapter 2 on Biomechanics). For the patient who has had a crush-type injury to the anterior knee (such as the dashboard-type injury), exercise will be safer closer to

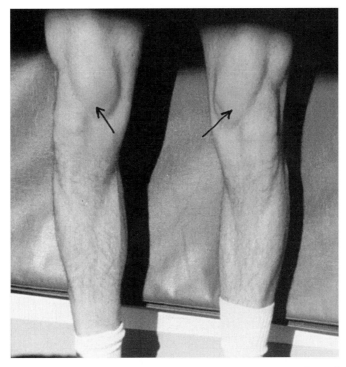

Figure 12.13. Regaining vastus medialis strength is important in most all patellofemoral rehabilitation.

full extension, where the proximal crushed portion of the patella does not experience contact. Leg press exercise in 0- to 30-degree knee range of motion is most appropriate here. The level of articular lesion is the single greatest factor in determining the degree of flexion in which exercises should be carried out.

Isometric quadriceps strengthening can also be highly effective. O'Neill et al (25) noted that patients with anatomically normal lower extremity alignment and no history of knee trauma or surgery responded favorably to isometric quadriceps strengthening as part of a structured exercise program in the treatment of anterior knee pain.

Ingersoll and Knight (26) emphasized the importance of VMO strengthening. Electromyographic (EMG) biofeedback training (Fig. 12.17) to selectively strengthen the VMO was effective in improving the patellofemoral congruence angle in their experience. Snyder-Mackler et al (27) have shown that electrical stimulation will improve quadriceps return.

Work on timing of quadriceps contraction, emphasizing VMO contraction earlier in the gait cycle to stabilize the patella, makes sense. Electrical stimulation of the VMO and biofeedback training to incorporate earlier VMO contraction and sustained contraction during the gait cycle should be a part of any complete patellofemoral rehabilitation program. It is interesting to note, however, that no difference in EMG patterns of quadriceps contraction in female runners with patellofemoral pain was noted by MacIntyre and Robertson (28). Also, Powers (29) has stated that selective VMO function has not been established. Nonetheless, emphasis on earlier VMO or overall quadriceps contraction may help to compensate for imbalance of the extensor mechanism.

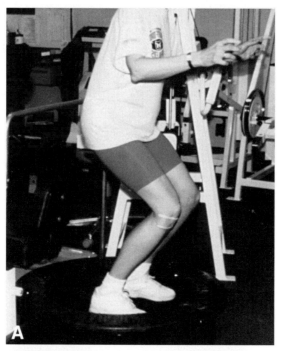

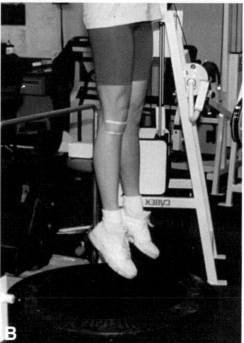

Figure 12.14. The trampoline is a convenient device for gaining both eccentric and concentric motor strength in both lower extremities.

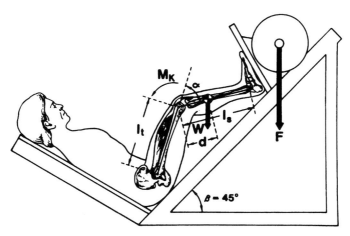

Figure 12.15. Leg-press exercise is most desirable in early range of motion from 0- to 30-degree knee flexion. Reprinted with permission from Steinkamp LA, Dillingham MF, Markel MD, Hill JA, Kaufman KR. Biomechanical considerations in patellofemoral joint rehabilitation. Am J Sports Med 1993;21(3):438–446.

General strengthening of other muscle groups around the knee should be introduced to *balance* quadriceps power and flexibility. Maintaining a normal hamstring–quadriceps ratio of approximately 65% is desirable. Much of this muscle balancing may be accomplished through *closed-chain* exercises and through the aerobic conditioning part of the rehabilitation process. Witvrouw (30) has pointed out that closed-chain exercise may

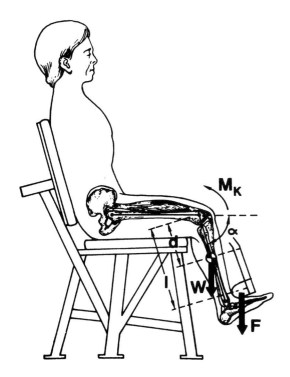

Figure 12.16. Knee-extension exercise against resistance is more desirable in the 60- to 90-degree range of motion. Reprinted with permission from Steinkamp LA, Dillingham MF, Markel MD, Hill JA, Kaufman KR. Biomechanical considerations in patellofemoral joint rehabilitation. Am J Sports Med 1993;21(3):438–446.

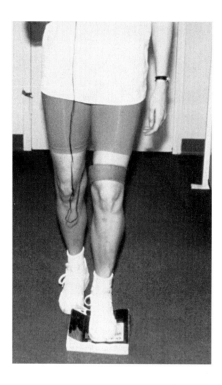

Figure 12.17. Biofeedback techniques help the patient to understand when the vastus medialis contracts and how to control it.

offer advantages in patellofemoral rehabilitation. Kibler and Livingston (31) have further emphasized this point.

Braces

There are a variety of braces that can lend a feeling of support to the patellofemoral joint. DJOrtho (Vista, California) produces the author's (JPF) Tru-Pull patella support (Fig. 12.18). Some patients find relief with a simple patellar strap. Elastic or neoprene knee braces with a patellar cut-out are useful in many patients. Almost any elastic support around the front of the knee can provide relief or an enhanced ability to exercise in selected patients. The type of brace may be chosen empirically, and some patients may try two or three braces before finding one that works well and is comfortable. The concept of proprioceptive feedback around the front of the knee, together with comfort and affordability, makes bracing desirable in patients who do not respond to exercise alone. Patellofemoral braces are particularly useful in athletes and for exercise during cold weather. Voight and Wieder (32) have emphasized that patients with patellofemoral mechanism dysfunction may have a neurophysiologic motor control imbalance, as demonstrated by a faster vastus lateralis response time in patients with patellofemoral dysfunction. As with taping, bracing may help to modify some of the feedback mechanisms in this neurophysiologic balance.

Cherf and Paulos (33) pointed out that orthotics and braces around the patellofemoral joint are helpful, particularly those applying a medially directed force on the patella. The Tru-Pull brace (DJOrtho, Vista, California) offers the most versatile, comfortable, and cost-effective alternative in the treatment of patients with patellofemoral pain or instability. Because the Tru-Pull wrap may be applied in a highly customized fashion by each

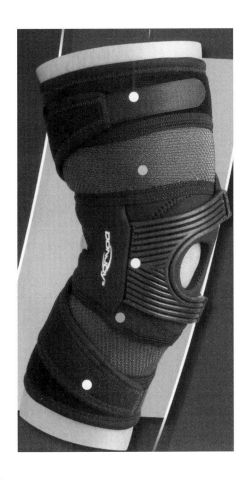

Figure 12.18. The Tru-Pull Advanced System (DJOrtho, Vista, California) is a sleeve that incorporates independent fixation points above and below the knee.

patient or therapist, it virtually eliminates the need for other patellofemoral braces and can offer a highly effective, easier to apply alternative to taping. The Tru-Pull wrap brace has also been very helpful in managing patellar tendonitis (Fig. 12.19).

Activity Modification

Although progression to an aerobic exercise program is desirable for most patients with anterior knee pain, some patients will require reduction of activities or withdrawal from sports participation. This tends to be more important in patients with posttraumatic pain or patellofemoral degeneration after anterior cruciate ligament reconstruction (34). If the problem is one of *overuse*, excessive metabolic activity in the *patella* or *surrounding structures*, acute damage, or chronic pain that has not responded to rehabilitative exercise, reduction of activity, splinting for short periods of time, ice application, and relative rest must be seriously considered. When rest of the patellofemoral joint is necessary, it is advisable to think in terms of 6 to 8 weeks minimum, using cryotherapy and antiinflammatory treatment simultaneously. It is usually possible to maintain some muscle tone and flexibility during this period of relative rest while cutting back on the more extreme levels of physical activity, which may be aggravating the knee. This is particularly true if there has been effusion. In this case, antiinflammatory treatment, rest, ice, and reduction of aggravating stresses will be important to bring the joint into balance.

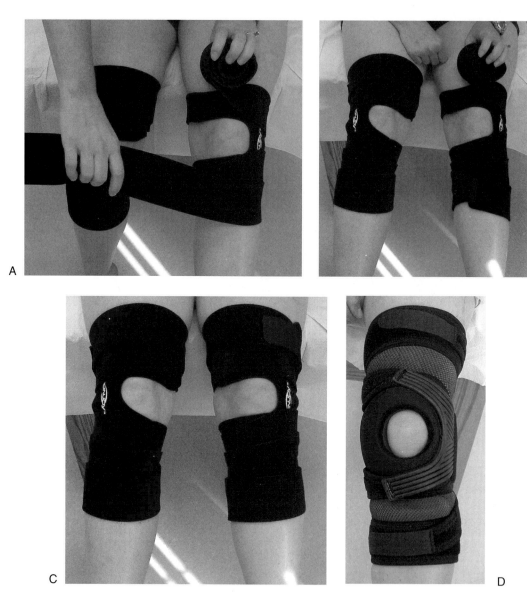

Figure 12.19. A–C, The Tru-Pull wrap is versatile and permits the patient or therapist to customize the application. **D,** Tru-Pull Advanced System Brace (DJ Ortho, Vista, CA).

When effusion and pain have been eliminated for 7 to 14 days, *gradually* increasing activity may be reintroduced, using cryotherapy after activity. The goal is to move each patient into normal activities of daily living and then to introduce a tailored aerobic conditioning program that is structured to avoid aggravating the pain problem while gaining aerobic capacity as tolerated, emphasizing home programs.

REFERENCES

1. Fulkerson JP, Kalenak A, Rosenberg TD, Cox JS. Patellofemoral pain (review). Instr Course Lect 1992;41:57–71.
2. Scuderi GR. Surgical treatment for patellar instability (review). Orthop Clin North Am 1992;23(4):619–630.

3. Ruffin MT 5th, Kinningham RB. Anterior knee pain: The challenge of patellofemoral syndrome (see comments) (review). Am Fam Physician 1993;47(1):185–194.

4. LaBrier K, O'Neill DR. Patellofemoral stress syndrome. Current concepts (review). Sports Med 1993;16(6): 449–459.

5. Doucette SA, Goble EM. The effect of exercise on patellar tracking in lateral patellar compression syndrome. Am J Sports Med 1992;20(4):434–440.

6. Scuderi G, ed. The Patella. New York: Springer-Verlag; 1995.

7. Fox J, Del Pizzo W. The Patellofemoral Joint. New York: McGraw Hill; 1992.

8. Fisher RL. Conservative treatment of patellofemoral pain. Orthop Clin North Am 1986;17(2):269–272.

9. Goldberg B. Chronic anterior knee pain in the adolescent. Pediatr Ann 1991;20(4):186–187, 190–193.

10. Jensen DB, Albrektsen SB. The natural history of chondromalacia patellae. A 12-year follow-up. Acta Orthop Belg 1990;56(2):503–506.

11. Crossley K, Bennell K, Green S, Cowan S, McConnell J. Physical therapy for patellofemoral pain: a randomized, double-blind, placebo-controlled trial. Am J Sports Med 2002;30(6):857–865.

12. Thomee R, Augustsson J, Karlson J. Patellofemoral pain syndrome: a review of current issues. Sports Med 1999;28:245–262.

13. Wilk KE, Davies GJ, Mangine RE, Malone TR. Patellofemoral disorders: a classification system and clinical guidelines for nonoperative rehabilitation. J Orthop Sports Phys Ther 1998;28:307–322.

14. Paulos LE, Wnorowski DC, Greenwald AE. Infrapatellar contracture syndrome. Diagnosis, treatment, and long-term follow-up. Am J Sports Med 1994;22(4):440.

15. Witvrouw E, Lysens R, Bellemans J, Cambier D, Vanderstraeten G. Intrinsic risk factors for the development of anterior knee pain in an athletic population. Am J Sports Med 2000;28:480–489.

16. Hopkins JT, Ingersoll C, Krause B, Edwards JE, Cordova ML. Effect of knee joint effusion on quadriceps and soleus excitability. Med Sci Sports Exerc 2001;33(1):123–126.

17. Wilk K, Reinold M. Principles of patellofemoral rehabilitation. Sports Med Arthrosc Rev 2001;9:325–336.

18. McConnell J. The management of chondromalacia patellae. J Physiotherapy 1986;32:215–223.

19. Cushnaghan J, McCarthy C, Dieppe P. Taping the patella medially: A new treatment for osteoarthritis of the knee joint? BMJ 1994;308(6931):753–755.

20. Bockrath K, Wooden C, Worrell T, Ingersoll C, Farr J. Effects of patella taping on patella position and perceived pain. Med Sci Sports Exerc 1993;25(9):989–992.

21. Ernst GP, Kawaguchi J, Saliba E. Effect of patellar taping on knee kinetics of patients with patellofemoral pain syndrome. J Orthop Sports Phys Ther 1999;29:661–667.

22. Natri A, Kannus P, Jarvinen M. Which factors predict the long-term outcome in chronic patellofemoral pain syndrome? A 7-year prospective study. Med Sci Sports Exerc 1998;30:1572–1577.

23. Werner S. An evaluation of knee extensor and knee flexor torques and EMGs in patients with patellofemoral pain syndrome. Knee Surg Sports Traumatol Arthrosc 1995;3:89–94.

24. Steinkamp LA, Dillingham MF, Markel MD, Hill JA, Kaufman KR: Biomechanical considerations in patellofemoral joint rehabilitation. Am J Sports Med 1993;21(3):438–446.

25. O'Neill DB, Micheli LJ, Warner JP. Patellofemoral stress. A prospective analysis of exercise treatment in adolescents and adults. Am J Sports Med 1992;20(2):151–156.

26. Ingersoll CD, Knight KL. Patellar location changes following EMG biofeedback or progressive resistive exercises. Med Sci Sports Exerc 1991;23(10):1122–1127.

27. Snyder-Mackler L, Ladin Z, Schepsis AA, Young JC. Electrical stimulation of the thigh muscles after reconstructing the anterior cruciate ligament. J Bone Joint Surg 1991;73:1025–1036.

28. MacIntyre DL, Robertson DG. Quadriceps muscle activity in women runners with and without patellofemoral pain syndrome. Arch Phys Med Rehabil 1992;73(1):10–14.

29. Powers C. Rehabilitation of patellofemoral disorders: a critical review. J Orthop Sports Phys Ther 1998;28(5): 345–354.

30. Witvrouw E, Lysens R, Bellemans J, Peers K, Vanderstraeten G. Open versus closed kinetic chain exercises for patellofemoral pain. A prospective, randomized study. Am J Sports Med 2000;28:687-694.

31. Kibler WB, Livingston BP. Closed chain rehabilitation for upper and lower extremities. J Am Acad Orthop Surg 2001;9:412–421.

32. Voight ML, Wieder DL. Comparative reflex response times of vastus medialis obliquus and vastus lateralis in normal subjects and subjects with extensor mechanism dysfunction. An electromyographic study. Am J Sports Med 1991;19(2):131–137.

33. Cherf J, Paulos LE. Bracing for patellar instability (review). Clin Sports Med 1990;9(4): 813–821.

34. Shino K, Nakagawa S, Inoue M, Horibe S, Yoneda M. Deterioration of patellofemoral articular surfaces after anterior cruciate ligament reconstruction. Am J Sports Med 1993;21(2):206–211.REF:

=13=
Surgical Treatment of Patellofemoral Articular Lesions

"Act as the creator of a statue that is to be made beautiful: cut away here, smooth there, make this line lighter, the other purer, until a lovely face has grown upon the work."

Plotinus, 270 AD

"To the creator there is no poverty and no poor, indifferent place."

Rilke, 1934

Historically, there have been many operations designed to treat patients with recalcitrant patellofemoral pain emanating from articular lesions. Surgical alternatives range from arthroscopic debridement to total joint arthroplasty. The primary goal of this chapter is to enhance accurate decision making before any treatment for a patellofemoral disorder, with emphasis on surgical procedures that are likely to correct a specific, defined mechanical disorder as determined by careful clinical evaluation and appropriate studies. In every case the surgeon must exhaust nonoperative, conservative measures before considering any surgical intervention.

Expanded knowledge of anatomy, physiology, and disease process permits improved surgical care of patients with patellofemoral disorders. New imaging techniques have enhanced the understanding of patellofemoral dysfunction from the mechanical and anatomic perspectives. Arthroscopy is helpful in the diagnosis and treatment of some patellofemoral disorders. Surgical intervention can be tailored more specifically now to each patient, thanks to improved diagnostic techniques. Although a surgeon can determine appropriate surgical correction of patellofemoral disorders more accurately than in the past, it is perhaps even more important that he/she can cure more patients without surgery and avoid operating on patients with patellofemoral pain who do *not* have a specific, correctable, mechanical disorder.

It is imperative that a full course of nonoperative treatment has been tried before contemplating surgery. Nonetheless, persistent pain or instability despite good nonoperative treatment may make surgical treatment desirable.

Surgical treatment alternatives are different for patients with patellofemoral pain with advanced patellar arthrosis as compared with patients with minimal cartilage disease or chronic instability. One can best evaluate patellofemoral articular cartilage condition by radiographic studies, particularly magnetic resonance imaging, and arthroscopy. Radiographic evaluation of such patients has been reviewed in Chapter 4.

PATELLOFEMORAL ARTHROSCOPY

In general, most patients with anterior knee pain will not need arthroscopy. Precise radiographs (Fig. 13.1), including a true lateral computed tomography and radionuclide scanning, permit the physician to gain considerable understanding of the patellofemoral joint without introducing instruments. The arthroscope, nonetheless, is a powerful tool and may be helpful in both adults and children (1) before performing definitive procedures such as lateral retinacular release, anteromedial tibial tubercle transfer, patellar debridement, or tibial tubercle anteriorization. I use the superomedial approach described by Schreiber (2) and an inferolateral approach to view the patellofemoral joint. It helps to view the patella from both above and below in more difficult cases, and it is usually better to do patellofemoral arthroscopy with the patient supine and without a leg holder.

There are patients who have normal patellar alignment (sometimes as a result of earlier corrective surgery), yet there is patellar articular fibrillation (Fig. 13.2) causing mechanically induced and enzyme-induced (3) aggravation of the entire knee joint. In

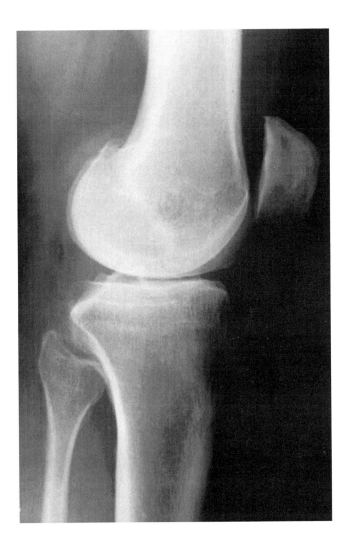

Figure 13.1. The true lateral radiograph (posterior condyles superimposed) helps in detecting patellar tilt and dysplasia of the trochlea (see Chapter 4).

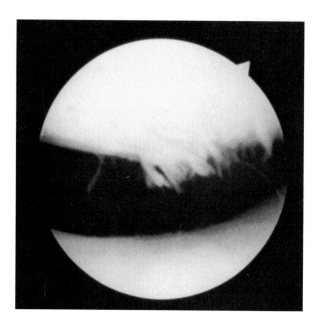

Figure 13.2. Patellar articular cartilage fibrillation may follow blunt trauma, and isolated debridement of such lesions may bring symptomatic relief when there is no ongoing overload to the affected surface.

such cases, arthroscopic debridement of the fibrillated articular surface may provide symptomatic relief and joint preservation. On occasion, there may be a finite area of exposed bone, and microfracture arthroplasty may give relief, particularly when combined with a specific procedure to unload the affected area.

Abnormal patellar alignment will usually be apparent at the time of arthroscopy, but there is some risk of *creating* distortion of patellar alignment at the time of arthroscopy. Anesthesia, paralysis, tourniquet pressure, intraarticular fluid, and distension may create an *impression* of malalignment in some patients who have functionally normal alignment. Therefore, patellofemoral arthroscopy should confirm preoperative clinical radiographic findings and quantitate articular damage, but one need not rely on arthroscopy alone to evaluate patellofemoral alignment.

The arthroscope is helpful in identifying a pathologic plica semilunaris or synovial shelf (4–6), and arthroscopic resection of a painful snapping shelf may be very helpful in the appropriate patient. Munzinger et al (7) and Broom and Fulkerson (8) noted residual problems in some patients after plica resection, although Richmond and McGinty (9) reported 86% good and excellent results after resection of a hypertrophic medial plica in 64 knees. Residual problems after plica resection may result from articular lesions or associated patellar imbalance. The true symptomatic plica is fairly uncommon, and diagnosis can generally be made preoperatively when a painful snapping band is palpable in the infrapatellar areas. Rarely, the arthroscopic surgeon may encounter synovial thickening proximal to the medial femoral condyle, and resection of this mass may give symptomatic relief as long as the clinical examination correlates with the arthroscopic finding (10).

Lindberg et al (11) noted the importance of recognizing the relationship between chondral damage and patellar malalignment. Most often, however, an arthroscope will help in defining the extent of articular degeneration (12, 13) before definitive surgery. The difference between Outerbridge Grade 2 fibrillation and Outerbridge Grade 4 exposed bone on the lateral facet may be the difference between a lateral retinacular release and an anteromedial tibial tubercle transfer in some patients. One can distinguish such lesions using the arthroscope.

Resection of chondral flaps may be helpful in relieving anterior knee pain. One must question, however, the reason for articular cartilage breakdown and decide if more definitive treatment is necessary to correct a causative mechanical abnormality. Ogilvie-Harris and Jackson (14) specifically emphasized the importance of resecting loose articular cartilage in patients with posttraumatic patellar lesions.

PATELLOFEMORAL RECONSTRUCTION

Particularly important are findings such as those reported by Leslie and Bentley (15), in which normal patellar articular cartilage (Fig. 13.3) was found in many patients with patellofemoral pain. The peripatellar retinaculum may be a primary source of pain in many of these patients (16). The same patellar imbalance that causes retinacular stretching and injury may lead later to articular cartilage breakdown and arthrosis because of abnormal contact pressure distribution. Lateral release alone often will help the patient with patellar tilt and minimal arthrosis, which have not responded to nonoperative rehabilitation. The approach to such patients has been reviewed thoroughly in Chapter 8.

When advanced arthrosis accompanies patellar instability, the treatment becomes more difficult. Grana et al (17) pointed out that unsatisfactory results of arthroscopic treatment are related to painful crepitation. In such patients, extensor mechanism realignment or decompression by anteriorization of the extensor mechanism may be necessary. There are some patients with patellar arthrosis in whom extensor mechanism anteriorization may be desirable at the same time as realignment, particularly when the painful articular lesion is distal on the patella (painful in early flexion), such that anteromedial or anterolateral tibial tubercle becomes necessary.

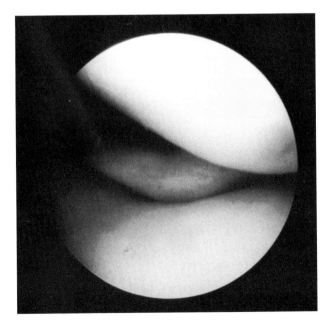

Figure 13.3. Normal patellar articular cartilage as seen with an arthroscope. Photo courtesy of Dandy D. Arthroscopy of the Knee slide collection, Gower Medical Publishing.

Whereas some patients develop patellar arthrosis after trauma to the patella, patellar arthrosis is frequently caused by longstanding extensor mechanism malalignment and poor distribution of articular contact pressures. Fortunately, many such patients will respond to nonoperative treatment or lateral retinacular release. When lateral facet arthrosis is severe (Outerbridge Grades 3–4), however, and pain is attributed to articular breakdown with resulting subchondral bone irritation, realignment and/or anteriorization of the patella may be indicated (18). Kolowich et al (19) have pointed out that the most predictable indicator of a good result from lateral release is a chronic tilt of the patella associated with a tight lateral retinaculum.

Anteromedial tibial tubercle transfer (20) achieves both unloading of the patella and improved alignment in one operation, assuming that there is preoperative lateral patellar tilt and/or subluxation. Although the same mechanical result is possible using bone graft behind an elevated tibial tubercle, as described by Bandi (21), Maquet (22), Ferguson (23, 24), and Radin (25, 26), similar benefit may be achieved with anteromedial tibial tubercle transfer, which does not require bone graft or distraction of the osteotomized tibial tubercle.

Selecting Appropriate Patients for Lateral Release

When there is significant malalignment and clinically evident chondromalacia or arthrosis, surgical treatment will be determined best using simple logic. One must correct malalignment by realigning the joint and treating the effect (articular degeneration), when significant, by unloading and either debriding or resurfacing the deficient area. Tables 13.1 and 13.2 present an overview of my classification and treatment program.

Simple *lateral retinacular release* will usually reduce abnormal patellar tilt, particularly if articular cartilage softening has not progressed to the point of joint collapse. Many patients with Outerbridge Grades 1 and 2 lesions of patellar articular cartilage and associated *tilt* respond well to lateral retinacular release, particularly if pain is most prominent in the lateral retinaculum. Patients with Outerbridge Grades 3 to 4 arthrosis of the lateral facet must be evaluated carefully, and if lateral release is chosen as the treatment, the patient should be warned that there is some risk of recurrent pain, particularly if the arthrosis itself is symptomatic. One must be particularly *wary* of lateral release when there is articular breakdown on the *medial* patella.

TABLE 13.1. *Fulkerson-Schutzer Classification of Patients with Patellofemoral Pain*

Type I	*A,* Patellar subluxation, with no articular lesion
	B, Patellar subluxation with Grades 1 to 2 chondromalacia
	C, Patellar subluxation with Grades 3 to 4 arthrosis
	D, Patellar subluxation with a history of dislocation and minimal or no chondromalacia
	E, Patellar subluxation with a history of dislocation, with Grades 3 to 4 arthrosis
Type II	*A,* Patellar tilt and subluxation with no articular lesion
	B, Patellar tilt and subluxation with Grades 1 to 2 chondromalacia
	C, Patellar tilt and subluxation with Grades 3 to 4 arthrosis
Type III	*A,* Patellar tilt with no articular lesion
	B, Patellar tilt with Grades 1 to 2 chondromalacia
	C, Patellar tilt with Grades 3 to 4 arthrosis
Type IV	*A,* No malalignment and no articular lesion
	B, No malalignment and Grades 1 to 2 chondromalacia
	C, No malalignment and Grades 3 to 4 arthrosis

TABLE 13.2. *Treatment Recommendations (Failed Conservative Treatment and Intolerable Patellofemoral Pain or Instability not Complicated by Reflex Sympathetic Dystrophy)*

Type I	*A and B,* Lateral retinacular release and VMO advancement
	C, Lateral retinacular release and anteromedial tibial tubercle transfer
	D, Acute dislocation—selective arthroscopy and reconstruction of osteochondral damage; consider lateral retinacular release; delay reconstruction. Recurrent dislocation—lateral retinacular release and either VMO advancement or tubercle realignment
	E, Lateral retinacular release and anteromedial tibial tubercle transfer (minimizing elevation by making a flatter cut)
Type II	*A and B,* Lateral retinacular release and careful VMO advancement or anteromedial tibial tubercle transfer
	C, Lateral retinacular release, careful debridement, and anteromedial tibial tubercle transfer
Type III	*A and B,* Lateral retinacular release
	C, Lateral retinacular release, careful debridement, and anteromedial tibial tubercle transfer
Type IV	*A,* Continue nonoperative treatment; look for another pain source
	B, Consider arthroscopic debridement of Grade 2 lesion
	C, Arthroscopic debridement and possible tibial tubercle anteriorization—when the lesion(s) are distal

Key: VMO = vastus medialis obliquus.

Anteromedial Tibial Tubercle Transfer

As the preceding chapters have already shown, lateral subluxation and tilt of the patella frequently lead to arthrosis. The usual patient who enters the physician's office with anterior knee pain has structural malalignment, either traumatic or congenital. Although lateral retinacular release is particularly helpful in relieving tilt, subluxation responds less consistently to lateral release, and patients with progressive arthrosis may not gain any prolonged benefit, particularly if advanced (Outerbridge Grades 3–4) degeneration has developed. Lateral retinacular release in patients with patellar arthritis but no retinacular tightness is analogous to cutting the medial collateral ligament in a patient with medial knee arthritis.

Bandi (21), Maquet (22), Ferguson et al (23, 24), Radin (25, 26), Schepsis et al (27), and others (28–34) have studied extensor mechanism anteriorization in the reduction of contact pressure on the patella or in the treatment of patellofemoral pain. Combining realignment of the malaligned extensor mechanism with anterior placement of the tibial tubercle may be extremely helpful in the management of patients with patellar arthrosis related to malalignment (20, 34–37). Hejgaard and Watt-Boolsen (33) noted that tibial tubercle anteriorization alone will not correct abnormal patellar tracking. Some very serious complications have been reported with straight tibial tubercle anteriorization using bone graft (38). The less secure fixation of some procedures has led to refinement of the "anteromedialization" concept such that early motion might be possible with better mechanical fixation.

Anteromedial tibial tubercle transfer permits the surgeon to achieve anteriorization of the extensor mechanism while improving patellar balance in the trochlea with medialization. Koshino (39) has shown also that the quadriceps lever arm and strength of knee extension can be improved with this procedure. Because of the frequent association between patellar malalignment and arthrosis, this procedure has been particularly useful in the management of patients with patellofemoral pain. It is important, however, to know the correct indications for anteromedial tibial tubercle transfer and to master the details of surgical technique.

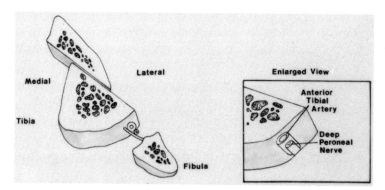

Figure 13.4. Anteromedial tibial tubercle transfer along an oblique osteotomy plane as described by Fulkerson (20). Note particularly that the deep peroneal nerve and the anterior tibial artery must be avoided and protected at all times. Illustration by Joyce Willis.

Indications

Anteromedial tibial tubercle transfer (20) (Fig. 13.4) might be understood best as a surgical alternative to the Maquet procedure in patients with malalignment and distal or lateral facet arthrosis (Fig. 13.5). Because lateral retinacular release will relieve abnormal tilt of the patella when there is minimal or no arthrosis, it should be the procedure of choice in such patients. At times, however, lateral facet degeneration progresses to a point that simple lateral release will be ineffective (Fig. 13.6), and it is such patients who might be considered for anteromedial tibial tubercle transfer (40–42). Some patients with distal patellar arthrosis (Fig. 13.7) may benefit from this procedure because contact stress is relieved, balanced, and moved proximally on the patella, essentially tipping up the "nose"

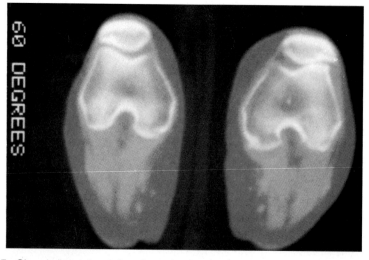

Figure 13.5. Chronic lateral patellar tilt and subluxation can cause lateral facet breakdown and arthrosis. Anteromedial tibial tubercle transfer will unload the lateral facet and realign the patella.

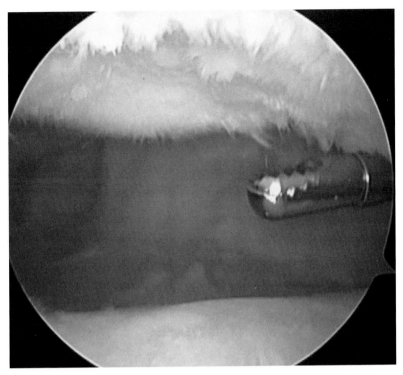

Figure 13.6. Extensive lateral facet patella chondral breakdown, with bone exposed on the lateral trochlea.

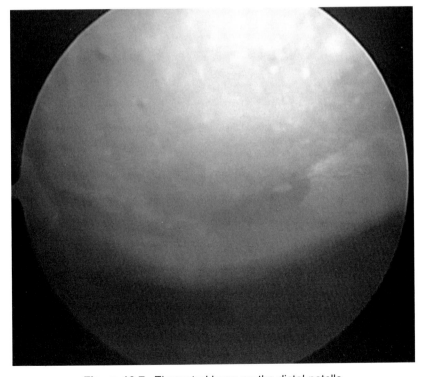

Figure 13.7. Eburnated bone on the distal patella.

of the patella. It is a particularly good alternative for patients who have patellar arthrosis secondary to malalignment. In most of the patients, the *proximal medial facet* escapes breakdown. This is the region that receives loading following anteromedialization. As with any surgical procedure, however, it is important to screen out patients who are seeking secondary gain or who have more severe problems, such as reflex sympathetic dystrophy, which will preclude a good result. Also, those patients with a *dashboard or crush injury* of the proximal patella are less likely to do well because the proximal patella is injured.

Fulkerson's Technique of Anteromedial Tibial Tubercle Transfer (20, 42–44) (Figs. 13.8–13.37)

An anterolateral skin incision extends from the midlateral patella to a point approximately 5 cm distal to the tibial tuberosity. Sharp dissection is used to the lateral retinaculum, which is released completely from the patella only to the level of the vastus lateralis. If further release appears to be necessary, it may be extended proximally to release the vastus lateral obliquus of Hallisey (see Chapter 1) only—being sure to preserve the

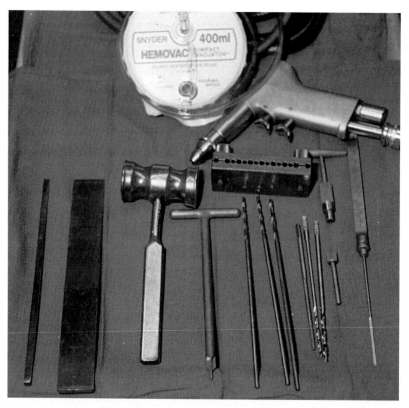

Figure 13.8. Instruments necessary to do an anteromedial tibial tubercle transfer include wide and ¼-inch Lambotte osteotomes; a mallet; extra-long drill bits; a drill guide (Howmedica Hoffman Drill Guide or DePuy Tracker Guide); drill bits for cortical screw fixation; depth gauge; tap; power drill; Hemovac, and, alternatively, an oscillating saw (not shown).

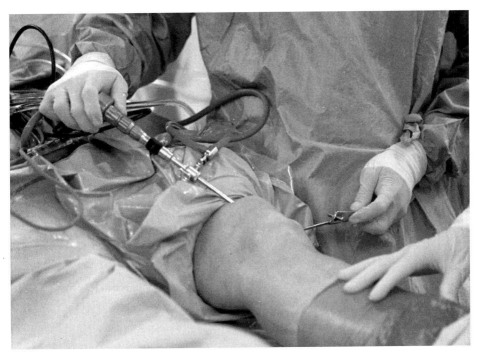

Figure 13.9. Before each anteromedial tibial tubercle transfer, routine arthroscopy is performed using a superior approach to view patella tracking and precise description of patella articular lesions as to extent and location. Routine arthroscopy of the entire knee is important to identify any associated or concomitant lesions.

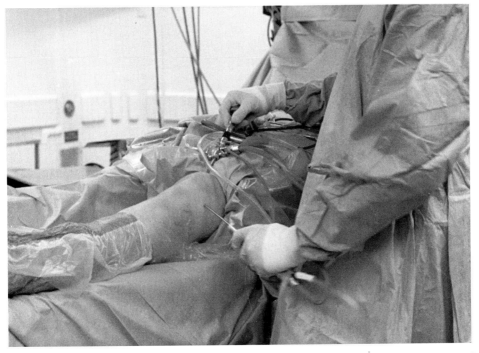

Figure 13.10. Debridement of lesions may be accomplished most effectively with arthroscopic visualization in many cases.

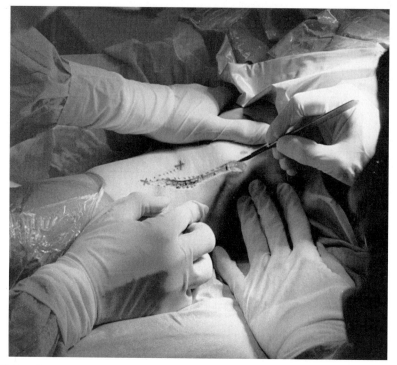

Figure 13.11. The incision is just lateral to midline and extends from the midpatella level to a point located 5 to 9 cm distal to the tibial tubercle.

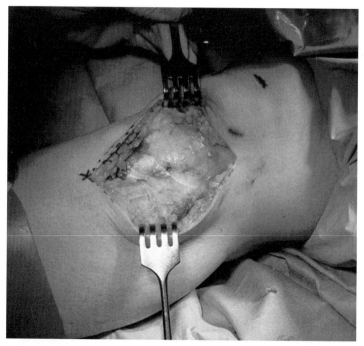

Figure 13.12. Sharp dissection, with minimal undermining, is used to expose the lateral side of the knee, including the patellar tendon.

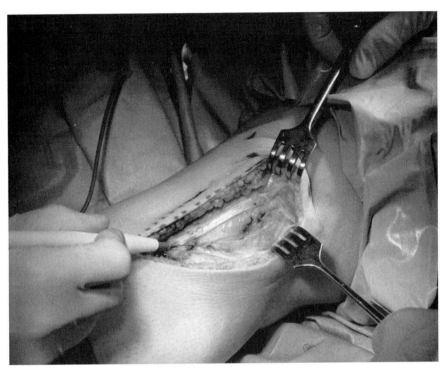

Figure 13.13. The patellar tendon is carefully identified as the retinacular fibers along its lateral edge are released while obtaining hemostasis.

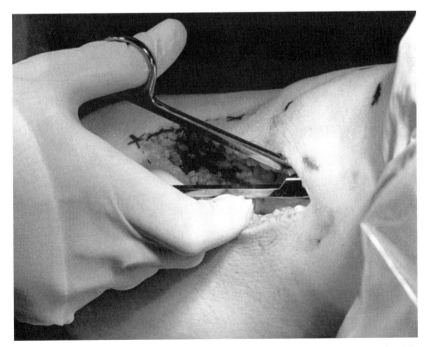

Figure 13.14. Lateral retinacular release may be accomplished by the surgeon using Mayo scissors after spreading subcuticular tissue. Again, careful attention must be paid to hemostasis. Also, the surgeon must avoid the main vastus lateralis tendon. Retractors are used as necessary.

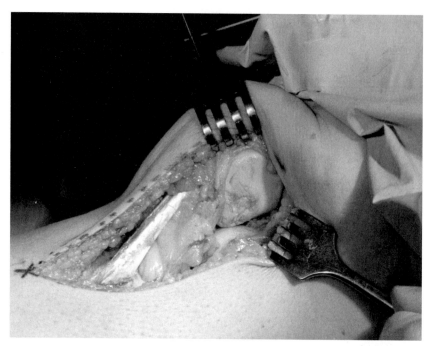

Figure 13.15. After lateral release, the surgeon can view the patella completely. Any infra-patellar contracture should be released so that the patella can be everted a full 90 degrees. A precise description of the articular lesion should be recorded in the operation report. This patella demonstrates typical lateral facet and central ridge (Ficat's critical zone) erosion. Note that the proximal patella is intact.

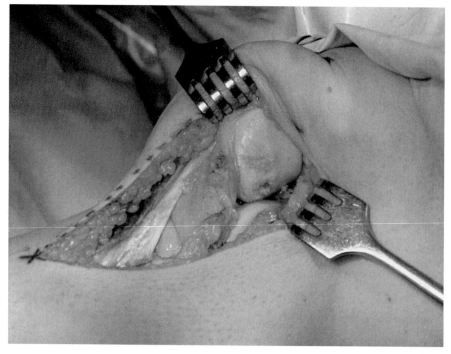

Figure 13.16. Another view more clearly demonstrating a Ficat's critical zone lesion and the intact proximal medial facet.

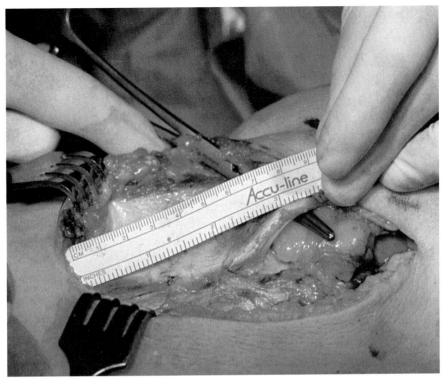

Figure 13.17. The patellar tendon is completely mobilized and released, if necessary, from any posterior contracture. The anterior tibial crest is exposed for a full 5 cm at least.

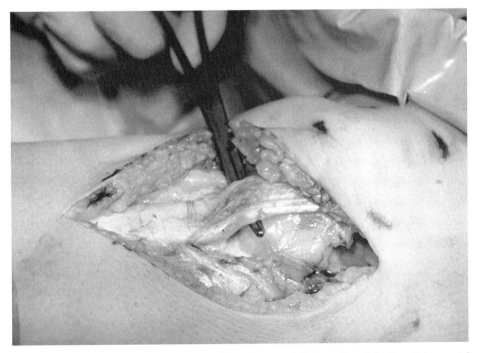

Figure 13.18. The patellar tendon should be free, and its insertion into the tibia must be clearly delineated.

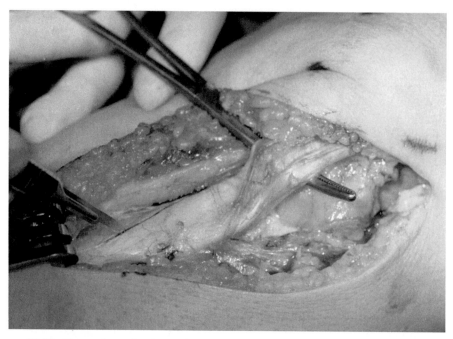

Figure 13.19. Sharp dissection is used to incise the periosteum just medial to the patellar tendon and extending distally just medial to the anterior tibial crest.

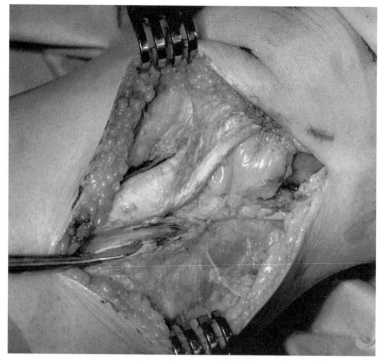

Figure 13.20. After incising the fascial insertion of the tibialis anterior muscle, the anterior tibial muscle is reflected sharply through the use of an elevator off the lateral side of the tibia, such that the entire lateral tibia may be viewed all the way to the posterolateral corner.

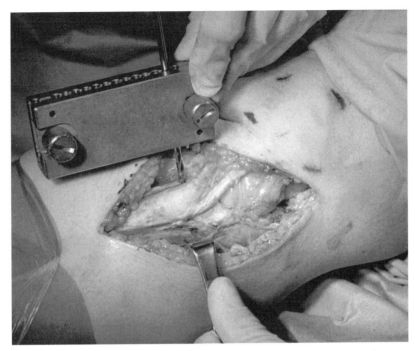

Figure 13.21. Using the drill guide, the surgeon fashions an oblique osteotomy, directing the drill bits posterolaterally and being sure to view the exiting drill bit tip at the posterolateral tibia just anterior to the posterolateral corner. A steep osteotomy permits maximal anteriorization and requires that the initial drill bit be placed immediately medial to the patellar tendon insertion.

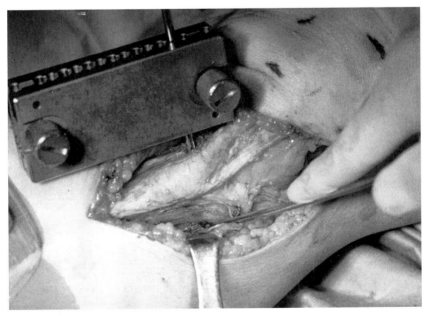

Figure 13.22. Note that the exiting drill bit tip is visualized fully, and a retractor is kept at this point to avoid any problem related to the drill bit passing posteriorly where the anterior tibial artery and deep peroneal nerve are located.

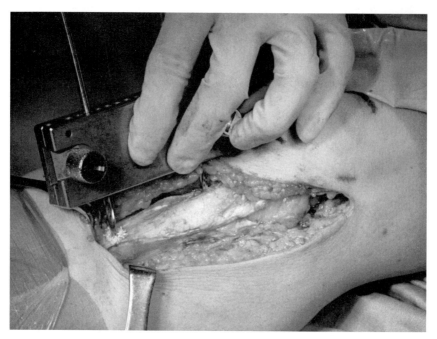

Figure 13.23. The distal drill bit is placed precisely parallel to the first drill bit, using the drill guide to assure parallelism. The guide should be slipped up and down on the two drill bits to avoid any binding or lack of parallelism. Some time is taken to assure this precise parallel placement of the second drill bit at the distal extent of the osteotomy. This distal drill bit must be *just behind* the anterior crest of the tibia, such that it is significantly more *anterior* than the initial drill bit. There is dense cortical bone at this point, and the drill bit will normally pass exclusively through cortex if it is properly placed. Once the two drill bits are in place, the drill guide is secured, and the two drill bits are left in place. The Mitak (Norwood, MA) Tracker guide uses two 2.0 pins for fixation of a cutting block with a slot for an oscillating saw.

main vastus lateralis tendon. The patella should be everted 90 degrees and examined carefully to determine how much debridement or arthroplasty to perform. Similarly, the surgeon should establish if any resurfacing of the trochlea is necessary and employ debridement, microfracture arthroplasty, osteochondral core transfer, or articular cartilage cell transplantation as indicated. In general, lesions 1 to 2 cm in diameter are treated by microfracture arthroplasty into subchondral bone. Larger lesions may require osteochondral or cellular resurfacing. Soft but intact articular cartilage is left alone. Loose flaps or fibrillations of articular cartilage are resected. The lesions are measured and described as to extent and location in the operative note. At this point, if there has been clear retinacular pain, a segment of the painful portion of lateral retinaculum may be excised and sent for Gomori's trichrome stain and histologic evaluation.

The proximal anterior compartment musculature (tibialis anterior) is released sharply from the lateral tibia and reflected posteriorly with a periosteal elevator. It is best to avoid traumatizing this muscle and to use careful subperiosteal dissection without cutting muscle. The junction of the lateral and posterior cortices is exposed. The anterior tibial artery and deep peroneal nerve are at this level and *must* be protected. A Kelly clamp is placed behind the patellar tendon, and the medial and lateral borders of the tendon are identified. After making a linear incision just medial to the anterior tibial crest, a periosteal ele-

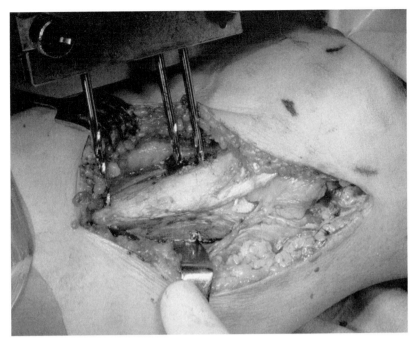

Figure 13.24. With the drill guide fixed in place, multiple drill holes are placed between the proximal and distal drill bits to create an osteotomy plane. Both cortices are drilled. A retractor is used to protect the lateral side of the knee from drill bit penetration past the lateral cortex, as noted in this illustration. Several unicortical drill holes are made proximal to the upper drill bit to a level above the patellar tendon insertion medially.

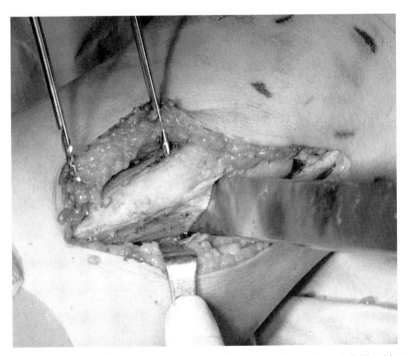

Figure 13.25. A wide Lambotte osteotome connects the most proximal drill bit with a point 5 mm above the patellar tendon insertion laterally. This cut is unicortical and is made to permit freeing of the osteotomy laterally once the osteotomy is complete, such that the bone pedicle may be displaced without fracturing into the metaphysis.

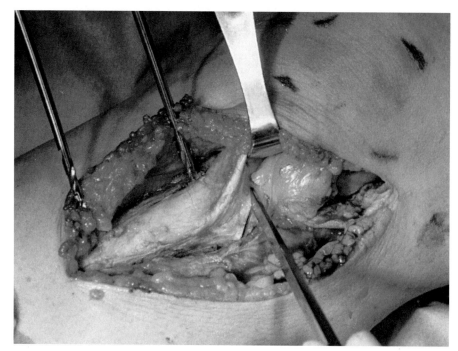

Figure 13.26. A ¼-inch osteotome completes the cortical cut 5 mm proximal to the patellar tendon insertion and is carried all the way to the medial cortex. A wide osteotome will complete the osteotomy. An oscillating saw may be used here alternatively. It is critically important that this cut be precisely between the proximal and distal drill bits along the osteotomy plane. Once the osteotome or saw is placed into the bone, it is *kept in* the osteotomy to complete the osteotomy with careful visualization of the lateral side to avoid damage to the tibialis anterior muscle. The surgeon should avoid removing the osteotome or saw to start a new osteotomy in another location in order to avoid disparate osteotomy planes. Careful attention to detail and patience are necessary at this point. Be sure that the osteotomy tapers anteriorly as it is created distally.

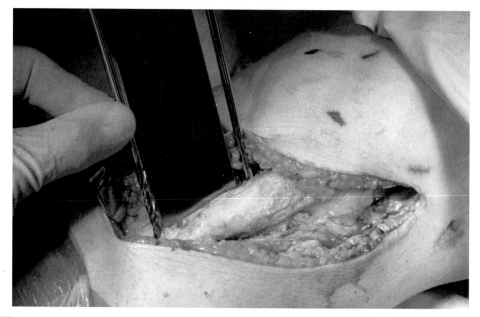

Figure 13.27. Large Lambotte osteotome makes the bone cut. An oscillating saw may also be used.

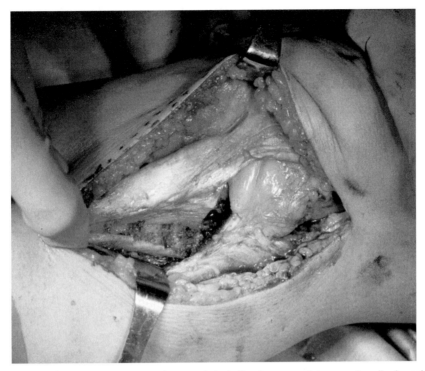

Figure 13.28. Once the osteotomy is completed, the bone pedicle may be displaced in an anterior and medial direction along the osteotomy plane. Notice the tapering of the osteotomy anteriorly at its distal extent.

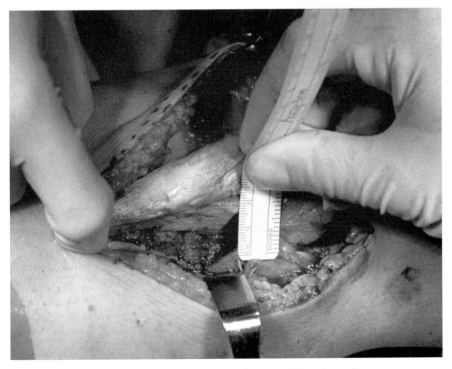

Figure 13.29. Anteriorization of 1.3 to 1.7 cm is routine.

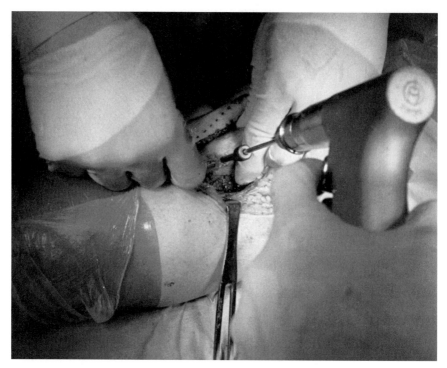

Figure 13.30. Holding the displaced pedicle in the desired location, after testing the patella alignment and anteriorization, cortical screw fixation will achieve stability of the osteotomy pedicle. The proximal cortex is overdrilled to allow a slight lag effect for compression across the osteotomy site. Notice that this drill hole is placed perpendicular to the osteotomy plane.

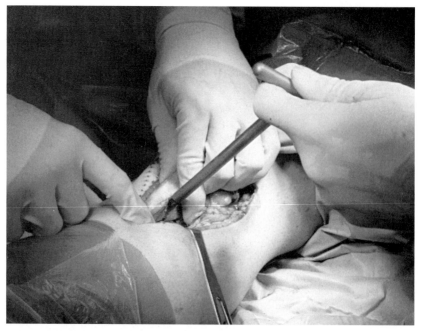

Figure 13.31. A countersink will assure that the screw head seats securely into the cortical bone with minimal risk of fracturing the pedicle.

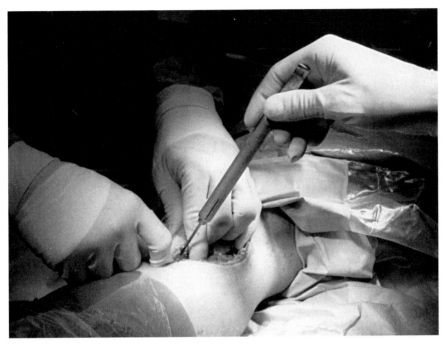

Figure 13.32. A depth gauge is used after the countersink to assure fixation to the posterior cortex.

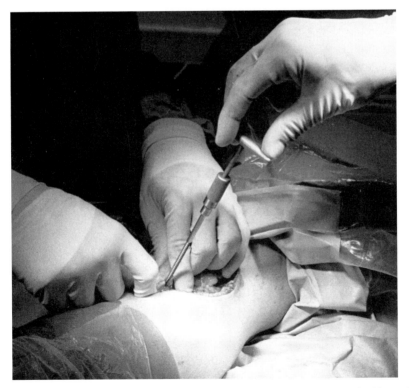

Figure 13.33. A tap just through the posterior tibial cortex assures secure cortical bone fixation.

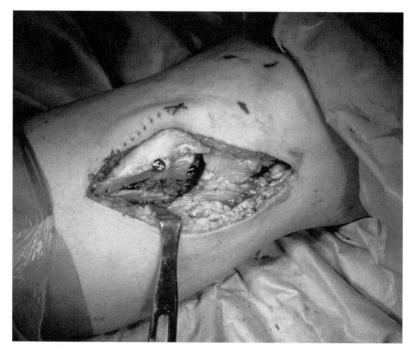

Figure 13.34. The first screw is perpendicular to the osteotomy plane and permits further testing of the patella alignment to assure that the distal patella is elevated and the alignment is optimal.

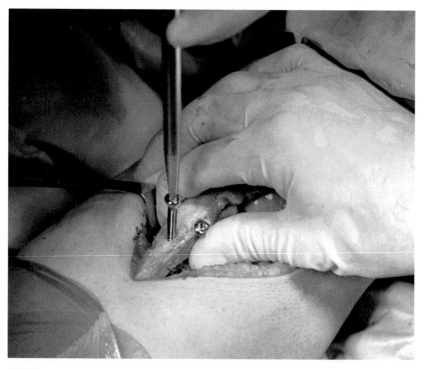

Figure 13.35. A second cortical screw is placed into the posterior cortex to maximize stability of the transferred bone pedicle.

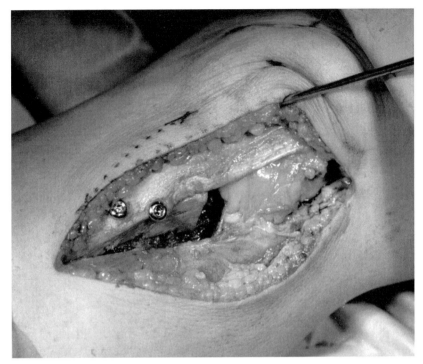

Figure 13.36. The completed anteromedial tibial tubercle transfer before release of the tourniquet and obtaining hemostasis.

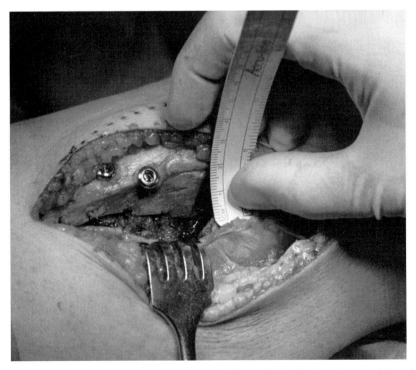

Figure 13.37. In this case, at least 1.5 cm of anteriorization has been achieved.

vator is used to expose bone from the level of the tibial tuberosity to 5 to 7 cm distal. The Hoffman drill guide or a suitable alternative (the Mitek Tracker guide, Norwood, Massachusetts, works very well) is used to place several long 3.2-mm drill holes parallel to each other but in a plane that extends from the anteromedial tibia in a posterolateral direction such that the drill bits enter the tibia just medial to the anterior tibial crest and exit just anterior to the posterolateral corner of the tibia. As the osteotomy plane is designed, it is *tapered* distally such that only 2 to 3 mm of bone are left on the bone pedicle at the distal hinge, approximately 5 to 7 cm distal to the tibial tuberosity. Great care is taken at all times to preserve the patellar tendon insertion into the tibial tuberosity. *Care is also taken to create a perfectly flat osteotomy plane.* This is possible if the surgeon spends some time assuring that the guide pins are parallel. Once the osteotomy plane has been demarcated with the long drill bits, the surgeon should assess the alignment of the osteotomy and assure that it will give the obliquity necessary to achieve significant anteriorization of the tibial tubercle (see Fig. 13.4). The Tracker guide mentioned earlier (Mitek, Norwood, Massachusetts) provides a cutting slot for creating the anteromedialization osteotomy and is an excellent alternative system that can improve the accuracy of this bone cut.

At this point, the surgeon may use an oscillating saw or broad flat osteotomes to complete the osteotomy through the defined plane. A cut is also made on the lateral side of the tibia to shorten the osteotomy such that it will not extend proximally (Fig. 13.38). Also, a small, half-inch osteotome is needed to cut the cortical bone proximal to the patellar tendon insertion. Once the osteotomy is complete, the bone pedicle is hinged distally, as in the Trillat procedure, and the bone pedicle is displaced in an anteromedial direction along the osteotomy plane. The knee may be placed through a range of motion

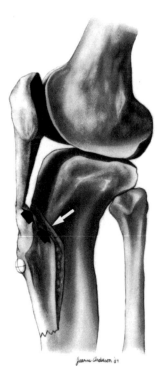

Figure 13.38. *Arrows* indicate the bone cut necessary to prevent extension of the osteotomy into the lateral tibial metaphysis. A second screw must be added.

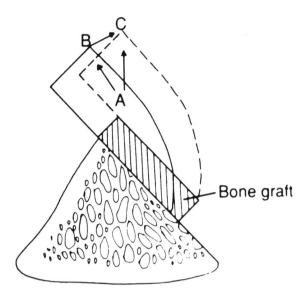

Figure 13.39. Offset bone graft to create straight anteriorization using an oblique osteotomy and local bone graft from the lateral metaphysis.

at this point with the osteotomy held in the desired alignment. Twelve to fifteen mm of anteriorization is routine without bone graft, but a small bone graft from the metaphysis may be added to neutralize medialization and add anteriorization in selected cases (Fig. 13.39). The patella is observed to check patellar alignment, load distribution, and tracking. The bone pedicle is generally locked in place with two screws, at least one of which should be placed carefully into the posterior tibial cortex. This fixation prevents rotation, and if the osteotomy is flat, the bone will be quite stable, permitting early motion of the knee and prompt healing. A Hemovac drain may be left in place for 2 to 24 hours and removed as the drainage diminishes. Assuming stable fixation of the bone pedicle, active and passive motion are started soon after surgery and most patients are discharged the day of surgery or the next morning, non-weight bearing on crutches with a knee immobilizer and ice wrap, which are removed daily for motion exercises. Patients are encouraged to remove the knee immobilizer at least once a day and bend the knee to 90 degrees. Otherwise, patients keep the knee immobilizer in place for 4 weeks. Crutches are used for at least 6 weeks and until full weight bearing and reasonable quadriceps support can be achieved. Early full weight bearing predisposes the patient to tibia fracture.

Results of Anteromedial Tibial Tubercle Transfer

O'Hara and Fulkerson (unpublished data) noted that a steep, oblique osteotomy will allow up to 17 mm of tibial tubercle anteriorization without using any bone graft. This procedure provides consistent long-term relief in appropriate patients. Unlike other extensor mechanism alignment techniques, 90% of patients more than 5 years after anteromedialization have had stable results without evidence of deterioration. Complications are less common and less severe than those reported after tibial tubercle advancement using bone graft. Skin slough, compartment syndrome, and avascular necrosis have been avoided using this technique. With early motion, stiffness has not been a problem. Less than 2% of patients have developed a clinically detectable postoperative deep venous thrombosis. Eight tibial tubercle avulsions or tibia fractures have occurred in more than 500 cases (less than 2%). It is now apparent that obese females are at particular risk for this complication. It is also apparent that early full weight bearing (before the seventh postoperative week) predisposes patients to tibia fracture. Of all patients followed for at least 2 years, 89% have had an objectively good or excellent result. Of those patients with *severe* patellar arthrosis, 75% have had a good result. Contact pressure studies in cadaver knees have shown substantial reduction of patellar contact pressures consistent with findings in other series of tibial tubercle anteriorization.

Buuck and Fulkerson (45) reviewed the long-term results of anteromedial tibial tubercle transfer patients (4 to 12 years, mean 8 years). The long-term satisfaction was consistently good (91%). As anticipated, worker's compensation insurance patients did less well as did those with dashboard and crush injuries. Pidoriano et al (46) correlated results of anteromedialization patients with location and severity of articular disease. Those patients with distal, central articular lesions (Ficat's critical zone) and lateral facet lesions did best after anteromedial tibial tubercle transfer, presumably because of preservation of the proximal medial facet, which receives load at the time of anteromedial tibial tubercle transfer. Patients with proximal crush lesions and diffuse articular changes generally did poorly. Consequently, it appears that anteromedial tibial tubercle transfer is best suited to those patients with distal and lateral facet lesions. Also, Pidoriano noted that patients with central trochlea lesions and worker's compensation issues did less well with the anteromedial tibial tubercle transfer procedure.

This procedure should be used very selectively in patients receiving worker's compensation and in patients who are overweight. Weight reduction is a reasonable prerequisite to doing this surgery.

OTHER SURGICAL ALTERNATIVES FOR THE PATIENT WITH PATELLAR ARTHROSIS

Patellectomy

Although it is rightfully considered the end of the line, patellectomy can lead to satisfactory results. These are better if the patellofemoral joint alone is affected (47–52). For older patients, not needing full quadriceps power and more likely to have loss of flexion, the patellar splitting technique (53) offers the advantage of immediate mobilization. Debeyre et al (54) have also reported good results with patellectomy for arthrosis, but Ackroyd and Polyzoides (55) reported only 53% good results after patellectomy. It is important when reviewing the literature on patellectomy to remember that results may be different for different conditions treated [chondromalacia (56), fracture, arthrosis (48)]. Nonetheless, patellectomy is a more questionable alternative (57) now that other techniques are available for the patient with patellar arthrosis. Kelly and Insall (58) emphasized that alternatives to patellectomy can usually be found. However, a good patellectomy may be the best way to reduce pain in selected patients. Lennox et al (59) found 76% good results following patellectomy at 12- to 48-year follow-up. Patients with osteoarthritis, however, did less well. In an unpublished series (1999), Richard Zell found that patellectomy enabled many worker's compensation patients, including a farmer, two truck drivers, a maintenance worker, and a corrections officer (of 20 patients), to return to work.

The essentials of the technique we use were reported by Boyd and Hawkins (53). The patella is approached through a vertical midline anterior incision (Fig. 13.40). The midportion of the quadriceps tendon and the patellar tendon are carefully identified and incised in the direction of their fibers into the joint. The insertion of the extensor appa-

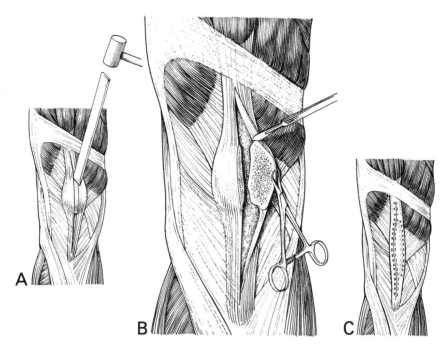

Figure 13.40. Patellectomy demonstrating the technique of Boyd and Hawkins. Reprinted with permission from Boyd H, Hawkins B. Patellectomy—A simplified technique. Surg Gynecol Obstet 1948;86:357.

ratus into the patella is incised in the midpatellar line, taking care that the patella is divided into equal halves. A malleable retractor is introduced into the joint proximally and distally to protect the trochlear surface, and the patella is divided longitudinally with an osteotome. The patella is now enucleated by grasping each half in turn with a towel clip and working from the undersurface of the quadriceps expansion from superior to the midportion of the patella and then inferiorly to the midportion of the patella. This facilitates a clean division of the fibers and preserves an intact, tough fascial covering that is in continuity from the quadriceps tendon to the patellar tendon. Depending upon what is necessary intraarticularly, the quadriceps tendon can be split in the midline proximally as far as 10 cm and the patellar tendon can be split down to the tibial tubercle. The wound is closed by imbricating one side over the other in a double row of interrupted sutures. Flexion on the table to 90 degrees without stressing the suture line is possible and should be carried out. If necessary, the lateral retinaculum can be divided at the level of the anterior border of the iliotibial tract to help centralize the extensor mechanism. It is extremely important to imbricate adequately to avoid impingement of the lateral extensor mechanism over the lateral condyle. *Snapping* in this region can cause postoperative pain.

Postoperatively, the patient is managed in a compression dressing and posterior splint. Quadriceps exercise is possible immediately, and the patient is encouraged to straight leg raise in the splint. The splint may be removed daily starting on the fifth postoperative day for a single cycle of flexion daily, as long as there is reasonable integrity of the extensor mechanism. Most patients achieve 90 degrees of flexion 2 weeks postoperatively. This technique is particularly advantageous if other intraarticular surgery has been necessary.

In one study on the mechanical function of the patella, there was a reduction of 15% of extensor power with patellectomy and transverse closure but a 30% reduction with longitudinal closure (59). However, their longitudinal closure was side-to-side without imbrication and it is likely that the quadriceps power was being transferred to the tibia through the retinacula, rather than through a central tendon with consequent reduction in extensor moment arm. In those cases in which we have employed the longitudinal imbricated closure, there has been no extension lag. Also, mobilization of the knee has been much less of a problem with the longitudinal closure technique.

Butler-Manuel et al (60) have noted increased uptake in the femoral groove on scintigraphy of postpatellectomy patients. This raises some questions regarding the long-term fate of the femoral trochlea post patellectomy but does not negate the validity of the procedure as a salvage operation.

Tibial Tubercle Anteriorization with Bone Graft

Bandi (21) and Maquet (61) proposed improving the effectiveness of the extensor mechanism by transposing the patellar tendon anteriorly. Bandi demonstrated, in his experimental model, up to 33% reduction in patellofemoral loading forces for a 10-mm anterior displacement (Fig. 13.41). Unit load reduction may be even greater if contact area is increased. It is important to release the lateral retinaculum at the time of anterior transposition. Several authors have reported impressive short-term results. Unfortunately, longer follow-up has shown far less desirable long-term results. Engebretsen et al (62) noted that only 10 of 33 patients showed overall improvement at 3 to 9 years of follow-up. He found also that patients with low-grade chondromalacia did least well with the Maquet procedure. Certainly, this is not a procedure for patients with minimal patellar arthrosis! Hehne (63) found that centralization of the tibial tubercle does not reduce overall load on the patella. However, Hirokawa (64), using a mathematic model, did find 20% to 30% reduction of patellofemoral stress with tibial tubercle elevation. We believe the benefits of anteriorization are related to shifting of load as well as load reduction. This load shift involves shift onto the more proximal patellar articular surface, particularly when using a shorter anterior tibial shingle (65).

Sasaki et al (66) noted that anterior displacement of the tibial tubercle in conjunction with high tibial osteotomy may be beneficial in patients with medial and patellofemoral joint arthrosis. Although bone graft may be necessary in some cases, direct anterior displacement of the osteotomized tibia may be preferable.

The anteromedial tibial tubercle osteotomy procedure, as described in this chapter, can give straight anteriorization of the tibial tubercle if a small amount of bone (usually local from the lateral metaphysis) is placed into the osteotomy site (see Fig. 13.39). Another approach has been to do a sagittal or near sagittal plane cut at the level of the medial patellar tendon, cutting in from the lateral tibia to create a shingle of bone that can be mobilized and secured anteriorly with screws placed from lateral to medial (Fig. 13.42) holding the anteriorized tibial tubercle anteriorly. In this situation, the bone fragment is fairly large, so secure fixation and protected weight bearing are imperative.

Unfortunately, there have been disastrous complications after straight anterior displacement of the tibial tubercle with bone graft (Maquet procedure). Skin sloughs, compartment syndromes, amputation, and mechanical failure (Fig. 13.43) have been reported after straight anteriorization with bone graft. Radin and Labosky (67) have written a helpful article on avoiding such complications. Preoperative use of Silastic skin expanders helps in avoiding skin problems. Also, the surgeon must be careful not to create undue

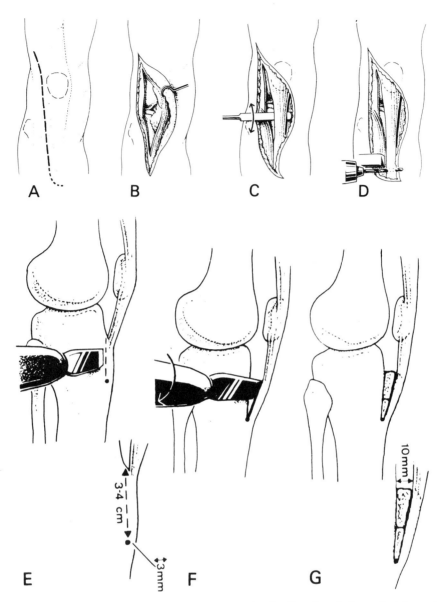

Figure 13.41. Anterior tibial tubercle displacement by the Bandi technique. **A,** Adequate lateral parapatellar incision is necessary. **B,** Lateral retinacular release and arthroscopy of the joint for removal of loose bodies, trimming of osteophytes, and any indicated ancillary intraarticular procedure is obligatory. **C,** Retropatellar tendon area of the tibia is exposed to determine the proximal margin of the insertion of the tendon into the tubercle. **D,** At 3 cm distal to this proximal border and 3 mm posterior to the anterior cortex, a drill hole is made in order to prevent inadvertent extension of the osteotomy. **E,** Position of the drill hole and the osteotomy are demonstrated. **F,** Osteotomy is carried out, and the anterior fragment is levered anteriorly. **G,** Bone graft is wedged in the opening using a cortical cancellous wedge from the iliac crest. Because the distal cortex has not been broken, the position is stable and does not usually require internal fixation. Reprinted with permission from Bandi W. Chondromalacia patellae and femoro-patellare arthrose. Helv Chir Acta (suppl) 1972;1:3–70.

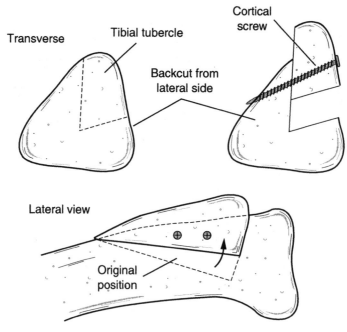

Figure 13.42. Sagittal plane osteotomy permits straight or near-straight anteriorization without bone graft but requires a large cut. Secure fixation and protected weight bearing are imperative.

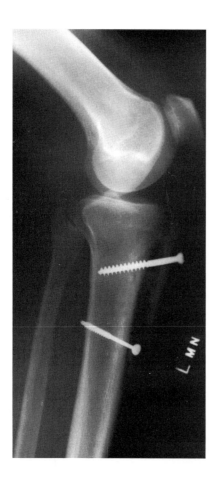

Figure 13.43. Mechanical failure of a tibial tubercle anteriorization using bone graft distraction of the osteotomy.

skin tension by placing too much bone graft behind the tubercle. On the whole, the Maquet procedure should be avoided, opting instead for more controlled and less profound anterior tibial tubercle transfer.

Cellular Resurfacing

Pridie's (68) original concept for the treatment of bone eburnation was to remove all of the dense subchondral bone, thereby exposing cancellous bone. During the 1980s, surgeons favored arthroscopic abrasion or microfracture arthroplasty into subchondral bleeding bone (67), thereby bringing new undifferentiated marrow cells onto the surface in the hope of gaining an improved articular surface with cartilage characteristics

Osteochondral transfer to the patella using a core transfer system (OATS, Arthrex, Naples, Florida) has been disappointing for the patella articular surface but quite successful for trochlear lesions (Fig. 13.44).

Cellular resurfacing of the patella may be possible as well as resurfacing other articular cartilage defects (Fig. 13.45). Brittberg et al (69) have demonstrated that it is possible to culture autologous articular cartilage cells and transplant the chondrocytes for treatment of knee cartilage defects. With regard to the patella, it is likely that normalization of stresses on the area of cartilage transplantation would be necessary for long-term viability of transplanted chondrocytes. Consequently, appropriate realignment and decompression surgery for the patella is often appropriate at the time of resurfacing.

OATS (autologous osteochondral transplantation) transplantation to the patella is difficult because of the unusual contours and dense bone of the patella. After bone surfaces are congruous, articular cartilage typically will be prominent and vulnerable (Fig. 13.46).

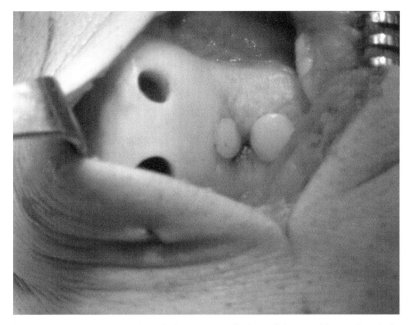

Figure 13.44. Autologous osteochondral core resurfacing of the trochlea using Arthrex OATS system (Arthrex, Naples, Florida)

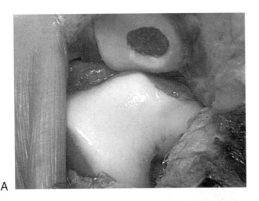

A

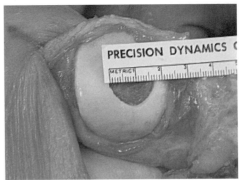

B

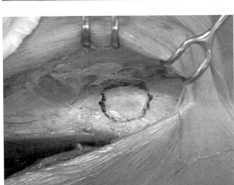

C

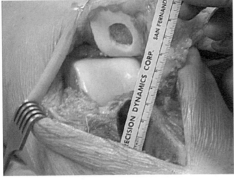

D

Figure 13.45. Carticel resurfacing of the patella. Concomitant unloading is necessary. **A,** Diseased cartilage resected. **B,** 1.7-cm diameter lesion. **C and D,** Periosteal flap. **E and F,** Periosteal free flap sutured to defect. Illustration courtesy of Jack Farr, MD.

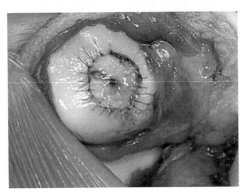

E

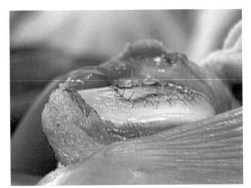

F

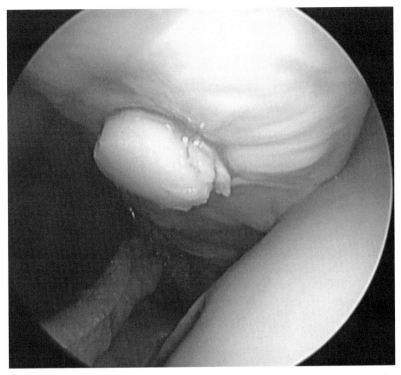

Figure 13.46. Osteochondral autograft core transfer to patella. Cartilage is prominent when bone is congruous. Concomitant unloading is necessary.

Our experience to date with osteochondral transplant to the patella has been disappointing. Results of OATS or articular cartilage cell transplantation to the patella may be enhanced by the concomitant use of tibial tubercle anteriorization or anteromedialization. Minas and Peterson (70) have combined articular cartilage implantation with anteromedial tibial tubercle transfer.

Infrapatellar Contracture Syndrome

Paulos (71) reviewed the infrapatellar contracture syndrome (ICS), a condition that can occur following cruciate ligament reconstruction, trauma, or other surgery around the anterior knee. Since Shelbourne and Nitz introduced accelerated rehabilitation after cruciate ligament reconstruction, ICS has been far less common as a complication of cruciate ligament surgery when the graft is positioned correctly. Nonetheless, there are many patients who are left with chronic scar behind the patellar tendon after trauma or surgery to the knee, and they will ultimately develop anterior knee pain as well as stiffness.

As a consequence of infrapatellar contracture, anterior knee pain may become intractable, and abnormally increased contact stress on patellofemoral articular surfaces is common. It is important to release this contracture, using an open technique to assure complete release of all tight, tethering bands. Early motion following this type of release is imperative.

Although most patients respond very favorably to complete release of an infrapatellar contracture, I have noted that some problems with anterior knee pain continue in many of these patients. The patient frequently may be happy with improved motion after the contracture release and experience reduction of pain but may be left with some functional loss and may return to the office requesting additional treatment for residual pain. Depending on the amount of actual articular damage, anteriorization of the tibial tubercle may be appropriate in some of these patients, provided there is good proximal articular cartilage on the patella. McMahon et al (72) have noted that resection of the retropatellar tendon fat pad will not compromise vascularity of the patella, so pain must be attributed to other factors. It is likely that some irreversible damage occurs to articular cartilage of the patella with infrapatellar contracture.

Patellofemoral Replacement

Many materials have been tried in the past, both artificial and natural. Arthroplasties with skin, fascia, fat pad, and bursa have been tried (73–77). Polyethylene replacement of the patella alone has been less successful than metal on articular cartilage (Fig. 13.47). McKeever (78) introduced a metal resurfacing prosthesis that has been reported to give reasonable results (78–80). In 1992, Harrington (81) reviewed the long-term (5–8 years) results of McKeever patella resurfacing in 28 patients (mean age, 36 years). Nineteen of the patients had normal trochlear cartilage. Seventeen of the 28 patients had a good or excellent result. There were three patients with poor results, which were attributed to tricompartmental arthritis. Harrington (81) noted a need for prolonged physical therapy after patella resurfacing, but had no problems of instability or prosthetic loosening.

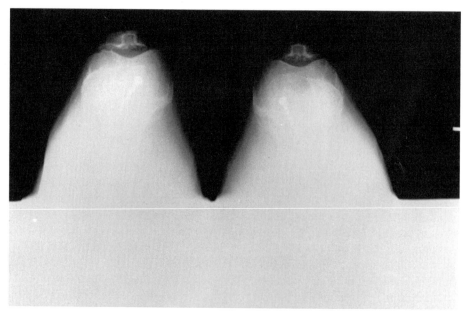

Figure 13.47. Polyethylene replacement of the patella is less desirable than metal because of poor polyethylene wear characteristics on articular cartilage.

Worrell (82) reported a redesigned version of the McKeever prosthesis in 1975 and published his results in young patients in 1986. Pickett and Stoll (83) reported better results with patellar replacement than with patellectomy. Blazina et al (84) recommended patellofemoral replacement particularly for patients with severe femoral groove degeneration. Worrell (82) suggested that prosthetic resurfacing of the patella is most appropriate for patients with Grades 3 or 4 chondromalacia of the patella and poor quadriceps function. Scott (85) has cautioned that there are numerous potential serious complications of prosthetic patellar replacement surgery including patella fracture and prosthesis loosening.

There has been a recent resurgence of interest in patellofemoral replacement, but no one prosthesis has emerged as definitive. There are many questions remaining to be answered about the use of patellofemoral replacement. What seems clear is that this is one alternative when articular preservation alternatives are exhausted or inappropriate. I have done ten patellofemoral replacements and have had better results when there are no compensation issues involved. Currently, I do not recommend patellofemoral replacement in patients receiving worker's compensation.

If isolated patellofemoral replacement is chosen, the surgeon must be sure that the extensor mechanism is centralized, there is no patella alta, the patient is fit enough to recover, the remainder of the knee is satisfactory, and the patient is motivated.

There are several unicompartmental patellofemoral prostheses available, and these are still evolving. Criteria for selecting the prosthesis should include a smooth transition from the trochlea component to the intercondylar notch area, adequate but not excessive trochlear depth, accurate and easy-to-use instrumentation, minimized bone resection, and minimal polyethylene-articular cartilage contact upon knee flexion.

Allograft replacement of the patella articular surface has been attempted (86). This alternative offers promise for the future (Fig. 13.48).

A 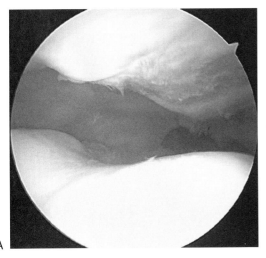 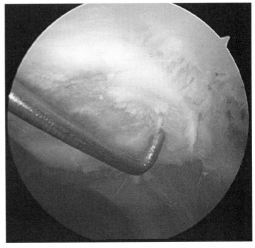 B

Figure 13.48. Osteochondral allograft resurfacing of the patellofemoral joint. **A,** Grade 4 patella cartilage loss viewed arthroscopically. **B,** Full-thickness loss of patella cartilage. *Continued on next page.*

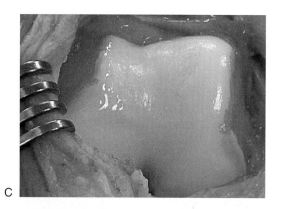

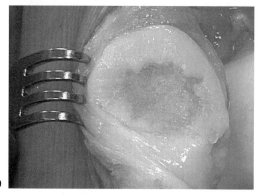

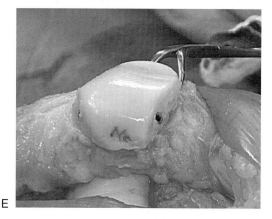

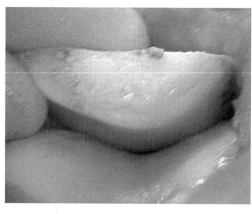

Figure 13.48. *Continued.* **C,** Intact trochlea. **D,** Lesion exposed. **E,** Osteochondral patella allograft. **F,** Nearly congruent allograft patella prepared for fixation to dorsum of host patella.

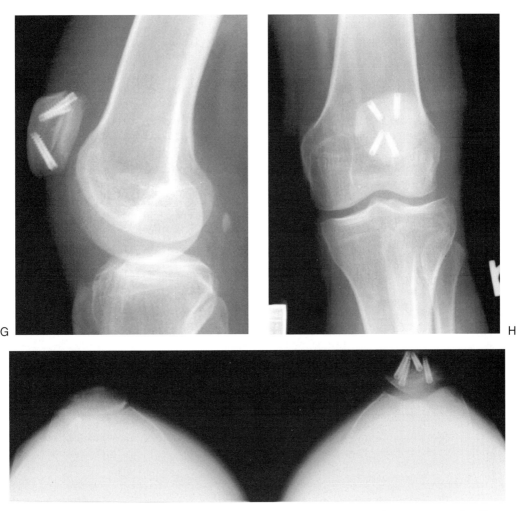

Figure 13.48. *Continued.* **G,** Patella allograft secured in place. **H,** Four fixation screws for allograft patella surface. **I,** Axial view of patella allograft. Illustrations courtesy of Jack Farr, MD.

PATELLOFEMORAL JOINT RESURFACING IN KNEE JOINT REPLACEMENT SURGERY

Rand (87) has pointed out that extensor mechanism problems are the most common cause of reoperation after total knee replacement. Problems include instability of the patella, patella fracture, wear debris, soft-tissue impingement, rupture of the patellar ligament, loosening of the patellar implant, and infection. He has also pointed out that there is a very high incidence of complication following isolated revision of a total knee patellar component (88). Consequently, precision in resurfacing the patellofemoral joint is extremely important at the time of knee replacement. Debate continues regarding the relative merits of a mobile bearing patella versus fixed polyethylene.

Koshino et al (89) have noted some tendency to develop mild patella baja following knee joint replacement. In 56 kinematic knee replacements, Johnson and Eastwood (90) noted 50% patellofemoral problems postoperatively, with 13 subluxations and 15 patients with anterior knee pain. Postoperative patellar tilt and displacement are common postoperatively (91) following knee replacement. Kirk et al (92) reported his results following realignment of the unstable extensor mechanism after patellar dislocation as a complication of total knee replacement. Using a Trillat procedure in 15 patients, there were no recurrent dislocations 2 years following revision.

Knee replacement without resurfacing the patella in selected patients with good cartilage yields satisfactory results (93). In many patients, however, patellar resurfacing will be necessary at the time of knee joint replacement. A minimum of 15 mm of patellar thickness should be maintained at the time of patellar resurfacing, according to Reuben et al (94). Rand (95) has reported that patellofemoral problems can be markedly reduced by using precise techniques, reducing patellar height 2 mm from the preoperative level, and taking care to balance the patella in the prosthetic trochlea.

Medial placement of the patellar component on the excised patellar surface creates better tracking, and slight external rotation of the femoral component appears to enhance patellar component stability (96). These authors also pointed out that in-setting of the patellar implant may provide greater stability and better alignment of the patellofemoral joint than on-laying the prosthesis.

There are some who say that total knee joint replacement is preferable to isolated patellofemoral resurfacing, particularly in elderly patients. When there is generalized or two-compartment arthritis (Fig. 13.49), this approach has merit. When disease is restricted to the patellofemoral joint, however, most patients will respond favorably to treatment of the one compartment without resurfacing in most cases. If resurfacing is

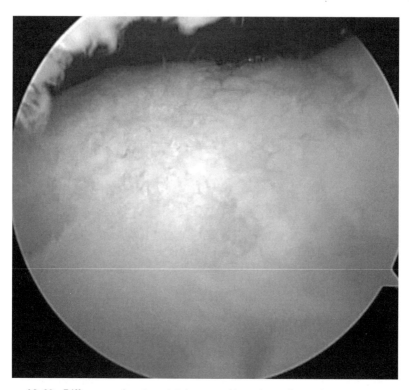

Figure 13.49. Diffuse grades 3 and 4 (exposed bone) cartilage damage on trochlea.

necessary, the surgeon may consider replacement of the patellofemoral joint alone in carefully selected patients or total knee replacement in elderly patients.

Osteotomy of the Patella

Hejgaard and Arnoldi (97) reported that simple longitudinal osteotomy of the patella may give significant relief of patellar pain associated with increased intraosseous pressure. Further confirmation of such findings is necessary before advocating this technique.

Vaquero and Arriaza (98) described a thinning osteotomy of the patella. By taking a 7 mm segment out of the midpatella, they reported a 16% to 27% reduction of contact pressure in the patellofemoral joint in 13 cadaver knee specimens. They refer to this as a "double parallel coronal osteotomy of the patella." I have no experience with this technique.

Anterolateral Transfer of the Tibial Tubercle

I have done more than 20 anterolateral tibial tubercle transfers to correct an overly medialized tibial tubercle (most commonly following a failed Hauser procedure). These patients have excessive medial contact stress on the patella, which can result in a bone-on-bone medial patellofemoral arthrosis. Such patients benefit from transferring the patellar tendon anterolaterally. A tibial pedicle similar to that used for anteromedial tibial tubercle transfer, but angling the osteotomy to permit anterolateral shift of the patellar tendon, has been helpful in the management of these difficult patients (Fig. 13.50). A back cut to release the osteotomy shingle is frequently necessary on the medial side, depending on the obliquity of the osteotomy cut. This procedure has been extremely helpful as a salvage procedure in the very troubled patients with intractable pain following excessive medial or posteromedial tibial tubercle transfer. This is a good salvage procedure (99). The pes anserinus must be reflected and a cut must be made from the lateral patellar tendon directed posteromedially to create an osteotomy that will produce a bone pedicle to slide in an anterolateral direction.

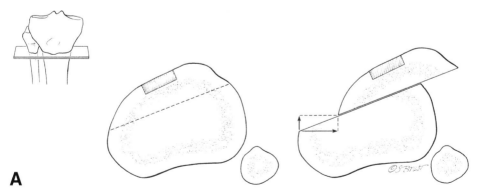

A

Figure 13.50. A, Anterolateral tibial tubercle transfer is possible by creating an osteotomy oriented from the anterolateral side of the tibia, directing it posterolaterally to include the posteromedially placed bone block of a previous Hauser procedure. Illustration by Susan Brust. *Continued on next page.*

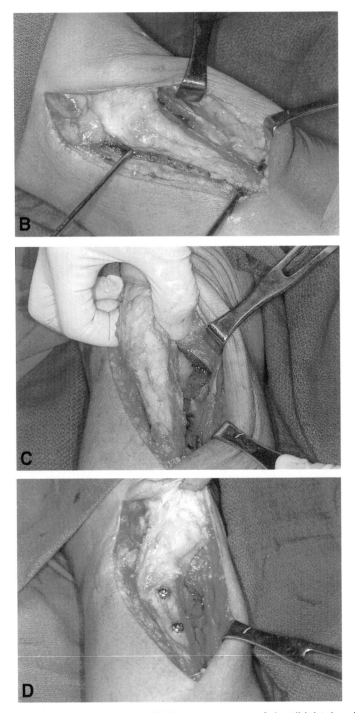

Figure 13.50. *Continued.* **B, C, and D,** Oblique osteotomy of the tibial tubercle will permit anterolateral shift of the tibial tubercle.

REFERENCES

1. Bergstrom R, Gillquist J, Lysholm J, Hamberg P. Arthroscopy of the knee in children. J Pediatr Orthop 1984;4(5): 542–545.
2. Schreiber SN. Proximal superomedial portal in arthroscopy of the knee. Arthroscopy 1991;7(2):246–257.
3. George R, Chrisman OD. The role of cartilage polysaccharides in osteoarthritis. Clin Orthop 1968;57:259.
4. Patel D. Arthroscopy of the plical-synovial folds and their significance. Am J Sports Med 1978;6:217–225.
5. Jackson RW, Marshall D, Fujisawa Y. The pathological medial shelf. Orthop Clin North Am 1982;13:307–312.
6. Vaughn-Lane T, Dandy D. The synovial shelf syndrome. J Bone Joint Surg 1982;64B:475–476.
7. Munzinger U, Ruckstuhl J, Scherrer H, Gschwend N. Internal derangement of the knee joint due to pathologic synovial folds: The mediopatellar plica syndrome. Clin Orthop 1981; 155:59–64.
8. Broom M, Fulkerson J. The plica syndrome: A new perspective. Orthop Clin North Am 1986;17(2):279–281.
9. Richmond JC, McGinty JR. Segmental arthroscopic resection of the hypertrophic mediopatellar plica. Clin Orthop 1983;178:185–189.
10. Rydholm A. Pseudochondromalacia patellae. Acta Orthop Scand 1978;49(2):205–210.
11. Lindberg U, Lysholm J, Gillquist J. The correlation between arthroscopic findings and the patellofemoral pain syndrome. Arthroscopy 1986;2(2):103–107.
12. Casscells SW. The arthroscope in the diagnosis of disorders of the patellofemoral joint. Clin Orthop 1979;144: 45–50.
13. Lund F, Nilsson BE. Anterior displacement of the tibial tuberosity in chondromalacia patellae. Acta Orthop Scand 1980;51(4):679–688.
14. Ogilvie-Harris D, Jackson R. The arthroscopic treatment of chondromalacia patellae. J Bone Joint Surg 7.984; 66B:660–665.
15. Leslie IJ, Bentley G. Arthroscopy in the diagnosis of chondromalacia patellae. Ann Rheum Dis 1978;37(6): 540–547.
16. Fulkerson J. Evaluation of the peripatellar soft tissues and retinaculum in patients with patellofemoral pain. Clin Sports Med 1989;8(2):197–202.
17. Grana WA, Hinkley B, Hollingsworth S. Arthroscopic evaluation and treatment of patellar malalignment. Clin Orthop 1984;196:122–128.
18. Fulkerson JP. Operative management of patellofemoral pain. Ann Chir Gynaecol 1991; 80(2):224–229.
19. Kolowich PA, Paulos LE, Rosenberg TD, Farnsworth S. Lateral release of the patella: Indications and contraindications. Am J Sports Med 1990;18(4):359–365.
20. Fulkerson J. Anteromedialization of the tibial tuberosity for patellofemoral malalignment. Clin Orthop 1983; 177:176–181.
21. Bandi W. Chondromalacia patellae and femoro-patellare arthrose. Helv Chir Acta (suppl 1) 1972;3–70.
22. Maquet P. Advancement of the tibial tuberosity. Clin Orthop 1976;115:225–230.
23. Ferguson AB Jr. Elevation of the insertion of the patellar ligament for patellofemoral pain. J Bone Joint Surg (Am) 1982;64(5):760–771.
24. Ferguson AB Jr, Brown TD, Fu FH, Rutkowski R. Relief of patellofemoral contact stress by anterior displacement of the tibial tubercle. J Bone Joint Surg (Am) 1979;61(2):159–166.
25. Radin EL. Anterior tibial tubercle elevation in the young adult. Orthop Clin North Am 1986;17(2):297–302.
26. Radin EL. The Maquet procedure—Anterior displacement of the tibial tubercle. Indications, contraindications, and precautions. Clin Orthop 1986;213:241–248.
27. Schepsis A, DeSimone A, Leach R. Anterior tibial tubercle transposition for patellofemoral arthrosis. Am J Knee Surg 1994;7:13–20.
28. Waisbrod H, Treiman N. Anterior displacement of tibial tuberosity for patellofemoral disorders: A preliminary report. Clin Orthop 1980;153:180–182.
29. Mendes DG, Soudry M, Iusim M. Clinical assessment of Maquet tibial tuberosity advancement. Clin Orthop 1987;222:228–238.
30. Nakamura N, Ellis M, Seedhom BB. Advancement of the tibial tuberosity. A biomechanical study. J Bone Joint Surg (Br) 1985;67(2):255–260.
31. Hadjipavlou A, Helmy H, Dubravcik P, Heller L, Kerner M. Maquet osteotomy for chondromalacia patellae: Avoiding the pitfalls. Can J Surg 1982;25(3):342–345.
32. Bessette GC, Hunter RE. The Maquet procedure. A retrospective review. Clin Orthop 1988;232:159–167.
33. Hejgaard N, Watt-Boolsen S. The effect of anterior displacement of the tibial tuberosity in idiopathic chondromalacia patellae: A prospective randomized study. Acta Orthop Scand 1982;53(1):135–139.
34. Cameron HU, Huffer B, Cameron GM. Anteromedial displacement of the tibial tubercle for patellofemoral arthralgia. Can J Surg 1986;29(6):456–458.
35. Rauschning W, Amici F Jr. Surgical treatment of recurrent subluxation of the patella in athletes. Ital J Orthop Traumatol 1982;8(2):167–174.
36. Beckers L. Displacement osteotomy of the tibial tuberosity. Acta Orthop Belg Tome 48 Fasc 1982;1:190–193.
37. Blauth W, Mann M. Medialversetzung der tuberositas tibiae and gleichzeitige vorverlagerung. Z Orthop 1977; 115:252–255.
38. Karrison J, Bunkertorp O, Lansinger O, Romanus B, Sward L. Lowering of the patella secondary to anterior

advancement of the tibial tubercle for the patellofemoral pain syndrome. Arch Orthop Trauma Surg 1986;105(1): 40–45.

39. Koshino T. Changes in patellofemoral compressive force after anterior or anteromedial displacement of tibial tuberosity for chondromalacia patellae. Clin Orthop 1991;266:133–138.
40. Post WR, Fulkerson JP. Distal realignment of the patellofemoral joint. Orthop Clin North Am 1992;23(4): 631–643.
41. Cautilli RA, Fulkerson JP. Operative treatment of patellofemoral disorders: Distal realignment. Sports Med Arth Rev 1994;2:250–262.
42. Fulkerson J. Anteromedial tibial tubercle transfer. In Jackson D, ed. Master Techniques in Orthopedic Surgery: Reconstructive Knee Surgery. New York: Raven Press; 1995.
43. Fulkerson J, Shea K. Current concepts review: Disorders of patellofemoral alignment. J Bone Joint Surg 1990; 72A:1424–1429.
44. Fulkerson J, Becker G, Meaney J, Miranda M, Folcik M. Anteromedial tibial tubercle transfer without bone graft. Am J Sports Med 1990;18(5):490–497.
45. Buuck D, Fulkerson J. Anteromedialization of the tibial tubercle: a 4 to 12 year follow up. Op Tech Sports Med 2000;8(2):131–137.
46. Pidoriano A, Weinstein R, Buuck D, Fulkerson J. Correlation of patellar articular lesions and results from anteromedial tibial tubercle transfer. Am J Sports Med 1997;25:533–537.
47. Burton VW, Thomas HM. Results of excision of the patella. Surg Gynecol Obstet 1972;135:753–755.
48. Dinham JM, French PR. Results of patellectomy for osteoarthritis. Postgrad Med J 1972;48:590–593.
49. Geckeler EO, Quaranta AV. Patellectomy for degenerative arthritis of the knee; Late results. J Bone Joint Surg 1962;44A:1109.
50. Stougard J. Patellectomy. Acta Orthop Scand 1970;41:110–121.
51. Tibermont G. La Patellectomie. Thesis, Bordeaux, France; 1958.
52. West FE. End results of patellectomy. J Bone Joint Surg 1962;44A:1089–1108.
53. Boyd HB, Hawkins BL. Patellectomy—A simplified technique. Surg Gynecol Obstet 1948; 86:357.
54. Debeyre J, Levernieux J, Patte D. Gonarthroses traitees par patellectomie, dont quelques-unes suivies depuis 10 ans. Presse Med 1962;70:2775.
55. Ackroyd CE, Polyzoides AJ. Patellectomy for osteoarthritis. A study of eighty-one patients followed from two to twenty-two years. J Bone Joint Surg 1978;60(B):353–357.
56. Bentley G. Chondromalacia patellae. J Bone Joint Surg 1970;52A:No. 2.
57. Insall J, Tria A, Aglietti P. Resurfacing of the patella. J Bone Joint Surg 1980;62A:933–936.
58. Kelly M, Insall J. Patellectomy. Orthop Clin North Am 1986;17(2):289–295.
59. Lennox IA, Cobb AG, Knowles J, Bentley G. Knee function after patellectomy. A 12- to 48-year follow-up. J Bone Joint Surg (Br) 1994;76(3):485–487.
60. Butler-Manuel PA, Guy RL, Heatley FW, Nunan TO. Scintigraphy in the assessment of anterior knee pain. Acta Orthop Scand 1990;61(5):438–442.
61. Maquet P, Biomechanische Aspekte der Femur-Patella-Beziehungen. Z Orthop 1974;112:620–623.
62. Engebretsen L, Svennengsen S, Benum P. Advancement of the tibial tuberosity for patellar pain. A 5 year follow-up. Acta Orthop Scand 1989;60(1):20–22.
63. Hehne H-J. Biomechanics of the patellofemoral joint and its clinical relevance. Clin Orthop 1990;258:73–85.
64. Hirokawa S. Three-dimensional mathematical model analysis of the patellofemoral joint. J Biomech 1991;24(8): 659–671.
65. Pan HQ, Kish V, Boyd RD, Burr DB, Radin EL. The Maquet procedure: Effect of tibial shingle length on patellofemoral pressures. J Orthop Res 1993;11(2):199–204.
66. Sasaki T, Yagi T, Monji J, Yasuda K, Tsuge H. High tibial osteotomy combined with anterior displacement of the tibial tubercle for osteoarthritis of the knee. Int Orthop 1986;10(7.):31–40.
67. Radin EL, Labosky D. Avoiding complications associated with the Maquet procedure. Complic Orthop Mar/Apr 1989;48–57.
68. Pridie KH. A method of resurfacing osteoarthritic knee joints. J Bone Joint Surg 1959;41B:618.
69. Brittberg M, Lindahl A, Nilsson A, Ohlsson C. Cellular aspects on treatment of cartilage injuries (review). Agents Actions Suppl 1993;39:237–241.
70. Minas T, Peterson L. Autologous chondrocyte transplantation. Op Tech Sports Med 2000;8(2):144–157.
71. Paulos L, Ownorowski D, Greenwald A. Infrapatellar contracture syndrome. Am J Sports Med 1994;22: 440–449.
72. McMahon M, Scuderi G, Glashow J, Scharf S, Meltzer L, Scott W. Scintigraphic determination of patellar viability after excision of infrapatellar fat pad and/or lateral retinacular release in total knee arthroplasty. Clin Orthop 1990;260:10–16.
73. Judet R, Judet J, Lord G, Roy-Camille R, Boutelier P. La patelloplastie a la peau conservé. Presse Med 1962;70: 983–986.
74. Albee FH. Original features in arthroplasty of the knee with improved prognosis. Surg Gynecol Obstet 1928;47: 312.
75. Murphy JB. Arthroplasty. Ann Surg 1913;57:593.
76. Campbell WC. Arthroplasty of the knee; report of cases. Am J Orthop Surg 1921;19:430.

77. Goymann V, Bopp HM. Chondrektomie and gelenktoilette bei schween arthrosen des femuropatellaren gleitweges. Z Orthop 1973;111:534–536.
78. McKeever DC. Patellar prosthesis. J Bone Joint Surg 1955;37A:1074.
79. DePalma AF, Sawyer B, Hoffman DJ. Reconsideration of lesions affecting the patello-femoral joint. Clin Orthop 1960;18:63
80. Levitt RL. A long-term evaluation of patellar prostheses. Clin Orthop 1973;97:153.
81. Harrington KD. Long-term results for the McKeever patellar resurfacing prosthesis used as a salvage procedure for severe chondromalacia patellae. Clin Orthop 1992;279:201–213.
82. Worrell R. Resurfacing of the patella in young patients. Orthop Clin North Am 1986;17(2):303–309.
83. Pickett JC, Stoll DA. Patelloplasty or patellectomy? Clin Orthop 1979;144:103–106.
84. Blazina ME, Fox JM, Del Pizzo W, Broukhim B, Ivey FM. Patellofemoral replacement. Clin Orthop 1979; 144:98–102.
85. Scott RD. Prosthetic replacement of the patellofemoral joint. Orthop Clin North Am 1979;10(1):129–137.
86. Bugbee W. Fresh osteochondral grafting. Op Tech Sports Med 2000;8(2):158–162.
87. Rand JA. The patellofemoral joint in total knee arthroplasty. J Bone Joint Surg 1994;76A:612.
88. Berry DJ, Rand JA. Isolated patellar component revision of total knee arthroplasty. Clin Orthop 1993;286: 110–115.
89. Koshino T, Ejima M, Okamoto R, Morii T. Gradual low riding of the patella during postoperative course after total knee arthroplasty in osteoarthritis and rheumatoid arthritis. J Arthroplasty 1990;5(4):323–327.
90. Johnson DP, Eastwood DM. Patellar complications after knee arthroplasty. A prospective study of 56 cases using the kinematic prosthesis. Acta Orthop Scand 1992;63(1):74–79.
91. Bindelglass DF, Cohen JL, Dorr LD. Patellar tilt and subluxation in total knee arthroplasty. Relationship to pain, fixation, and design. Clin Orthop 1993;286:103–109.
92. Kirk P, Rorabeck CH, Bourne RB, Burkart B, Nott L. Management of recurrent dislocation of the patella following total knee arthroplasty. J Arthroplasty 1992;7(3):229–233.
93. Levitsky KA, Harris WJ, McManus J, Scott RD. Total knee arthroplasty without patellar resurfacing. Clinical outcomes and long-term follow-up evaluation. Clin Orthop 1993;286:116–121.
94. Reuben JD, McDonald CL, Woodard PL, Hennington LJ. Effect of patella thickness on patella strain following total knee arthroplasty. J Arthroplasty 1991;6(3):251–258.
95. Rand JA. Patellar resurfacing in total knee arthroplasty. Clin Orthop 1990;260:110–117.
96. Gomes A, Bechtol DJ, Gustillo R. Patellar prosthesis positioning in total knee arthroplasty. Clin Arthroplasty 1988;236:72–81.
97. Hejgaard N, Arnoldi CC. Osteotomy of the patella in the patellofemoral pain syndrome. The significance of increased intraosseous pressure during sustained knee flexion. Int Orthop 1984;8(3):189–194.
98. Vaquero J, Arriaza R. The patella thinning osteotomy. An experimental study of a new technique for reducing patellofemoral pressure. Int Orthop 1992;16:372–376.
99. Fulkerson J. Anterolateralization of the tibial tubercle. Tech Orthop 1997;12(3):165–169.

Subject Index

A

Abnormal bony relationships, in patellar dislocation, 213

Abrasion arthroplasty, of grade 4 patellar lesion, 113*f*, 114

Achondroplasia, superior/inferior patella malposition and, 138, 138*f*

ACL deficiency/reconstruction. *See* Anterior cruciate ligament deficiency/reconstruction

Acute patellar dislocation, 216–220
  clinical presentation of, 216–217
  Fulkerson's approach to, 219–220
  pathoanatomy of, 218, 218*f*
  radiologic features of, 217–218
  treatment for, 219

Aerobic exercise, as nonoperative treatment, 304

Alpine hunter's cap dysplasia
  as partial hypoplasia, 132*f*, 133
  patellar subluxation and, 193, 193*f*

AMZ. *See* Anteromedialization

Anterior cruciate ligament (ACL)deficiency/reconstruction, nonarthritic knee pain and, 154

Anterior knee trauma, 77

Anterior patellar surface, 2, 2*f*

Anterior tibial tubercle displacement, Bandi technique of, 346, 347*f*

Anterior trochlear line, patellar tilt angles and, 90, 91*f*

Anterolateral transfer of tibial tubercle, patellofemoral joint resurfacing and, 357, 357*f*, 358*f*

Anteromedial tibial tubercle transfer
  arthroscopy in, 326, 327*f*
  cortical bone fixation in, 339*f*, 340*f*
  diagram of, 324, 324*f*
  dissection for, 328*f*
  Ficat's critical zone lesion in, 331*f*
  Fulkerson's technique of, 326, 327*f*, 328*f*, 329*f*, 340*f*, 341*f*
  incision location for, 328*f*
  indications for, 324, 324*f*, 325*f*

instruments for, 326, 326*f*
  lateral retinacular release in, 329*f*
  offset bone graft in, 342, 343*f*
  osteotomy plane in, 335*f*
  patellar tendon identification in, 329*f*
  patellofemoral reconstruction and, 323, 324, 326, 327*f*, 328*f*, 329*f*, 340*f*, 341*f*
  results of, 343–344
  using drill guide in, 333*f*, 334*f*, 335*f*

Anteromedialization (AMZ)
  for patellar subluxation, 208, 208*f*
  patellar tilt compression syndrome after, 167, 168*f*

Anteroposterior (AP) view
  of patellofemoral joint imaging, 76–77, 77*f*
  standing, 76, 77*f*

Anteversion examination, rationale for, 68

AP view. *See* Anteroposterior view

Aplasia, as patellar dysplasia, 129, 129*f*

Apprehension sign, 57
  in recurrent patellar dislocation, 222, 222*f*

Arterial supply, of patellofemoral joint, 20–21, 20*f*

Arthrography, 97, 97*f*

Arthroscopic arthroplasty, 122, 124*f*, 125*f*

Arthroscopic debridement, 118

Arthroscopic lateral release, 119–122. *See also* Lateral release
  advantages of, 119, 119*f*
  decision for, 120
  results of, 121, 122
  spinal needle for, 120, 120*f*, 121
  techniques for, 120, 120*f*, 121

Arthroscopic medial imbrication, 122, 123*f*, 124*f*
  for patellar subluxation, 206*f*, 207

Arthroscopic proximal imbrication, 122, 123*f*

Arthroscopy
  articular lesions and, 110
  entry point for, 108, 108*f*, 109*f*
  in anteromedial tibial tubercle transfer, 326, 327*f*
  lateral trochlea lesions and, 110, 111*f*
  medial facet lesions and, 110, 111*f*